Prevent Alzheimer's, /
With 7 Supplements, 7 Lifestyle Choices, and a Dissolved Mineral

Author: Dr. Dennis N. Crouse, BSc Biochemistry, - Harvard College, Ph.D. Organic Chemistry - Harvard University Chemistry Department, Post-graduate courses: Understanding Dementia - Wicking Faculty of Health, University of Tasmania, Fundamentals of Neuroscience - Harvard.

Copyright © 2016 by Dennis N. Crouse
All rights reserved. This book or any portion thereof
may not be reproduced or used in any manner whatsoever
without the express written permission of the publisher
except for the use of brief quotations in a book review.

Printed in the United States of America

First Printing, 2016

Second Edition Printing, 2018

ISBN 978-1535183161

Etiological Publishing

Legal Disclaimer: The information in this book is provided for general educational purposes only and is not intended to constitute (i) medical advice or counseling, (ii) the practice of medicine or the provision of health care diagnosis or treatment, (iii) or the creation of a physician-patient relationship. If you have or suspect that you have a medical problem, contact your doctor promptly.

No one paid the author to write this book and he receives no financial reward for any product herein recommended.

Dedication

This book is dedicated to my mother and father: Beulah J. and Norman G. Crouse

Forward

This book is written so that you can understand how best to take care of your brain, and the brains of those you love, in order to prevent Alzheimer's disease, autism, and stroke. For the last 50 years, in spite of excellent research, the causes of Alzheimer's, autism, and stroke have remained controversial. It may be years before all needed research is performed and the controversy ends. But a tipping point has been reached and there is convincing evidence that aluminum accumulation in our bodies and brains can cause Alzheimer's, autism, and stroke. This book describes this evidence and gives you a course of action to decrease aluminum accumulation in your brain. This book also gives you recommendations on how to keep the brain chemically fit. Making a decision to adopt these recommendations requires balancing the benefits of taking action versus the risks of not taking action. After reading this book I think you will agree that the benefits of preventing Alzheimer's, autism, and stroke make following these recommendations worthwhile.

Acknowledgements

I appreciate the support and encouragement of my wife Laurie Adamson. Special thanks to Dr. Christopher Exley, Dr. J.R. Walton, Dr. Christopher Shaw, Dr. John Rockstroh, and Amy Yasko for fact checking and Jere Beasley, Melissa Easter, and Patrice Morrow for copy editing and suggestions. Thanks to David Adelizzi, Susan Doubler, Gary Marshall, Bill Hamilton, and Donna Safreed for useful comments.

Table of Contents

About the Author 8
Introduction 10
    Chapter Preview 12
Chapter 1 – Alzheimer's Disease 13
    What Causes Alzheimer's Disease? 13
    The Case for Aluminum Being the Cause of AD 33
    Aluminum an Unrequired and Unwanted Intruder 48
    Prevalence of Alzheimer's Disease 49
    Symptoms of Alzheimer's Disease 50
    Diagnosis of Alzheimer's Disease 51
        Biochemistry and Neurochemistry of AD 55
        Neurochemistry of Memory Impairment by Aluminum 58
Chapter 2 – Stroke and Vascular Dementia 61
    Aluminum a Causal Factor for Stroke 64
    Homocysteine Metabolism 66
    Three Pathways of Homocysteine Metabolism 67
    Additional Factors Linked to Elevated Total Serum Homocysteine 68
    Additional Causes of Stroke 72
    Visiting my Doctor 75
    Biochemical Mechanism of Supplements to Lower Homocysteine 77
Chapter 3 – Preventing and Possibly Reversing Dementia with 7 Supplements 80
    PQQ as an Oral Supplement to Prevent Dementia and Possibly Autism 80
    PQQ as an Oral Supplement for Reversing Brain Ageing 83
        Biochemistry of PQQ Stimulating NGF Production 84
    CoQ10 as an Oral Supplement for Brain Energy 85
    Vitamin D3 as an Oral Supplement 86
        Vitamin D Increases Glutathione 93
    Taurine Improves and Protects the Ageing Brain 94
        Mystery of How Taurine Protects Against Metal Toxicity 96
    Vitamin K2-MK-4 for Preventing Stroke and Possibly Reversing aFib 97
        Vitamin K2-MK-4 Prevents Osteoporosis 99

Vitamin K2-MK-4 Activates Proteins to Prevent MAC 99

Vitamin B12 and B6 as a B100 Supplement to Keep Homocysteine Levels Low 99

5-MTHF Supplement as Insurance to Keep Homocysteine Levels Low 102

DHA in a Healthy Diet for Memory Improvement 103

Biosynthesis of Taurine and Glutathione 108

Chapter 4 - Controlling Aluminum Ingestion 109

Aluminum in Food 110

SALPs and Alumsb as Major Sources of Aluminum in Food 111

Alum as a Source of Aluminum in Food 112

Aluminum in Pharmaceuticals 112

Colorants for Food, Drugs, and Cosmetics that Contain Aluminum 113

Aluminum in Vaccines 114

Aluminum in Infant Formula 114

Absorption of Aluminum in Antiperspirants and Astringents 115

Aluminum in Beverages 116

Alum Fertilizer as a Source of Aluminum in Beverages 116

Aluminum Beverage Cans as a Source of Aluminum in Beverages 116

Aluminum in Drinking Water 118

Cement as a Source of Aluminum in Drinking Water 119

Alum Pretreatment as a Source of Aluminum in Drinking Water 122

Defluoridation as a Source of Aluminum in Drinking Water 122

Enhancement of Aluminum Corrosion by Fluoride 123

Fluoride Increases Aluminum Absorption 126

Coffee Percolators and Tea Warmers as an Aluminum Source 127

Chapter 5 – Controlling Your Aluminum Retention with a Dissolved Mineral 129

Preparation of Silicade 134

Chemistry of Orthosilicic Acid Complexation with Aluminum 138

Siliceous Organisms and their Contribution to OSA in Drinking Water 140

Chapter 6 – Seven Lifestyle Choices to Prevent Alzheimer's, Autism, and Stroke 142

Stop Smoking 142

Decrease Daily Moderate Alcohol Consumption 144

Avoid Aluminum Ingestion 145

- Increase Dissolved Silica in Your Diet 153
- Aerobically Exercise 159
  - *Neurochemistry of Memory Improvement by Exercise* 163
- Avoid Lack of Sleep 165
- Avoid Head Trauma 168
  - Acute Traumatic Encephalopathy 168
  - Chronic Traumatic Encephalopathy (CTE) 169

Chapter 7– Drugs for Alzheimer's Disease 172
- Drugs for Slowing or Reversing the Progression of AD 173
- Future Drugs for Curing AD 179

Chapter 8 – Alzheimer's and Stroke as Mismatch Diseases 181
- Geochemical Evolution 181
- *Homo Sapiens* Evolution 182
- Geochemical Dysevolution 183
- *Homo Sapiens* Dysevolution 184
  - Pellagra as an Ancient Mismatch Disease 185
  - Lead Poisoning as an Ancient Mismatch Disease 185
  - Alzheimer's and Stroke as Modern Mismatch Diseases 188

Chapter 9 – Autism as a Mismatch Disease 191
- *Homo Sapiens* Evolution 192
- *Homo Sapiens* Cultural Evolution 193
- Aluminum a Causal Factor of Autism 194
- *Homo Sapiens* Cultural Dysevolution and Autism 198
  - Increased Baby Formula Usage 199
  - Increased Vitamin D Deficiency 204
  - Increased Air Pollution 207
  - Increased Use of Sunblock and Sunscreen 208
  - Increased Premature Birth 208
  - Increased Number of Infant Vaccinations 209
- Cures for Autism 216

Conclusion of Prevent Alzheimer's, Autism, and Stroke 222
- Recommendations for Preventing Alzheimer's, Autism, and Stroke 223

Appendix I	229
Dementia with Lewy Bodies and Parkinson's Disease	229
Appendix II	232
Metabolic Dementia	232
Appendix III	236
Hippocampal Sclerosis	236
Appendix IV	239
Cerebral Amyloid Angiopathy	239
Appendix V	240
Blood-Brain Barrier's Role in Alzheimer's Prevention	240
Appendix VI	245
Epidemiology Supporting Aluminum's Causal Role in Alzheimer's Disease	245
References	249

Table of Figures

Figure 1 - STDP in rat cortical slices	57
Figure 2 – Atherogenesis and aluminum's role as a cause of stroke	64
Figure 3 – Metabolism of homocysteine	67
Figure 4 – Effect of OSA on aluminum in blood plasma	139
Figure 5 – Global ocean conveyor belt	140
Figure 6 – Box plot of serum silicon content of various groups	154
Figure 7 - Lead in old bones	187
Figure 8 – Formula-fed as a percentage of infants versus age in the U.S.	200
Figure 9 – Vitamin D lowers elevated aluminum levels in children	206

About the Author

Of all the books I read in college, the three most significant in shaping my career were: "Silent Spring" by Rachel Carson, "The Fitness of the Environment" by L. J. Henderson and "The Immense Journey" by Loren C. Eiseley. These books describe how our planet evolved to become an ideal environment for life and how our species, *Homo sapiens,* evolved to unwittingly upset this environment by introducing chemicals, such as DDT and aluminum.

After graduating from college I co-founded a company to analyze the chemicals in food and water. In less than a year the company became the only one in New England approved by the FDA to analyze meat products for toxic chemicals, such as PCB's and pesticides. The company tested and approved these products for sale to the public.

With my two business partners, I later purchased a company that produced isotopically labeled chemicals. With the help of a group of talented chemists, I developed a series of stable isotopically labelled toxic chemicals and pesticides that were sold and used worldwide for quantifying these chemicals in food and water.

I developed the first computerized instruments to measure the corrosion rate of metals in contact with liquids. These rates are important when storing food and water in metal containers for long periods of time. These rates become even more important when cooking food in contact with metal surfaces, since heat usually increases the rate of metal corrosion.

Working with a dedicated group of people, I helped develop a new type of detector for toxic and flammable gases. Thousands of these detectors were manufactured and are currently used by gas utility leak technicians for finding toxic and flammable gas leaks in homes.

Since 2012 I have taken courses at the University of Tasmania on dementia and at Harvard on neurochemistry along with studying the scientific literature relating to the neurochemistry of the brain. This book is the result of this study.

Also results of this study include four videos on You Tube:

- "Brain Fitness in the Aluminum Age – Preventing Alzheimers"
- "Brain Fitness in the Aluminum Age - Eliminating Aluminum"
- "Brain Fitness in the Aluminum Age – Coffee Makers"
- "Silica Water – How to Make it at Home"

Up to date information is available at my Blog: http://prevent-alzheimers-autism-stroke.blogspot.com/ and my website: http://prevent-alzheimers-autism-stroke.com

My wife and I enjoy hiking and leading others hiking. We often hike in a 2,500 acre wooded nature sanctuary called the Middlesex Fells near our home. We particularly enjoy leading children on hikes and encouraging them to observe and inquire into their natural world.

Introduction

I have found a surprising connection between Alzheimer's, autism, and stroke and this groundbreaking book describes their common causal factor. These diseases are ***modern mismatch diseases*** created by our brains attempting to function in the presence of a chemical monster at levels not experienced during the brain's evolution. This book describes specific preventative measures to be taken by you and your family to rid yourself of this chemical monster. It also encourages cultural changes that will allow our society to prevent these mismatch diseases. Most importantly a preventative system for individuals is described in this book involving 7 specific supplements, 7 lifestyle choices, and a dissolved mineral that will prevent Alzheimer's, autism, and stroke. This is also a combination therapy that has been shown to reverse the cognitive decline seen in early-stage Alzheimer's disease. Elements of this combination therapy have also been found to reverse the course of autism in the very young and the course of hardening of the arteries and stroke in the very old.

My interest in dementia started after an acquaintance died of the after-effects of a stroke and my mother and a friend's mother, both 86 years old at the time, began suffering severe frustration and panic attacks due to short term memory failure. Having no preconceived notions about dementia and autism, I spent a number of years reading research articles in scientific journals. The search for the causes of Alzheimer's and stroke started as a mystery and led to a surprising connection with the cause of autism. Once the mystery was solved it transformed into a crusade. I found this monster lurking in my medicine cabinet, food pantries, refrigerator, and the water pipes leading into my home. This monster has been damaging the brains of newborn infants, elderly family members, and everyone in between for years. It is time to take on this monster as both individuals and as a culture. Reading the book will allow you to make an informed decision about what recommendations you will use to prevent this monster from claiming your brain and the brains of those you love.

Being a biochemist I am naturally suspicious of supplementing my diet with impure herbal extracts. Small traces of toxic impurities in these extracts can do damage to your body and especially your brain. Therefore this book only recommends supplements containing purified biochemicals and a dissolved mineral all of which are commonly found in your body.

The Alzheimer's Association finds that Alzheimer's disease is grossly misunderstood and underestimated. When they surveyed people in 12 countries they found:

"59 percent of people surveyed incorrectly believe that Alzheimer's disease is a typical part of ageing and 40 percent of people believe that Alzheimer's is not fatal".

Alzheimer's (AD) is currently a terminal disease but it is not an inevitable part of aging. The following table will give you some "food" for thought. Does this table suggest that AD is a typical part of ageing?

Life Expectancy and AD Death Rate by Country		
Country	**Life Expectancy (yrs.)***	**AD Death Rate (per 100,000)****
Iceland	83.3	34.1
United States	79.8	45.6
Malaysia	75.7	0.7
Singapore	84	0.2

*Life expectancy data from WHO 2014, **AD death rate data 2016 worldlifeexpectancy.com

There are countries in the world, such as Malaysia and Singapore, where people with similar life expectancy to the U.S. have much less AD. This book explains why AD is not prevalent in some parts of the world and how countries like the U.S. can lower their rate of AD. This book also explains how individuals can take steps to lower their risk of AD and work toward cultural changes in their countries to lower the rate of AD. True prevention is only possible by first discovering the cause of a disease such as Alzheimer's. The book begins as I did, searching for the cause of Alzheimer's. I hope you join me in this exciting search by reading Chapter 1.

Chapter Preview

- **Chapter 1** – As a modern Sherlock Holmes the cause of Alzheimer's disease is subjected to the scrutiny of a detective's mind. Also the case for aluminum being the cause of Alzheimer's disease is presented.
- **Chapter 2** – Explores the causes of stroke and the process of atherogenesis that leads to atherosclerosis or hardening of the arteries. Surprisingly the same factor that causes Alzheimer's disease also causes stroke.
- **Chapter 3** – Describes how 7 supplements and a good diet work together to provide neuroprotection from the causes of Alzheimer's, autism, and stroke.
- **Chapter 4** - Explains how your ingestion of the common causal factor of Alzheimer's, autism, and stroke can be controlled by diet.
- **Chapter 5** – Explains how your excretion of the common causal factor of Alzheimer's, autism, and stroke can be controlled by a dissolved mineral.
- **Chapter 6** – Explores 7 lifestyle choices that can improve the chemical fitness of your brain and avoid the common causal factor of Alzheimer's, autism, and stroke.
- **Chapter 7** – Describes currently available supplements that reverse the progression and postpone the onset of Alzheimer's and drugs under development to possibly provide palliative relief to Alzheimer's patients in the future.
- **Chapter 8** – Looks at the bigger picture of how both the earth and human cultures have evolved to make us more susceptible to the neurotoxicity of the common causal factor of Alzheimer's and stroke. And how this has led to modern mismatch diseases such as Alzheimer's and stroke.
- **Chapter 9** – This chapter looks at why autism is also a modern mismatch disease, what causes autism, and how to prevent and cure autism.
- **Conclusion** – Recommendations for individual and collective actions that improve brain fitness and help to prevent Alzheimer's, autism, and stroke.

The information presented in italics with gray background goes into greater depth on relevant topics for readers who share my interest in how the neurochemistry of the brain works. Reading this information is not required to understand the thesis and conclusions of this book.

Chapter 1 – Alzheimer's Disease

"... anatomically it provided a result which departed from all previously known disease pathology." L. Alzheimer 1907[1]

What Causes Alzheimer's Disease?

The book begins as I did, searching for the cause of Alzheimer's. I initiated this search when simultaneously my mother and a friend's mother began having panic attacks due to short term memory failure at age 86. The progression of short term memory loss had been slow and steady and was just beginning to impact their daily living skills. Routine things they had done on a daily basis, such as grocery shopping, balancing the checkbook, and sewing, had become impossible tasks. I hoped that learning what was known about the cause of Alzheimer's would allow me to help these women slow the progression of the disease and possibly prevent further erosion of their memories.

I quickly discovered that finding the cause versus symptom of a disease like Alzheimer's is a tricky business. It takes a sleuth with the knowledge and cunning of Sherlock Holmes. Being a chemist I have always had a fascination with Mr. Holmes, probably because he was portrayed as a chemist by Sir Arthur Conan Doyle. Young Stamford said Holmes was a "first-class chemist" when he first introduced Watson to Holmes in "A Study in Scarlet". In order to understand my search for a cause of Alzheimer's (AD) please follow Mr. Holmes and Doctor Watson and read "The Case of the Cloaked Assassin".

The Case of the Cloaked Assassin

Watson we may have a killer loose on the streets! I just read on the internet in the Journal of Medical Case Reports 8:41 (2014) of the strange death of a 58 year old man with no prior medical history who was diagnosed with early-onset AD. Ten years prior to his diagnosis he began working on a daily basis handling alum dust in order to develop a new insulation for the nuclear and space industry. He was working with minimal respiratory protection. After six years performing this work he began suffering from memory loss and depression. In 2011, after his death due to AD at age 66, the frontal lobe of his brain was analyzed for aluminum. It contained approximately 3mcg (3 micrograms) of aluminum per gram of dried brain tissue (3mcg/gr. dry wt.)[2]. This is more than three times higher than the median concentration of aluminum (e.g. 0.87mcg/gr. dry wt.) found after death in the frontal lobes of people 60-70 years old[3]. In addition, an abundance of beta-amyloid (Aβ) plaque and a profusion of neurofibrillary tangles (NFTs), hallmarks of AD, were found in his frontal cortex.

So Watson what is coincidence and what caused AD in this case of strange death? There are four possibilities:

- The victim was genetically predisposed toward AD
- Aβ plaques were the cause of AD
- NFTs were the cause of AD
- Alum was the cause of AD

The first question – what are Aβ plaques and NFTs? These plaques and NFTs are insoluble protein molecules that are three dimensional aggregates of smaller soluble molecules called peptides and oligomers that are comprised of amino acids. An amino acid is a molecule with at least one each of an amine and acid.

Amyloid beta (Aβ) plaques are made from Aβ oligomers that are aggregates of Aβ peptides that are in turn fragments enzymatically cleaved from a larger protein called amyloid precursor protein (APP).

NFTs are filaments of a phosphoprotein called tau that stabilizes structural elements in neurons called microtubules. Tau has 79 potential sites for phosphorylation. Thirty of these sites are usually phosphorylated in normal tau proteins giving them an overcoat of phosphorus, oxygen and hydrogen. The tau in NFTs is more highly phosphorylated than normal and is called hyper-phosphorylated tau.

The second question - what is in alum? Alum is a word that describes both specific compounds and a class of compounds. The specific compounds "alum" describes are sulfate salts that contain either aluminum and potassium, or aluminum and sodium ions. Members of the class of alum sulfate salts are additionally described by ions other than aluminum, potassium, or sodium that they contain. Such as "ammonium alum" (a.k.a. ammonium aluminum sulfate).

After hearing this definition of "alum" as being an aluminum salt, Doctor Watson became agitated and said: "Wait just a minute Holmes, as a medical doctor I believe aluminum should not be on the list of suspects for AD!" Watson pointed out that according to the Alzheimer's Association "… studies have failed to confirm any role for aluminum in causing Alzheimer's"[4]. Holmes turned to Watson and replied: I applaud you, your profession, and the Alzheimer's Association for their dedication to caring for and supporting those with illnesses and their mission to eliminate Alzheimer's disease through the advancement of research and the promotion of brain health. But historically there have been examples when the medical profession has not been sufficiently open-minded to explore all the potential causes of a disease.

One such example of a missed opportunity to save lives was the prevention of pellagra. Pellagra results in dementia, painful disfigurement, and death and is now known to be caused by a lack of niacin in the diet. Niacin is concentrated in the outer-most layer of the endosperm and germ layers of the corn kernel that are removed by milling. In 1901 the Beall Degerminator was patented that could mill the corn removing the outer endosperm and germ layers from the kernels for improved storage. In the southern part of the U.S. between 1906 and 1940 mechanical corn milling resulted in 3 million people sickened by pellagra and more than 100,000 deaths due to pellagra. In 1913 Casmir Funk wrote an article suggesting that the new procedure for corn milling was causing pellagra, but he was ignored[5]. The medical profession in the U.S. firmly believed a toxin in rancid unripe corn was the cause of pellagra[6]. It took a number of years after the connection between niacin deficiency and pellagra was discovered for the medical profession to finally abandon their toxin theory. So as you can see Watson we should remain open-minded and leave aluminum on the list of suspects for AD so we do not repeat any missed opportunities to save lives.

Watson, who was still pondering this dilemma regarding aluminum as a suspect, responded: "I am all for saving lives and I know that aluminum is a proven to be toxic to neurons but I have read and believe the following:"

- Aluminum compounds are inert or insoluble preventing entry into the body.
- Any aluminum that does get into the body is immediately excreted.
- Any aluminum that is not excreted is deposited in biologically inert stores such as bone.

Well Watson we may find comfort in believing this dogma but these are untrue myths that give us a false sense of security. Aluminum can cloak itself in a variety of chemical disguises and enter the body through the gut, skin, lung, and nose. Acidification of aluminum compounds in the environment by acid rain and in the gut by stomach acid solubilizes these compounds and allows aluminum the freedom to change its chemical disguise. Once in the body some of the disguised aluminum finds its way to the brain and accumulates in our brain during our lifetime. I know these facts are unpleasant to deal with, but facing reality is better than keeping our heads in the sand. So Watson let's proceed ahead with aluminum on the suspect list and see where this investigation takes us.

The third question that begs an answer is how old is Alzheimer's disease? Is AD an ancient disease that happened to finally get a diagnosis or is it a modern disease? In 1888 Doctor Alois Alzheimer began working at a psychiatric hospital in Frankfort Germany. Thirteen years later at age 35 Doctor Alzheimer started observing a hospital patient named Auguste Deter. She had strange behavioral symptoms and had lost her short term memory. After she died in 1906 her brain was autopsied by Dr. Alzheimer. Using special stains he found amyloid plaques and neurofibrillary tangles. So let's ask the doctor himself if AD is a modern disease. After an exchange of letters, Holmes had the answer. In a translation of Dr. Alzheimer's words:

> *"The case presented even in the clinic such a different picture, that it could not be categorized under known disease headings, and also anatomically it provided a result which departed from all previously known disease pathology"*[1].

Doctor Alzheimer believed AD is a modern disease but did anyone else share his opinion? The mental health of older people living between 1886 and 1889 is described in the monograph "Old Age" published in Cambridge England in 1889[7]. The monograph summarizes the results of British general practitioners studying the mental health of their oldest patients during the mid-1880s. The study group was 900 subjects who were 80 or older including 74 centenarians. The monograph's author concludes that dementia:

> *"... was witnessed only in two of our centenarians ... indeed the brain held out as well or better than other organs"*

This 3% rate of dementia among centenarians in the mid-1880s can be compared with a study 111 years later. In 2000 a study was done of people in three Dutch towns with populations greater than 250,000. Of the 17 centenarians found in this more recent study 15 had dementia for an 88% rate of dementia. The other 2 centenarians could not be examined[8].

From Doctor Alzheimer's comments in 1907 and comparing these two studies of dementia among centenarians done 111 years apart, it is obvious Watson that AD is a modern disease that is between 110 and 180 years old. So now Watson let us look at the first suspect: genetics.

Is there a genetic defect that could be responsible for AD? Yes Watson, there are two types of AD: familial and sporadic. Familial AD is believed to have a genetic link but accounts for only 1-2% of AD cases[9]. Sporadic AD accounts for the remaining 98-99% of AD cases and after extensive searching only the apoE4 gene has been found to increase the risk for sporadic AD[9]. Carriers of the apoE4 gene, about 20% of the population, have a 60% chance over age 80 of having AD versus a 10% overall risk of AD over age 80 in the general population. Therefore the difference in risk for AD between carriers and non-carriers of this gene is 50%. In 2002 there were 9 million people in the U.S. who were 80 years of age or older[10]. A 50% chance of AD in the 20% of those over 80 with the apoE4 gene corresponds to 10% of 9 million people or 0.9 million cases of AD. There were 2.7 million AD cases in the U.S. in 2002[11]. This means approximately 1/3 (33%) of the sporadic AD cases in the U.S. could be due to genetics involving the apoE4 gene.

Carriers of the apoE4 gene are more vulnerable to AD because they have higher than normal levels of Aβ peptides that can result in higher levels of Aβ oligomers and Aβ plaques. ApoE proteins are chaperones that complex with Aβ peptides and facilitate their transfer across the blood-brain-barrier and out the brain. Carriers of the apoE4 gene may be more vulnerable to AD because they produce an Aβ peptide chaperone molecule apolipoprotein E4 (apoE4). This chaperone works with a slow receptor that slows Aβ peptide clearance from the brain[12]. Also carriers of the apoE4 gene have less apoE protein in their serum and this also slows Aβ peptide clearance from the brain[9]. Therefore carriers of the apoE4 gene have higher than normal levels of Aβ peptides in their brains that can result in higher levels of Aβ oligomers and plaques in their brains.

Is there any other indication that AD is caused by a genetic defect? In 1987 L.E. Nee, et al. reported a clinical and family study of 22 twin pairs in which one or both twins had AD. In approximately 40% of the cases, AD affects both twins showing that about 40% of cases in the U.S. could be due to genetics (i.e. the apoE4 gene) [13]. Within experimental errors this 40% agrees with the 33% derived from the math based upon the frequency of the apoE4 gene in the U.S. population.

So as you can see Watson with the data agreeing from a risk analysis and a study of twin pairs we can conclude that greater than 50% of AD is not related to genetics and likely caused by environmental factors. But before turning our back on genetics, could it be possible there is a gene other than the apoe4 gene responsible for AD?

Could any dominant gene or genes spread through the population and cause a modern disease? If a dominant gene is inherited from either parent it is always expressed in that parent's children. For a recessive gene to be passed on, both parents must have it, so dominant genes spread more quickly through a population than recessive genes.

As we now know Watson, Alzheimer's disease is a modern disease first observed 110 years ago in a person 56 years old at the time of death. Since Alzheimer's is a modern disease, a mutation, such as the apoE4 gene, that could cause Alzheimer's would have had to occur approximately 180 years ago. A human generation lasted, on average, 30 years during the last 200 years[14]. A period of 180 years corresponds to 6 generations. But how many generations did this gene have to spread through the population by the time people were born who are currently over 80 years old? The 9 million people in the U.S. over 80 were born after approximately 3 of those 6 generations. Therefore the gene carrying the mutation would have had only 3 generations to spread through the population before those people currently over 80 were born.

Watson asked: "How many people can potentially carry a dominant gene three generations after the single mutation that created the gene?" Holmes answered: "If there was a single mutant and every one of the three succeeding generations had both a dominant gene and eight children, there would be only 512 carriers of the gene worldwide after three generations. As already mentioned there are 9 million people over age 80 in the U.S. and 20% (1.8 million) of them are carriers of the apo4 gene. The calculated 512 carriers are not even close to the estimated 1.8 million carriers of this gene in the U.S. population over age 80. So a mutation 180 years ago of the apo4 gene, or for that matter any gene, could not be the cause of AD".

At this point Holmes turned and noticed that Watson was madly calculating $8 \times 8 \times 8 = 512$ on a sheet of scratch paper and looking confused. Watson looked up and asked: "So can a modern disease as common as AD be due to a recent mutation?" Holmes replied: "No, it takes thousands of years to spread even a dominant mutation to a significant percentage of the population".

Since AD is a modern disease and not an ancient disease we now know three important facts from which we can draw a conclusion:

- Because of its prevalence the apoE4 gene as it exists today is an ancient gene not a modern gene
- Twenty percent of humans who have the apoE4gene have been living with higher than normal levels of Aβ peptides in their brains for thousands of years and did not get AD.
- Only one third of those with AD in the U.S. have the apoE4 gene.

This is the first crux of the case Watson! Because the apoE4 gene is ancient it alone can't be the cause of a modern disease like AD. Since the apoE4 gene causes higher than normal levels of Aβ peptides, a good percentage of people have lived with these high levels of Aβ peptides for thousands of years and not gotten AD. Therefore excessive levels of these Aβ peptides can't cause a modern disease like AD.

Watson looked startled and said: "Amazing Holmes this proves that AD is not caused by the ancient apoE4 gene or a recent genetic mutation or even higher than normal levels of Aβ peptides in the brain. So if not genetics and Aβ peptides, then what is the cause of AD?"

Is AD caused by high levels of Aβ plaque?

Watson noted: "Aβ plaque is a hallmark of AD and it is found in higher than normal levels in the brain of the case of strange death. This puts Aβ plaque on the list of suspects. But is there any evidence that Aβ plaque is harmful to the brain?" Holmes replied: "No, AD-related neuron loss and dementia are mediated by Aβ oligomers, not Aβ plaque[536]. This is because Aβ oligomers inhibit neuronal viability ten times more that Aβ plaque and forty times more than Aβ peptides[15]. Soluble Aβ oligomers (e.g. clusters of soluble Aβ peptides) are converted in the brain to insoluble Aβ plaque[16]. Metals, such as aluminum, facilitate the conversion of Aβ peptides to Aβ oligomers and then to Aβ plaque[16,17]. Aβ oligomers have been isolated from the cerebral cortex and cerebrospinal fluid in concentrations six times higher than normal in the brains of AD patients[18]".

Watson then suggested: "Since these findings suggest that Aβ oligomers rather than Aβ plaque might be a cause of AD, we should add Aβ oligomers to our list of suspects. After all it would appear that Aβ oligomers had to be present in order to make Aβ plaque observed in the brain of the case of strange death."

Holmes replied: "Excellent deduction Watson, our new list of suspects now includes:

- NFTs
- Aβ oligomers
- Aluminum"

How are NFTs formed in the brain?

NFTs are insoluble tangles of soluble phosphoproteins called tau. Because these tangles start forming inside neurons they are called neurofibrillary tangles or NFTs. The appearance in the brain of these NFTs as "tombstones" or "ghosts" is one of the hallmarks of AD. NFT formation requires two things:

- An above normal amount of phosphoryl groups (PO_3^{2-}) coated on the tau proteins. This phosphoryl coated tau protein is called hyper-phosphorylated tau.
- Metal ions that facilitate the formation and pairing of hyper-phosphorylated tau to form paired helical filaments (PHFτ) called NFTs.

Lesions in the brain caused by NFTs are better correlated with cognitive decline in AD than intracellular Aβ oligomer and extracellular Aβ plaque formation[19].

Does aluminum cause NFTs or does aluminum complex with NFTs after they form?

Some metal cations inhibit numerous key enzymes in the brain. One of these key enzymes is PP2A that keeps tau from being covered with too many phosphoryl (PO_3^{2-}) groups (i.e. over-phosphorylated). When PP2A is inhibited by zinc[20], mercury[21], or aluminum[22] ions the result is over-phosphorylation of tau leading to PHFτ formation, neuronal death, and ultimately neurofibrillary tangles in place of former neurons. Of the three cations that are known to inhibit PP2A, zinc is a neurotransmitter that is required by our brains and zinc and mercury are not on the list of suspects in the case of strange death as they are not contained in alum. Therefore Watson, zinc and mercury are "red-herrings" and this leaves aluminum in alum on the suspect list.

In 1988 aluminum chloride added to rat brain cells resulted in NFTs that were "distinct" immunochemically from human Alzheimer NFTs[23]. This resulted in more controversy but was resolved in 1998 when aluminum chloride was injected into the cerebrospinal fluid in the brains of New Zealand white rabbits[24]. The resulting NFTs were immunochemically identical to NFTs found in the brains of AD patients. In 1992 it was found that aluminum stimulates the interaction between filaments of hyper-phosphorylated tau. This interaction results in paired helical filaments of tau (PHFτ) and NFT formation[25].

Is aluminum linked to NFTs in neurons?

In 1973 levels of aluminum were found to be higher than normal in some regions of the brains of Alzheimer patients[26]. This finding remained controversial until 1980 when a combination scanning electron microscope and x-ray spectrometer analysis showed there was aluminum in neurons with NFTs in the brains of both Alzheimer and elderly non-Alzheimer patients and no aluminum in adjacent neurons without NFTs[27]. Since NFTs are a hallmark of AD, this finding was the first to link aluminum to AD at the neuronal level. Even more disturbing was the fact that aluminum and NFTs are in the neurons of the elderly in general not just those with an AD diagnosis. These findings are consistent with research that finds aluminum in the brains of the elderly in general[28,29].

Aluminum is a non-essential cation in our brains and an unwanted intruder. It is obvious Watson, since aluminum promotes the formation of paired helical filaments of tau and NFTs, NFTs are at best only a secondary cause or symptom and not the primary cause of Alzheimer's.

But Watson was looking skeptical and asked: "Since aluminum is looking more and more like the culprit in the case of strange death, why do people with the apoE4 gene have a 50% higher chance of getting AD than people without this gene?"

Holmes replied: Carriers of the apoE4 gene have lived with higher levels of Aβ peptides, oligomers, and plaque for thousands of years and not had AD. There must be an environmental factor that facilitates the formation of Aβ peptides, oligomers, or plaque to cause AD".

Watson asked: "Could this environmental factor be aluminum?"

Yes Watson aluminum is a likely environmental casual factor of AD. Metal cations such as aluminum, copper, zinc, and iron are known to complex with Aβ peptides to form Aβ oligomers[16,17]. However, only aluminum complexes of Aβ oligomers are neurotoxic[16]. Aluminum makes the degree of neurotoxicity worse because it has the unique property of "freezing" Aβ peptides in the oligomeric state, resulting in high concentrations of Aβ oligomers[16]. When these Aβ oligomers are complexed with aluminum they cause excess calcium to diffuse into neurons which can ultimately kill them. Therefore aluminum can cause AD both with and without the apoE4 gene but is 50% more likely to cause AD in carriers of the apoE4 gene. This is due to the carriers having higher levels of Aβ peptides in their brains making it possible for aluminum to freeze more Aβ peptides in the neurotoxic oligomeric state.

Aluminum acts in five ways to increase the accumulation of Aβ oligomers in the brain putting carriers of the apoE4 gene at greater risk of getting AD:

- Aluminum freezes Aβ peptides in the neurotoxic oligomeric state[16].
- Aluminum lowers gene expression of neprilysin, an enzyme that is the rate limiting step in Aβ peptide and oligomer degradation[30,31].
- Aluminum lowers gene expression of the LDL receptor LRP1, required for Aβ peptide clearance and the importation of cholesterol to neurons[30,32].
- Aluminum increases gene expression of BACE1, the β-secretase enzyme that cleaves the amyloid precursor protein (APP) to the precursor of Aβ peptides[30,31].
- Aluminum increases gene expression for the production of APP, the precursor of Aβ peptides[31].

Those with the apoE4 gene are also more likely to get AD due to head trauma or aluminum accumulation leading to an ischemic event, such as stroke. Ischemia occurs when blood flow is temporarily suspended to some regions of the brain. Sporadic AD is believed to be associated in some cases with an ischemic event[33]. Post mortem analysis of the brains of those with AD has shown that 30% have evidence of an ischemic event[33]. Shortly after an ischemic event there is increased genetic expression of an apoE protein, such as apoE4[33]. Also there is both an increased genetic expression of amyloid precursor protein (APP) and the enzyme β-secretase (BACE1) that cleaves APP to the precursor of Aβ peptides[33]. Those with the apoE4 gene have slower Aβ peptide clearance than normal. Because of this, after an ischemic event there is even less clearance than normal in the brains of those with the apoE4 gene and more production of Aβ peptides and Aβ oligomers.

Accumulation of aluminum in the brain increases the toxicity of Aβ oligomers, the amount of aluminum-complexed Aβ oligomers, and the likelihood of an ischemic event (see Chapter 2). Aluminum is a likely environmental causal factor for both toxic Aβ oligomers and ischemic events and puts people with the apoE4 gene at greater risk than normal for AD.

Watson, this is the second crux of the case. Since Aβ oligomers are only a facilitating factor for AD they can be removed from our list of suspects.

Watson looked alarmed for the first time and asked: "Is there aluminum in my brain that is 'freezing' neurotoxic Aβ peptides in the oligomeric state?" Holmes replied "I am afraid that we are all suffering from some frozen neurotoxic Aβ oligomers. But luckily we can control the amount of aluminum we ingest, absorb, and excrete. As you have sensed Watson, the sum total of this research has now reached a tipping point".

Aluminum is the only remaining suspect for causing the case of strange death. But before we can be certain that aluminum is the culprit we need to find if aluminum has the means and motive to cause AD in the case of strange death.

How does aluminum get into our bodies and brains?

Aluminum salts began to be used as a food preservative in the mid-1880's and that may be a reason why the first case of AD was discovered approximately 20 years later in 1907 by Doctor Alzheimer. The commercialization of aluminum salts, and products containing aluminum, has resulted in more aluminum being refined and made available every year. Currently we use aluminum in reduced metal, oxidized metal, and ionic chemical forms, such as salts. The ionic chemical forms of aluminum are neurotoxic. The reduced metal form of aluminum must be converted first by corrosion to the oxidized metal form and then by acidic conditions to the ionic form in order to become neurotoxic. The oxidized metal and ionic chemical forms of aluminum are found in a variety of pharmaceuticals, such as antacids, vaccines, food products, baking powder, drinking water, sunscreens, cosmetics, antiperspirants, astringents, and fertilizers.

Because of the amount of drinking water we consume daily, any aluminum in drinking water presents an opportunity for its absorption and accumulation in the body. The ionic form of aluminum is in drinking water due to acid-rain freeing bound aluminum from minerals in the ground, city water departments using alum to clarify drinking water, and mortar lined city water pipes leaching aluminum into drinking water.

There appeared to be no connection between aluminum in drinking water and AD until the data were reevaluated in 1996. This analysis revealed a correlation between aluminum in drinking water and AD when taking into consideration the concentration of fluoride and silicic acid as well as aluminum in the drinking water[34]. Fluoride ions facilitate the transfer of aluminum across the blood-brain barrier increasing aluminum absorption in the brain[35], while silicic acid facilitates aluminum removal from the blood by the kidneys decreasing aluminum absorption by the brain[36-38]. Therefore, Watson, drinking water is a common way that aluminum is ingested, absorbed by our bodies, and accumulated in our brains and silicic acid slows this accumulation.

The three points of entry for aluminum into the body are oral ingestion, inhalation, and absorption through the skin. We do not know which pathway was the major source of aluminum in the case of strange death. Due to the lack of proper respiratory protection, we might assume that inhalation was the point of entry. Inhaled aluminum can take a shortcut to the brain across the olfactory epithelium cells lining the nasal cavities and then diffusing through olfactory receptor neurons to enter the brain via both olfactory bulbs[39-41]. Organic complexes of aluminum have been found to readily enter the brain via this pathway[42]. The other two pathways require that aluminum crosses the blood-brain barrier in order to enter the brain. Once in the brain, some of the aluminum stays there throughout life[43] inhibiting numerous key enzymes and killing neurons[44].

Aluminum in the ionic form can form complexes with a wide variety of organic and inorganic ligands. Some of these complexes are optimal for absorption from the gastrointestinal track into the blood and others are optimal for crossing the blood brain barrier. Ionic aluminum is like a cloaked assassin using these ligands as disguises to cross two barriers: between the gut and blood and the blood and brain. The following organic ligands have an affinity for ionic aluminum and have been found to be present in the blood at the approximate concentrations indicated: citrate (ca. 250μM), pyroglutamate (ca. 180μM), glutamate (ca. 10μM), nucleotides ATP, ADP, and AMP (ca. 5μM), and transferrin (ca. 1μM)[45]. In addition to these organic ligands there are inorganic ligands that also have an affinity for ionic aluminum including: fluoride, silicic acid, hydroxide, and phosphate.

Transferrin receptors are more numerous in those areas of the brain that have the highest levels of aluminum accumulation[46]. For this reason transferrin has been theorized to be the primary (i.e. 90%) transporter of aluminum to the brain[43,47,48]. The problem with this theory is the molecular weight of the transferrin aluminum complex is four-fold higher than can be handled by the kidney's glomerulus[45]. This means that the rapid changes in urinary excretion of aluminum seen following exposure to aluminum can't be accounted for with such a large transporter. The rest of the previously mentioned ligands result in aluminum complexes that are small enough to be handled by the glomerulus of the kidney and are therefore more likely to comprise aluminum's cloak. But aluminum can change its disguise when reaching the blood-brain barrier and possibly transferrin is the best disguise for successfully crossing this barrier.

Watson had become agitated with worry. He asked Holmes: "So how long will it take to get the aluminum I consumed at breakfast out of my body? " Holmes' answer was discouraging: "Once aluminum is ingested and absorbed 64% will be excreted during the first day but the rest will be slowly excreted and even after 50 years 4% of what you ingested with breakfast this morning will remain in some parts of your body[43]."

As you can see Watson, aluminum has the means to get into the brain. But is aluminum normally found in the brain and is a higher level of aluminum in the brain associated with AD?

How much aluminum is in a normal brain?

It is calculated that the human brain accumulates aluminum at a rate of 10-70 billionths of a gram of aluminum per gram dry weight of brain per year during a lifetime. This amount is consistent with the 0.4 to 5.6mcg (1.08mcg mean across all 4 main lobes) aluminum per gram dry weight of brain as observed by autopsy of different regions of 60 human brains after a normal lifetime of exposure to aluminum[3]. It now appears likely that this slow aluminum accumulation may facilitate an increased incidence of a wide range of neurological diseases including AD[49].

Is there more aluminum in brains of those with AD?

From aluminum analysis of the brains of those who died of sporadic AD, familial AD, and occupational AD, it has been concluded that median levels of aluminum in excess of 2.0mcg per gram dry weight of brain across all four main lobes is both a common characteristic of AD and a contributor to its etiology[50]. Some people absorb and accumulate aluminum at higher rates than others and this may account for why some get AD earlier than others[3,51]. AD patients younger than 77 years old have a 64% greater gastrointestinal aluminum absorption rate than age-matched non-AD controls[52]. However both AD and non-AD people over 77 have similar high rates of gastrointestinal aluminum absorption[53]. These high rates of gastrointestinal absorption result in faster aluminum accumulation in elderly brains as compared with middle-age brains[28,29]. Also aluminum in the brain is not uniformly distributed. In the elderly, aluminum is highest in the hippocampus (5.6mcg/gr. dry wt.) and lowest in the corpus callosum (1.5mcg/gr. dry wt.)[3].

A meta-analysis of published studies involving 1,208 participants, including 613 AD patients, revealed that aluminum is significantly higher in brains, serum, and cerebrospinal fluid of AD patients compared with non-AD participants[54].

Therefore Watson, aluminum as the "cloaked assassin" has the means to get into the normal brain and more aluminum does get into the brain of those with AD. But does it have the motive or biochemical motivation to cause mitochondrial disease, a clinical symptom of AD?

How does aluminum cause mitochondrial disease?

Mitochondrial disease occurs when the mitochondria of the cell fail to produce enough energy for cell or organ function. This neuro-metabolic dysfunction has been theorized to be a factor in the causation of AD[55]. But it is hard to tell the difference between a cause and a symptom of a disease. Watson, here is why aluminum is the cause of mitochondrial disease and mitochondrial disease is not a cause but a symptom of AD.

Mitochondria are membrane bound organelles inside brain and muscle cells that produce stored energy in the form of ATP generated by combining oxygen with nutrients in food. The brain normally consumes 30% of the total energy produced from these nutrients by the body. This process is called bioenergetics and it requires using nutrients, such as sugar, to make ATP in a series of steps called the Krebs cycle (a.k.a. TCA cycle). Aluminum lowers the amount and activity of several Krebs cycle enzymes involved in ATP production[56,57]. So aluminum lowers the efficiency of ATP production in brain. This lowers the amount of energy available to the brain resulting in mitochondrial disease.

Aluminum facilitates the formation of reactive oxygen species (ROS) by glial cells in the brain that are toxic to mitochondria and neurons[58]. Aluminum also inhibits two enzymes in the Krebs cycle that are involved in NADH production[56,57]. NADH is used in the body for making reduced-glutathione[59]. Reduced-glutathione reduces cofactors in the body, such as pyrroloquinoline quinone (PQQ), that in turn reduce the reactive oxygen species (ROS) that are harmful to mitochondria and neurons. The inhibition of NADH production by aluminum decreases reduced-glutathione levels allowing ROS to harm mitochondria and neurons resulting in mitochondrial disease[60].

Therefore Watson, aluminum can cause mitochondrial disease by decreasing ATP production, increasing ROS production, and preventing cofactors, such as PQQ, from protecting the mitochondria from oxidative harm by ROS.

How does aluminum impair memory?

Some parts of the brain are more prone to absorb aluminum than others, possibly due to some cells having more transferrin receptors[46]. The main aluminum-affected brain regions in humans, rats, and rabbits exposed to aluminum in their diet include the entorhinal cortex (EC), hippocampus, and locus coeruleus (LC). The EC and the hippocampal regions (e.g. CA1 pyramidal cell layer) are the regions with most absorbed aluminum in rats chronically exposed to aluminum in their diet[44]. These are also regions of the brain most vulnerable to NFT formation and neuronal death in AD[61]. In fact the EC is the first area of the brain to be affected by AD[62].

The entorhinal cortex (EC) is a neuronal hub linking the hippocampus with the neocortex. The hippocampus plays a key role in declarative memories such as autobiographical, episodic, and semantic memory and spatial memories including memory formation and consolidation and memory evolution during sleep. The neocortex is involved with sensory stimuli, generation of motor commands, spatial reasoning, conscious thought, and language. A region of the EC (e.g. layer III) is connected to all regions of the hippocampal formation including the dentate gyrus, all CA regions, including the CA1 pyramidal cell layer, and subiculum. These connections are called the perforant pathway. Surgical destruction of the perforant pathway in rats results in memory impairment[44] and surgical destruction of the perforant pathway in humans results in impairment of short term memory[63]. Aluminum in the diets of rats results in both lesions in the perforant pathway and in memory impairment[44]. Therefore Watson, aluminum, like a surgeon's knife, can cause short term memory loss.

Conclusion of the Case of the Cloaked Assassin

Holmes and Watson, have methodically solved the case of the "Cloaked Assassin" by reaching the following conclusions:

- **Aluminum in alum is the cause of AD in the case of strange death.**
- **Aluminum is the only suspect capable of causing AD and has both means and motive to cause AD.**
- **Aluminum causes the two hallmarks of AD:**
    - **AB-plaques**
    - **NFTs**
- **Aluminum causes two symptoms of AD:**
    - **Mitochondrial disease**
    - **Memory impairment**

Watson, we need to inform Lestrade over at Scotland Yard so the police can regulate this evil monster before more harm is done.

Before leaving on his mission, Watson turned and asked Holmes: Why isn't aluminum regulated like other toxic chemicals?

Holmes replied: "Even though aluminum adversely influences more than 200 biological reactions and has various neurotoxic effects on the mammalian central nervous system, it has not been regarded as posing a health hazard[64]. As a consequence, aluminum compounds are used in food additives, food processing, water purification, pharmaceuticals, and inoculations[66]. These factors may account for why, in the U.S. by the year 2002, 2.7 million people had AD[11] and worldwide by the year 2005, 24 million people had AD[67]. "

The controversy surrounding aluminum being a cause of AD has impacted the regulations regarding aluminum exposure. In 2010 the World Health Organization (WHO) lowered the provisional tolerable weekly intake (PTWI) of aluminum per person from 7 mg/kg of body weight to 1 mg/kg based upon new data[68]. In both 1998 and 2003 WHO stated:

> *"The positive relationship between aluminum in drinking-water and AD ... cannot be totally dismissed."* World Health Organization 1998 and 2003

Since 2010, the European Aluminum Association with support from the aluminum industry has participated in the Codex process, submitting biased reviews of the scientific literature in order to have the new aluminum limit re-assessed[64]. In response to this lobbying by the aluminum industry a joint FAO/WHO Expert Committee on Food Additives recently established a PTWI of 2 mg/kg body weight, superseding the previous WHO PTWI of 1 mg/kg body weight[69].

The initial response of government agencies to commonly used substances found to be toxic by scientific researchers usually favors the industries producing the substances[70]. For example, in 1979 when lead exposure in children was found to be correlated with low IQ, the credibility of the researcher was questioned by psychologists hired by the tetraethyl lead industry. These psychologists publically accused the researcher of scientific misconduct[70]. The parallel between lead and aluminum is very strong as they are both neurotoxins with powerful industrial lobbies backing their continued use. The only difference is that lead has a much longer history than aluminum (see Chapter 8 for the history of lead poisoning).

Watson looked discouraged and said "If it can't be better regulated is there any hope for individuals to lower the aluminum levels in their bodies and possibly prevent AD?

Holmes suggested: "One method to lower your body burden of aluminum and possibly prevent AD is to routinely ingest or inject a metal chelator or complexing agent. Ideally this agent will only attach itself to aluminum and thereby facilitate the removal of aluminum from the body."

In 1991 McLachlen, et al. demonstrated for the first time that a chemical called desferrioxamine (DFO), when given by intramuscular injection 5 days a week for 24 months, led to a 50% decrease in the rate of decline of AD patients' daily living skills[71]. In 1998 Savory, et al. demonstrated that DFO could reverse the formation of NFTs in white rabbits from New Zealand that had been previously injected with aluminum[24]. DFO removes aluminum from the aluminum/PHFτ complex and allows PHFτ to be degraded reversing the formation of aluminum-induced neurofibrillary tangles (NFTs)[24]. The problems with DFO are the number of required injections and its ability to remove not only aluminum but also the required element iron from the body.

A more ideal candidate for preventing or reversing AD would be a complexing agent for aluminum that can be taken orally and does not complex iron. Such a candidate has been found to be the dissolved mineral orthosilicic acid (OSA) that will be discussed in Chapters 5, 6, and 7.

This concludes the case of the cloaked assassin.

The Case for Aluminum Being the Cause of AD

Proving that aluminum is the cause of AD and not just correlated with AD has been the subject of a long-term debate among scientists. In order to prove causality, established epidemiological and experimental criteria for causality must be met. These criteria were originally set out by Sir Austin Bradford Hill[72]. In addition, the application of Hill's criteria to neuropsychiatric conditions, such as AD, has been further developed by Robert Van Reekum[73]. Briefly stated these criteria for causality are:

1) **Strength** of association between aluminum and AD
2) **Consistency** of association between aluminum and AD
3) **Specificity** of association between aluminum and AD
4) **Temporality** of aluminum accumulation occurring before AD
5) **Biological gradient** with dose-response effects of aluminum on AD risk
6) **Biological plausibility** of aluminum neurotoxicity causing AD
7) **Coherence** of what we know about how aluminum causes AD
8) **Analogy** of metal neurotoxicity to diseases similar to AD
9) **Experimental evidence** showing that AD can be prevented

These nine criteria have been applied by Doctor J. R. Walton to testing the aluminum/AD relationship using data from human and animal studies[74]. The conclusions were that AD is caused by aluminum and AD is a human form of chronic aluminum neurotoxicity[74]. In this chapter the following 9 criteria have been applied using primarily data from human AD patients and not animal studies, with the same conclusions being reached.

1) Strength of association between aluminum and AD:

Populations exposed to high levels of aluminum in their drinking water have a higher risk of AD than those exposed to lower levels of aluminum in their drinking water.

- The most extensively controlled study of AD and aluminum in drinking water was based upon autopsy-verified brains from AD patients and non-demented controls donated to the Canadian Brain Bank between 1981 and 1991[75]. These brains were from people who had lived in 162 geographic locations in Ontario with recorded aluminum levels in their drinking water. This study found that the risk of developing AD is 2.6 times higher among those who drank water containing over 100mcg/L for at least 10 years versus those who drank water containing less than 100mcg/L[75].

- A 15 year study of 3,777 people 65 years or older living in France also found that those who drank water containing more than 100mcg/L of aluminum had a 3.3 times greater relative risk of developing AD versus those drinking water containing less than 100mcg/L[75,76].

- Another study of 1,924 people found a 2.7 times greater relative risk of AD after 44 years of exposure to high aluminum levels in drinking water[77].

These studies all indicate a strong association between aluminum and AD and also show that the association is dose dependent with more than 100mcg/L in drinking water increasing the risk of AD by a factor of 2.6 to 3.3.

2) Consistency of association between aluminum and AD:

The relationship between aluminum and AD has been consistently confirmed in independent investigations[78]. The consistency of the association between aluminum in drinking water and AD has been demonstrated by a number of epidemiological studies that are completely reviewed in Appendix VI of this book. A 2001 meta-analysis involving a comprehensive literature survey discovered that 9 out of 13 epidemiology studies had found a significant positive correlation between aluminum in municipal drinking water and AD[79]. For example, In 1989 a high incidence of AD was reported in areas with a high level of aiuminum in the drinking water in England and Wales[80]. In 1991 high levels of aluminum in drinking water were linked with high dementia mortality in an area of Norway[81]. In 1991 a positive relationship between aluminum in drinking water and AD risk was identified in Canada[82].

The consistency of these epidemiology studies led the World Health Organization to conclude in 1998 and 2003 drinking water standards: *"The positive relationship between aluminum in drinking-water and AD ... cannot be totally dismissed"*[83]. WHO recommended a limit of 100mcg/liter of aluminum in drinking water in 1998 and 2003[83].

Humans have been tested for their rate of aluminum absorption using an isotope of aluminum (e.g. ^{26}Al) that has identical properties to aluminum (e.g. ^{27}Al)[84]. After ingestion there was a three-fold variation in aluminum retention among those tested[51]. AD patients absorb on average 64% more aluminum than non-demented control subjects[52]. In 2015 a meta-analysis was performed on 34 published studies involving 1,208 participants, including 613 AD patients. Aluminum was measured in brain tissue in 20 studies involving 386 participants, serum in 12 studies involving 698 participants, and cerebrospinal fluid (CSF) in 4 studies involving 124 participants. AD sufferers had significantly higher aluminum levels in brain tissue, serum, and CSF than did controls[54]. Ferritin is an iron storage protein in the blood that is shaped like a hollow sphere that can hold 4,500 iron atoms. Aluminum and zinc in the blood compete with iron for binding sites inside ferritin. Serum ferritin of AD patients had on average 62% aluminum versus only 37% aluminum in non-demented controls[85].

Measuring aluminum levels in the brain was at first inconsistent and inconclusive. But recently improved analytical techniques are providing a more consistent picture of how aluminum accumulates in the brains of AD patients. In 2005 inductively-coupled plasma atomic emission spectroscopy was used by Andrasi et al. to measure aluminum levels in specific brain regions in three AD patients and three non-demented controls[86]. The data in the following table shows that there are aluminum "hot spots" in the brain where aluminum is preferentially absorbed at higher levels in AD patients than non-demented controls.

From aluminum analysis of the brains of those who died of sporadic AD, familial AD, and occupational AD, it has been concluded that median levels of aluminum in excess of 2.0mcg per gram dry weight of brain across all four main lobes is both a common characteristic of AD and a contributor to its etiology[50].

Brain Aluminum Measurements from Humans with AD and Non-demented Controls[86]		
Regions of Brain Analyzed	**AD** (Al mcg/g of brain tissue)	**Controls** (Al mcg/g brain tissue)
Entorhinal Cortex	10.2 ± 9.0	1.5 ± 0.6
Hippocampus	4.9 ± 3.0	1.4 ± 0.6
Frontal Cortex (caudal)	6.8 ± 4.3	1.8 ± 0.6
Frontal Cortex (basal/ventral)	6.4 ± 2.9	2.5 ± 0.7

In 2011 Rusina et al. measured both aluminum and mercury in the hippocampus and associated visual cortex of 27 controls and 29 histologically-confirmed AD cases. There was a four-fold increase in aluminum levels in the hippocampus of the AD cases versus the controls. There was no difference in mercury levels between the AD cases and controls[87]. Crapper et al. (1973) were the first to observe "hot spots" of aluminum in the brains of AD cases[26]. An amount as high as 8mcg/g of aluminum per gram dry weight of brain tissue has been found in the inferior parietal lobe[88]. Hot spots in human brains with AD typically are in excess of 4mcg/g dry weight of brain tissue[88]. They contain a large number of NFTs or large pyramidal cell with high levels of aluminum. Hot spots are not found in non-demented age-matched controls[88].

3) **Specificity of association between aluminum and AD:**

This criterion of specificity is based upon old beliefs that each disease results in only one outcome. As Van Reekum et al. has pointed out this criterion is invalid for exposures to toxic substances like aluminum that can cause a variety of outcomes[73]. In fact aluminum is the likely cause of at least five diseases depending upon the age of the patient and the amount of aluminum accumulation. In the unborn fetus and newly born infant aluminum causes autism. In middle and old age aluminum causes both AD and vascular disease leading to stroke. Also aluminum may be involved in α-synuclein aggregation that is a hallmark of Lewy Body dementia as described in Appendix I. Aluminum may also be a causal factor in hippocampal sclerosis as described in Appendix III and cerebral amyloid angiopathy as described in Appendix IV.

We have shown that the cause of sporadic AD is environmental and not genetic. Out of all environmental factors considered, only aluminum experimentally triggers all major histopathological events associated with Alzheimer's[67]. The "hot spots" in the brain where the highest levels of aluminum were found include the hippocampal complex, entorhinal cortex, and frontal cortex[86]. These areas of the brain are all important for memory. Impaired memory is the core clinical feature of AD. The entorhinal cortex had the highest overall aluminum levels, is amongst the earliest regions of the brain to develop NFTs, and is ultimately the most damaged region of the brain in AD[89-92]. Some brain atrophy in the hippocampal complex and the frontal cortex (i.e. 0.3-0.6%) is common with age in healthy adults[93]. In 2009 Fjell et al. studied brain atrophy in people 60-91 years old. The study included 142 healthy participants and 122 with AD. The four areas of the brain found to significantly atrophy during one year in AD patients were the same areas found to be "hot spots" for aluminum accumulation. Also rate of atrophy is much higher in AD brains than in healthy adult brains as shown in the following table[94]. Of course even healthy brains have accumulated some aluminum and that could account for the atrophy observed in the controls.

Brain Atrophy in Humans with AD and Non-demented Controls During 1 Year[94]		
Regions of Brain Analyzed	**AD Longitudinal % Change**	**Controls Longitudinal % Change**
Entorhinal Cortex	-3.75	-0.55
Hippocampus	-2.42	-0.84
Frontal Cortex (caudal)	-1.60	-0.40
Frontal Cortex (ventral)	-1.06	-0.38

Note: these are the same brain regions found to be "hot spots" for aluminum accumulation[86]

In the brains of those with autism it has been found that the brain regions most impacted include the hippocampal complex, entorhinal cortex, and amygdala. These areas of the autistic brain have smaller and less complex neuronal networks than normal suggesting a curtailment of normal neuron development[95]. These areas of the brain are also responsible for disturbances of memory, learning, and emotion and behavior that comprise the core clinical features of autism[96].

These are the same brain regions found to be "hot spots" for aluminum accumulation[86]. The specificity of aluminum accumulation in these brain regions may manifest itself as the clinical symptoms of AD in older people and autism in the very young.

The presence of mixed cerebral pathologies becomes more common in individuals with advancing age, particularly in those over 90[97]. Pathologies associated with dementia were studied in a group of 183 participants of "The 90+ Study". This clinical-pathology investigation involved longitudinal follow-up and brain autopsy. Six of the pathologies studied and the percentage of participants with both dementia and these pathologies were:

- Alzheimer's disease (AD) – 23%
- α-Synuclein aggregation (a.k.a. Lewy body disease – see Appendix I) – 1%
- Cerebral amyloid angiopathy (cause of some hemorrhagic strokes - see Chapter 2) – 3%
- Strokes due to 3 or more micro infarcts (see Chapter 2) – 6%
- White matter disease (see Chapter 2) – 4%
- Hippocampal sclerosis (see Appendix III) – 4%

All of these pathologies may be linked to aluminum accumulation in the brain. Supporting Van Reekum's claim that environmental toxins like aluminum can cause a variety of outcomes[73], 45% of the cases of dementia in the 90+ study had a multiple number of these pathologies. The presence of multiple pathologies is associated with increased likelihood and severity of dementia. AD as a single pathology is present in 28% without dementia and 23% with dementia. When a single additional pathology in addition to AD is present the chance of dementia is four times higher than with just AD pathology. When any three or more of these pathologies were present, the chance of dementia is 95% in those over 90[97].

Environmental factors, such as aluminum, can cause changes in the way genes are expressed. This process is called epigenetics and it does not involve changes in the genetic information stored as a DNA sequence. A gene is first expressed by messenger RNA (mRNA) being made from a small portion of the DNA sequence. Then mRNA is used to make a specific type of protein that may be used as an enzyme or factor in the body. This two-step process can be either slowed or increased in speed by aluminum binding to the phosphate groups of DNA and mRNA.

Trace amounts of aluminum (i.e. nanomoles) can affect the expression of genes that are responsible for brain function[98] resulting in the pathologies summarized in the following table:

Epigenetics of Aluminum (Al) in Humans and other Mammals		
Epigenetic Effect	**Epigenetic Outcome**	**Associated Disease**
Al Lowers Gene Expression for Protein Phosphatase 2A (PP2A)	Hyperphosphorylated Tau & NFTs - Hallmark of AD	AD[99,100]
Al Indirectly Lowers Gene Expression for Brain Derived Neuro Factor (BDNF)	Impairs Long Term Memory & Impairs Spatial Learning	AD[101-103]
Al Lowers Gene Expression for Neprilysin and LDL Receptor LRP1 and Increases Gene Expression for BACE1 and the Aβ peptide precursor APP	Aβ Oligomers and Plaques – Hallmark of AD	AD[30,31,104]
Al Lowers Gene Expression for Krebs Cycle Enzymes	Mitochondrial Disease – Symptom of AD	AD & Autism[57]
Al Lowers Gene Expression for DNA Repair Factor BRCA1*	Broken DNA	AD & Cancer[105-107]
Al Increases Gene Expression for TNF-α that in turn Decreases Gene Expression for the Enzyme MS	Increased Homocysteine	Stroke & Autism[108,109]

*BRCA1 gene mutations are common in AD[106] and in breast[110], ovarian[110], and prostate cancer[111]

The effect of aluminum accumulation in the brain manifests itself in a variety of pathologies dependent upon age and the amount of aluminum. Therefore aluminum lacks specificity to cause a single pathology due to its ability to complex with a wide variety of proteins and nucleic acids in the brain resulting in multiple pathologies.

4) Temporality of aluminum accumulation occurring before AD:

This criterion requires that the causative agent occurs prior to the outcome. Therefore chronic aluminum exposure must precede AD if chronic aluminum intake is the environmental cause of AD.

For the last 125 years we have lived in the "aluminum age" during which there has been a steady increase in our exposure to aluminum. We ingest food, pharmaceuticals, and drink water containing aluminum, we apply aluminum containing products to our skin, we are vaccinated with aluminum containing vaccines, and we inhale air containing aluminum[112]. This results in a slow accumulation of aluminum in our brains from the fetal stage to old age[3,28,113,114]. Therefore humans living in an industrialized society accumulate aluminum in certain regions of their brains many years before the onset of AD. There are three sub-cellular changes in brain physiology that occur prior to overt AD in humans and all three lead to AD:

- Progressive aluminum accumulation in neurons
- Hyperphosphorylation of tau due to aluminum inhibition of an enzyme
- Oxidative stress due to aluminum

Increasing aluminum exposure and accumulation is in lock-step with the increasing frequency of AD. AD was described as a rare disease in The Lancet fifteen years after Alzheimer's 1911 paper[115]. The reported number of AD cases rose from one in 1907 to more than 90 by 1935[116]. Subsequently the age-adjusted death rate for AD in the U.S. rose from 0.4 per 100,000 in 1979 to 25 per 100,000 in 2010[117,118]. In the 25 year span from 1980 to 2004 the annual U.S. death rate from AD in those over 65 rose from 1,037 to 65,313 per year[117].

It is estimated that in North America the mean aluminum intake is 24mg of aluminum per day, equivalent to more than 8.76 grams per year[118]. The demand for aluminum products has increased requiring more and more aluminum be extracted and refined from bauxite deposits. The current annual global demand for aluminum is 11 kg per person[119]. This means approximately 0.08% of the aluminum produced each year is ingested. Demand for aluminum has increased 30-fold since 1950 and is estimated to increase by 3-fold current levels by 2050[119].

Using these data on aluminum demand, it is estimated that human exposure to aluminum has and will continue to increase at a rate of 90 fold over the 100 year period from 1950 to 2050[39]. This means we only ingested 0.29 grams of aluminum per year in 1950 and by 2050 we will be ingesting more than 26 grams per year.

So temporality exists as aluminum accumulates in our bodies prior to the onset of AD. In addition the rate of ingestion and accumulation of aluminum is increasing and this accounts for the rising prevalence of AD.

5) Biological Gradient with Dose-response Effects of Aluminum and AD:

In 1996 McLachlan, et al. observed a dose-response in the amount of aluminum in drinking water with the risk of AD in humans[75]. Each subject's residential and drinking water history for the 10-year period prior to death was taken into account. The drinking water that subjects were exposed to varied from less than 100mcg/L to 175mcg/L. A single pathologist performed histopathological examinations of all 614 brains included in this study. The brains were assigned to AD or control groups based upon clinical history and the presence or absence of plaques and NFTs. The results in the following table demonstrate a dose-response relationship between aluminum in drinking water and AD.

Dose-response Relationship Between Aluminum in Drinking Water and AD[75]	
Aluminum in Drinking Water (mcg/L)	**Relative Risk of AD**
<100	1
>100	1.7
>125	3.6
>150	4.4
175	7.6

Several other epidemiological studies have also shown a dose-response effect of aluminum and AD risk[75-77,82,120].

6) Biological Plausibility of Aluminum Neurotoxicity Causing AD:

It is known that aluminum facilitates the formation of Aβ plaques and NFTs in the brain that are two hallmarks of AD[17,25]. Aluminum causes oxidative stress that kills mitochondria and ultimately kills neurons[53]. This results in mitochondrial disease and increased atrophy of some brain regions both of which are clinical symptoms of AD. Aluminum also disrupts memory storage that is a behavioral symptom of AD[44].

Some metal ions, such as aluminum, act as physiological stressors in the brain by stimulating brain cells to produce oxidizing chemicals (a.k.a. ROS)[121,122]. This ROS can damage and kill mitochondria and neurons creating inflammation in the brain. Aluminum tops the list of metal ion inducers of ROS in human brain's glial cells[58].

It has been observed from microscopic evidence that aluminum causes lesions in the brain's perforant pathway that result in short term memory loss[44]. Aluminum also acts as individual ions to block the neurochemistry of long and short term memory storage[123]. This mechanism of action explains why very small amounts of aluminum in the brain (i.e. on the order of several parts per million or micrograms per gram of brain on a dry weight basis) can have a very large impact on memory storage.

Calmodulin is a calcium-binding messenger protein required for memory formation and storage. Aluminum ions modify its structure thereby inhibiting its function[123]. This prevents calmodulin from regulating calcium levels in neurons and also prevents the activation of four key enzymes that control memory formation and storage in neurons.

The neurochemical explanation of how memories are stored in neural networks is still evolving. However considerable detail has already been discovered. The ground-work was laid by Donald Hebb in 1949[124] when he described a theory of neuronal learning as:

"Neurons that fire together - wire together and neurons that are out of sync - do not link".

The neurochemical mechanism that supports Hebbian Theory involves the synchronized firing of several different types of neuroreceptors at a synapse between two neurons. When this occurs in synchrony it leads first to stronger or potentiated neuronal connection between the two neurons. This connection is then made even stronger by several types of neuroreceptors moving their location in order to increase their density at the synapse. The theory that describes this two- step process of strengthening neuro-circuits is called spike-timing dependent plasticity (STDP)[125]. The successful result of this process is called long term potentiation (LTP). STDP and LTP are theorized to be the way memories are stored. A lack of synchrony in the process leads to no potentiation and is called long term depression (LTD) or lost memories. Aluminum ions inhibit calmodulin from activating four key enzymes involved in LTP[101,123,126-129]. Thereby aluminum ions encourage LTD and cause memory loss (see Neurochemistry of Memory Impairment by Aluminum for details on role of these four enzymes in memory storage).

The biological plausibility of aluminum causing AD is well established by those studies that have connected aluminum's neurotoxicity with the hallmarks and symptoms of AD.

7) Coherence of what we know about how aluminum neurotoxicity causes AD:

Aluminum taken in by ingestion alone is estimated to be 24mg a day of which approximately 0.2% is absorbed into our blood[118,130,131]. We know that aluminum accumulates more in some areas of the human brain such as memory processing regions[86]. This accumulation likely results in chronic aluminum neurotoxicity and the hallmarks and symptoms of AD. The cells in these regions have very high energy needs. The high rate of energy utilization increases the demand for iron. Transferrin is the molecule that carries iron to these cells. Therefore these cells have a high density of transferrin receptors on their membrane in order to facilitate iron uptake. Aluminum and iron ions are almost equivalent in size and can have the same ionic charge. This allows aluminum to be carried by transferrin into these cells in higher than normal amounts even though the cells have no need for aluminum.

Some metal ions act as physiological stressors in the brain by stimulating brain cells to produce oxidizing chemicals (a.k.a. ROS)[121,122]. The metal ions stimulate inducible nitric oxide synthase (iNOS) in microglial and astroglial cells of the brain to produce nitric oxide (NO) that reacts to produce ROS[122]. This ROS can damage and kill neurons creating inflammation in the brain. The following table shows how much ROS is produced from a cell culture of human glial cells exposed to 50nM aqueous solutions of various common metal ions[58]. Aluminum tops the list of metal ion inducers of ROS in human brain's glial cells.

Metal Ion Induction of ROS in Human Glial Cells[58]	
Metal Sulfate	**Relative Induction of ROS**
Aluminum	10
Iron	6
Manganese	4.5
Zinc	4
Nickel	3.5
Lead	3.5
Gallium	3
Copper	3
Cadmium	3
Tin	2
Mercury	1.5
Magnesium	0
Sodium	0

The brain damage caused by aluminum inducing ROS could partially account for the neuronal death that underlies brain atrophy. This atrophy is seen in those areas the brain that are aluminum "hot spots" and it parallels aluminum accumulation in those areas of our brains as we age[86,94].

Neurofibrillary tangle (NFT) formation in the brain is a hallmark of AD. Aluminum has been shown to participate in NFT formation in both pre-tangle and tangle-bearing cells[132]. Aluminum inhibits the activity of enzyme PP2A that clips off excess phosphoryl groups on a structural protein of the brain called tau[133]. Aluminum also inhibits the expression of a gene involved in making PP2A[100]. Aluminum creates a lack of active PP2A that results in tau being coated with more than the normal number of phosphoryl groups. This accounts for low PP2A activity and paired helical filaments (PHFτ) found in the brains of AD patients[133]. In AD brains aluminum secondarily aggregates the PHFτ into granules that fuse and grow into cytoplasmic pools of PHFτ and aluminum that give rise to NFT filaments[132]. Aluminum and PHFτ give rise to NFTs in brain cells, including large pyramidal and stellate cells, particularly in the brains of those with AD[132]. Pyramidal cells are found in many regions of the brain, including the hippocampus, entorhinal, and prefrontal cortex.

Aβ plaque formation in the brain is another hallmark of AD. Aβ plaques form from Aβ peptides that are cleaved from large Aβ precursor proteins (APP). This process is called amyloidogenic cleavage and alteration of this process is a key feature of AD[134]. Beneficial non-amyloidogenic cleavage of APP leads to a secreted product that is important for promoting neurite growth and maintaining brain tissue. Protein phosphorylation stimulates the beneficial non-amyloidogenic pathway. Both protein kinase C (PKC) activity that increases phosphorylation and protein phosphatase 2A (PP2A) activity that decreases phosphorylation are involved in the control of how much of each competing pathway is used for APP cleavage[135]. Activation of PKC decreases production of Aβ peptides by 50-80% and increases the beneficial non-amyloidogenic cleavage by 30-50%[135]. Nanomolar concentrations of aluminum reduce PKC activity by 90%[136]. Therefore inhibition of PKC activity by aluminum directs APP to the amyloidogenic pathway resulting in more Aβ peptide[135]. This situation is partially modulated by aluminum's inhibition of PP2A[135].

Microtubules are important neuronal structural features that are required for strength, rigidity, and transportation of cell constituents between the nucleus of the cell and the synapses. Human pyramidal cells that contain NFTs and/or high levels of aluminum accumulation are microtubule-depleted[44]. Aluminum-induced microtubule depletion is possibly more fundamental to AD neuropathology than Aβ oligomers, Aβ plaques, or NFTs[74]. This is because microtubule depletion is more damaging to neuronal connectivity and function than these hallmarks of AD neuropathology that may represent protective cell responses to aluminum [132,137]. Aluminum-induced microtubule depleted cells have axonal and dendritic dieback that is consistent with AD being associated with neuronal disconnection. In addition aluminum-induced microtubule depletion leads to synapse breakdown and depletion[44,138]. This explains why humans with AD have impaired axonal transport[139,140].

Neuronal death is marked in the brain by ghost NFTs that can be the result of aluminum accumulation in the neuron prior to death. NFTs inside the pyramidal cells tend to displace the cell nucleus to the periphery resulting in denucleation. The denucleated cell is unable to renew cellular membranes and eventually the cell membrane ruptures[74]. This results in an extracellular ghost NFTs that act as tombstones of former neurons and a hallmark of AD.

8) Analogy of metal neurotoxicity to diseases similar to AD:

The two best analogies for a trace metal in the environment causing a disease, such as aluminum causing AD, are the effects of lead or mercury accumulation in our brains. Like aluminum both of these metals slowly accumulate in our bodies over our lifetime and cause mental illness.

Low level lead exposure was common during the Roman Empire. The people of this period used lead to make water pipes, cookware, and cosmetics. Corrosion of lead in contact with their drinking water and application of leaded cosmetics to their skin resulted in lead accumulation in their bones and brains[141]. Judging from the amount of lead found in their bones, these people suffered from mild to severe lead poisoning resulting in brain swelling that caused severe headaches, confusion, irritability, seizures, and possibly death. Lead exposure continues today as there is lead in drinking water due to lead water pipes and lead pollution in ground water. For more information on the analogy between lead and aluminum exposure see Chapter 8.

Low level mercury exposure is currently common. Mercury gets into the environment from both human-generated sources, such as coal-burning power plants, and natural sources, such as volcanoes. Consumption of fish is the primary ingestion-related source of mercury in humans. The mercury in both salt and fresh water organisms is bio-concentrated in the food-chain that ends up in fish and humans. Symptoms of mercury poisoning typically include lack of coordination and sensory impairment, such as vision, hearing, speech, and sensation. Although these symptoms indicate brain damage, mercury also damages the kidneys and lungs and can lead to death.

9) Experimental evidence showing that AD can be prevented:

The primary goal of this book is to show that diseases caused by aluminum can be prevented by 7 supplements, 7 lifestyle choices, and a dissolved mineral. For example AD may be prevented by, antioxidants that counteract the oxidative effects of aluminum (Chapter 3), avoidance or minimization of aluminum exposure (Chapter 4), a complexation agent and vitamin that lower brain aluminum accumulation (Chapter 3 and 5), and a combination of aerobic exercise and sleep (Chapter 6).

- The antioxidant PQQ protects the brain from low level aluminum exposure by inhibiting the formation of reactive oxygen species (ROS) and reducing ROS as they form in the brain due to aluminum accumulation.
- Avoiding foods and pharmaceuticals, like antacids, that are high in aluminum, filtering drinking water, and cooking in non-aluminum cookware minimizes aluminum exposure.
- Orthosilicic acid taken orally is absorbed into the blood and complexes with aluminum facilitating its excretion by the kidneys.
- Vitamin D3 taken orally is converted by the body to vitamin D that facilitates the excretion of aluminum by the kidneys, even in the case of damaged kidneys due to kidney disease.
- Aerobic exercise and sleep help to cleanse the brain of Aβ peptides and oligomers that are complexed with aluminum.

The best evidence that AD can be prevented is comparing the AD rate in countries with high levels orthosilicic acid in their drinking water, such as Singapore and Malaysia, with countries with low levels of orthosilicic acid in their drinking water, such as the U.S. and Iceland.

Life Expectancy and AD Death Rate by Country		
Country	Life Expectancy (yrs.)*	AD Death Rate (per 100,000)**
Iceland	83.3	34.1
United States	79.8	45.6
Malaysia	75.7	0.7
Singapore	84	0.2

*Life expectancy data from WHO 2014, **AD death rate data 2016 worldlifeexpectancy.com

With comparable life expectancy and higher orthosilicic acid in their drinking water, people who live in Malaysia and Singapore have a much lower death rate due to AD. Since orthosilicic acid facilitates the excretion of aluminum by the kidneys, there is evidence that lowering aluminum will prevent AD.

Conclusion: The nine criteria of causality originally set out by Sir Austin Bradford Hill[72] and applied to neuropsychiatric conditions, such as AD, by Robert Van Reekum[73] have been applied using primarily human data taken from studying AD patients and controls. The conclusions are that aluminum is the likely cause of AD and AD is a human form of chronic aluminum neurotoxicity. Given these conclusions we as individuals and a society have a responsibility to take action. This book proposes what action can and needs to be taken to avoid or lower our exposure to aluminum and prevent diseases caused by aluminum.

Aluminum an Unrequired and Unwanted Intruder

People representing the aluminum industry routinely point to aluminum's omnipresence in our bodies as a sign of its essentiality. It is true that we all currently have a body-burden of aluminum but there has been no proven benefit of aluminum in our bodies. In fact aluminum is a neurotoxin and aluminum exposure is the known cause of a number human diseases[142].

The brain relies on a delicate balance of monovalent (e.g. potassium and sodium) and divalent (e.g. calcium, magnesium, and zinc) cations in order to function properly. These cations bind reversibly and not tightly with aminoacids, such as histidine and lysine that are involved in the active sites of key enzymes (e.g. protein phosphatase) or on the backbones of key proteins (e.g. β-amyloid and α-synuclein). Aluminum is a small trivalent cation that can bind tightly to both key enzymes and proteins in the brain. For instance magnesium regulates over 300 proteins and aluminum competes for magnesium binding. Aluminum binds to some of these proteins 10 million times stronger and dissociates 10 thousand times slower than magnesium[143]. This property results in aluminum's slow accumulation in select areas of the brain and aluminum's inhibition of enzymes that causes the onset and progression of AD and possibly other forms of dementia. Aluminum is an unrequired neurotoxic element and not a nutrient for normal body function. This makes aluminum an unwanted intruder.

Prevalence of Alzheimer's Disease

The 2002 ADAMS study of dementia in the U.S. estimated that 2.7 million people in the U.S. had Alzheimer's disease (AD)[11] and by the year 2005, 24 million people worldwide had AD[67]. AD prevalence is the highest in those 80 years of age and older. In 2002 there were 9 million people in the U.S. who are 80 years of age or older[10]. Therefore in 2002 approximately one in three people 80 years of age or older had AD. This means almost everyone over 80 will be impacted by AD as they age. Those of us who live to 80 and beyond will have at least a 1 in 3 chance of getting AD and, if we don't get AD, we have at least a 1 in 2 chance of caring for a friend or relative with AD.

The prevalence of AD is increasing both as the size of the population in the U.S. over age 65 continues to increase and as our exposure to aluminum continues to increase. Currently the Alzheimer's Association estimates that 5.3 million people in the U.S. have AD[4]. By 2025 the number of people 65 and older with AD is estimated to reach 7.1 million and by 2050 this number is projected to be 13.8 million, barring adoption of preventive measures, such as those described in this book, or the development of medical cures.

Symptoms of Alzheimer's Disease

The clinical symptoms that characterize AD are:

- Mitochondrial disease
- Decreasing Aβ peptides and Aβ oligomers in cerebrospinal fluid
- Increasing tau in the cerebrospinal fluid
- Shrinkage of the brain
- Olfactory dysfunction*

*Olfactory dysfunction or anosmia (i.e. the inability to smell) is among the first signs of AD and Parkinson's Disease[144,145].

The behavioral symptoms that are a result of cognitive impairment and characterize AD are[4]:

- Short term memory loss that disrupts daily life
- Difficulty in planning and problem solving
- Difficulty completing familiar tasks
- Confusion with time and place
- Confusion with visual and spatial relationships
- Difficulty with word finding during speaking and writing
- Increased daytime sleepiness*
- Changes in mood and personality
- Withdrawal from work or social activities
- Decreased or poor judgement

*Sleepiness is measured by timing how long it takes for an individual to fall asleep while laying on a bed in a quite dark room. The largest difference in sleepiness between non-AD (16min.), mild AD (11min.), and moderate AD (8min.) was observed at 10AM and 12PM[146]. In those with dementia, including AD, sleepiness should not be confused with 5 to 20 second long fainting spells, called syncope, that start abruptly and end with spontaneous recovery[147,148].

Diagnosis of Alzheimer's Disease

Alzheimer's disease (AD) is a chronic neurodegenerative disease that is a terminal illness with an average life expectancy of three to nine years post diagnosis. The AD process occurs in stages 5 to 20 years before the first symptom of cognitive impairment is observed. The stages of AD are as follows:

- The first stage of this process involves aluminum facilitating the formation of small soluble protein fragments from amyloid precursor protein (APP), such as Aβ peptides and Aβ oligomers, and insoluble Aβ plaques between neurons. Aluminum conjugates of Aβ oligomers are much more neurotoxic than any other APP metabolite[16]. Aluminum's epigenetic effect of lowering gene expression for both neprilysin and LDL Receptor LRP1, and increasing gene expression for both BACE1 and APP results in more Aβ peptides and Aβ oligomers, and insoluble Aβ plaques[30,31]. Aluminum chloride with D-galactose has been found to create predementia in a mouse model for AD[104]. The first stage of AD can be detected in humans as decreasing levels of Aβ peptides and Aβ oligomers in the cerebrospinal fluid. These levels decrease as the peptides and oligomers are formed into insoluble Aβ plaques.

- The second stage of this process involves aluminum facilitating tau protein clumping together in tangles (NFTs). Normally tau protein is used for microtubule assembly and stabilization in neurons. Aluminum's epigenetic effect of lowering the production of the enzyme PP2A and aluminum's inhibition of PP2A results in excess phosphoryl groups on tau[22,99,100,136]. Aluminum also facilitates the formation of NFTs from these over phosphorylated tau proteins[24,25]. NFT formation results in the death of neurons that are replaced with "tombstones" or "ghosts" of NFTs. The second stage can be detected as increasing levels of tau in cerebrospinal fluid.

- The third stage is called mild cognitive impairment (MCI) and it occurs 1 to 4 years prior to a person being diagnosed with AD. MCI is characterized by poor decision making and difficulty in remembering recent events and other lapses of memory. These symptoms are due to aluminum causing microtubule loss, dendritic die-back, and cortical atrophy resulting in slow loss of memory[149]. MCI can also be a symptom of metabolic (non-AD) dementia that may be curable (see Appendix II).

- The fourth stage is called Alzheimer's disease because it can be diagnosed as a slow loss of cognition with symptoms including difficulties with word recall and disorientation, such as getting lost, mood swings and behavioral issues. These symptoms are due to substantial neuron damage and loss, called lesions, in areas of the brain related to short term and long term memory and decision making. The severity of this stage can be gauged by performing either volumetric MRI to measure the shrinkages of the brain due to neurons expiring or FDG-PET that gauges the health of mitochondria in neurons.

If you are like me and have one or more aging parents, you may already have witnessed the slow decline of their short term memory. It is disturbing to realize they may have reached the 3rd stage of AD without even being aware their brains have the hallmarks of AD. Also if you are like me you may worry that your own brain is beginning that downward spiral into AD. Until recently it was only in the 4th stage that the disease could be diagnosed and called AD. This late stage diagnosis of AD requires two major symptoms with short term memory loss usually being one of the two symptoms.

According to the Alzheimer's Association only 45% of those with AD or their caregivers report being told of an AD diagnosis. In part this is due to the difficulty in making the diagnosis. Until recently examination of brain tissue after death was required for a definitive diagnosis of AD. The two hallmarks of AD histopathology are:

- Neurofibrillary tangles (NFTs) inside neurons and "tombstones" or "ghosts" of former neurons in between living neurons.
- Insoluble Aβ plaques formed from Aβ peptides and oligomers in between living neurons.

See sidebar on "Biochemistry and Neurochemistry of AD" for details on these two hallmarks.

One reason it has been difficult to prove what causes AD is that the symptoms of AD become apparent only in the 3rd and 4th stage and a definitive diagnosis of AD has required an autopsy. A new class of ligands has recently been developed that allows for brain imaging by PET scans of both NFTs[150] and Aβ plaques[151]. This allows researchers to follow the development of the hallmarks of AD histopathology in living patients. These tests should facilitate our understanding of how aluminum and possibly other environmental toxins cause AD. These tests should also allow faster testing of drugs under development that will provide palliative relief from the symptoms of AD, if not a cure for AD.

Conclusion of Alzheimer's Disease

For the last 50 years, in spite of excellent research, the cause of Alzheimer's has remained controversial. It may be years before all the needed research is performed and the controversy ends. But now a tipping point has been reached and as described in this chapter there is convincing evidence that aluminum accumulation in our brains can cause Alzheimer's disease. Aluminum absorption in select areas of the human brain can result in the cognitive deterioration and associated cerebral pathology seen in AD as described in the following list:

- Increased amyloid plaque formation in the brain that is a hallmark of AD

- Increased phosphorylation of tau protein leading to neurofibrillary tangles (NFTs) that are a hallmark of AD

- Inhibition of mitochondrial enzymes resulting in mitochondrial disease that is a clinical symptom of AD

- Lesions in the perforant neuronal pathway resulting in loss of short term memory that is a behavioral symptom of AD

The presence of mixed cerebral pathologies becomes more common in individuals with advancing age. Forty-five percent of those over 90 with dementia had a multiple number of cerebral pathologies[97]. The presence of multiple pathologies is associated with increased likelihood and severity of dementia. AD as a single pathology is present in 28% of those over 90 without dementia and 23% with dementia. When a single additional pathology in addition to AD is present the chance of dementia is four times higher than with just AD pathology. When any three or more of these pathologies is present, the chance of dementia is 95% in those over 90[97]. In addition to aluminum being a causal factor for AD, it has also been implicated as a casual factor for other cerebral pathologies (see Appendix I, III, and IV). For instance in Chapter 2 aluminum's role as a causal factor for strokes and white matter disease is discussed. This is not to say that aluminum is the only cause of cerebral pathologies. There are numerous environmental chemicals and several factors, such as head trauma, that have been implicated in cerebral pathologies (see Appendix I). Future research may find additional chemicals in our environment and additional factors that cause cerebral pathologies.

Since the commercial production of aluminum began, there has been a dramatic increase in AD cases worldwide. There are cases of accidental and occupational exposure to aluminum that have shown that aluminum can cause both early-onset AD and the hallmarks of AD.

The Alzheimer's Association finds that Alzheimer's disease is grossly misunderstood and underestimated. When they surveyed people in 12 countries they found:

> *"59 percent of people surveyed incorrectly believe that Alzheimer's disease is a typical part of ageing".*

As a society we have made an incorrect assumption:

> *"Because we now live longer, more of us will die of Alzheimer's disease"*

This assumption is a self-fulfilling prophecy unless action is taken by individuals to lower their exposure to aluminum and society to improve regulations on the amount of aluminum in food, drink, and pharmaceuticals. By lowering our aluminum ingestion and absorption we may be able to live longer without developing and suffering from AD.

The people of Malaysia and Singapore have a much lower death rate due to AD than the U.S even though they have a similar life expectancy. Could the people of Malaysia and Singapore be ingesting a dissolved mineral called OSA that increases aluminum excretion by their bodies? See Chapter 5 for the answers to these questions. In Chapter 4 we will discuss ways to avoid or lower aluminum ingestion and in Chapter 5 we will discuss how to decrease aluminum absorption by your brain after ingesting aluminum.

Biochemistry and Neurochemistry of AD

Aluminum's Impact on NFT and HPτ Accumulation

Memories are stored in your brain by persistent neural networks consisting of trillions of interconnection points called synapses. Microtubules inside neurons are required for these synapses to function. Normally tau interacts with tubulin to form microtubule associated protein (MAP). In brains of AD patients tau is hyperphosphorylated to form HPτ. HPτ is neurotoxic because it sequesters MAP's into cytosolic pools inside neurons inhibiting microtubule assembly and synaptic function[152,153]. HPτ can also self-assemble into paired helical fibers forming NFTs that provide the brain with some neuroprotection from excess HPτ[152]. Aluminum binds to HPτ in both NFTs and cytosolic pools aggregating the excess HPτ and slowing its degradation[44,154,155]. HPτ concentration is 4 - 8 times higher in brains of AD patients as compared with elderly without AD[152].

The amount of phosphorylation of tau protein is regulated by the activity of an enzyme called protein phosphatase 2A (PP2A) that catalyzes the de-phosphorylation of phosphorylated tau protein. Cations such as aluminum[20], zinc[21], and mercury[22] inhibit PP2A and promote HPτ formation, while methylation of PP2A increases its activity and inhibits HPτ formation[156]. Elevated total serum homocysteine levels can result in excessive homocysteine methylation by methionine synthase depleting available methylation sources, such as folic acid. This lack of methylation sources inhibits methylation of PP2A favoring formation of HPτ in neurons[157]. Therefore people with elevated homocysteine (e.g. tHcy = 13-20μM/L) have nearly twice the risk of AD as compared with those who have normal levels[158].

Aluminum's Impact on Hippocampal Memory

AD impacts those regions of the brain involved in creating new neurons that store both short and long-term memories. One such region is the hippocampal region of the brain where about 1,400 new neurons per day are created throughout our lives[159]. AD patients have hippocampal regions that are significantly smaller than average[160]. This shrinkage indicates a loss of neurons due to both NFTs, resulting from aluminum increasing $HP\tau$[161], and increased calcium diffusion into neurons caused by aluminum complexing with both Aβ oligomers, potentiating their neurotoxicity[16], and calmodulin, inhibiting the calcineurin calcium pump and increasing calcium levels in neurons[123]. Too much calcium both slows production of ATP by neuronal mitochondria[16] and activates an enzyme creating more toxic forms of $HP\tau$[162]. Hippocampal cells from both rats fed low-levels of aluminum and elderly humans with and without AD contain aggregates of aluminum/$HP\tau$ complex in intracellular cytosolic pools within the cell body (e.g.. somas) of hippocampal cells (i.e. CA1 pyramidal cells) and this complex is also seen in mature extracellular NFTs [44,132].

Areas of the brain used for synaptic plasticity and memory have neurons linked together by synapses. The synaptic cleft between two neurons is studded with a variety of receptors on the postsynaptic neuron. NMDA and AMPA receptors are excitatory receptors and $GABA_A$ receptors are inhibitory receptors. The NMDA receptor is a molecular coincidence detector because it is both ligand-gated and voltage-gated. The NMDA receptor requires two ligands for activation: either glutamate or homocysteine and D-serine or glycine or taurine [163,164]. In addition the NMDA receptor also requires an excitatory postsynaptic voltage (EPSP) for activation that can originate from the AMPA receptor. When the NMDA receptor is activated first by the presynaptic neuron releasing ligands (i.e. glutamate and zinc) into the synaptic cleft and then milliseconds later by an EPSP, it opens an ion channel allowing a small number of calcium ions to diffuse into the neuron. These calcium ions complex with calmodulin and this complex activates enzymes that increase (i.e. potentiate) the EPSP (see Figure 1).

When synchronized in this manner, early phase LTP occurs and is theorized to be how short-term memories are stored. When the EPSP arrives at the NMDA receptor too early, long-term depression (LTD) occurs as no calcium is released into the neuron and there is a decrease in the amplitude of the EPSP (see Figure 1). In LTD both synchrony and short-term memories are lost. In late phase LTP calcium ions increase the density of AMPA receptors at the synapse making a more potentiated EPSP. Aluminum ions modify the 3D shape of calmodulin inhibiting both the activation of enzymes and early stage LTP.

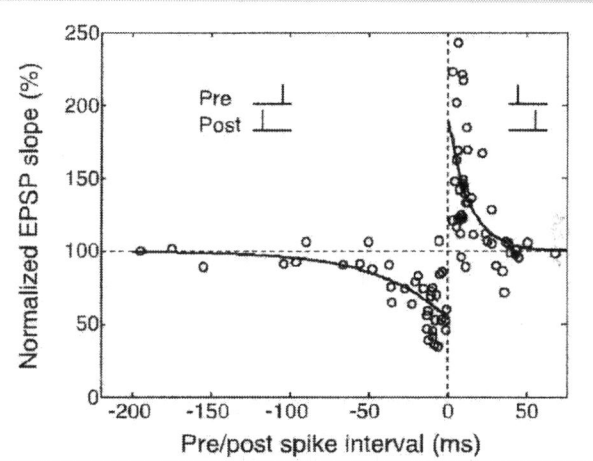

Figure 1 - STDP in rat cortical slices
Zero time is the release of glutamate and zinc ions into the synaptic cleft. Vertical axis is the strength of the resulting EPSP and horizontal axis is the timing of the EPSP as it arrives at the NMDA receptor. Each circle is one experiment[125].

$GABA_A$ inhibitory receptors in the synaptic cleft act as voltage filters inhibiting unsynchronized EPSPs by producing inhibitory postsynaptic potentials (IPSP's) when activated. Zinc ions released into the synaptic cleft by the presynaptic neuron prevent the production of IPSP's by the $GABA_A$ inhibitory receptors. This creates a 20 millisecond window of time for activation of NMDA receptors by an EPSP without inhibition[165,166]. This uninhibited window of time also allows for transmission of a potentiated EPSP down the axon[167]. In late phase LTP $GABA_A$

receptor density at synapses increases due to LTP that in turn decreases the chance of an unsynchronized IPSP from inhibiting a potentiated EPS[168].

In AD patients there is increased excitatory synaptic activity called excitotoxicity. This results in excess intracellular calcium ions inside neurons and excess extracellular zinc ions outside neurons. The excess calcium ions can kill neurons and the excess zinc ions can cause both the formation of Aβ oligomers in the synapse[169] and the inhibition of $GABA_A$ receptors preventing them from filtering out unsynchronized EPSPs, resulting in LTD and loss of short term memory.

Under conditions in the brain when simultaneously both:

- *Glycine levels are high, such as a stroke or head trauma*
- *Homocysteine levels are greater than 10μM/L*

The result can be excitotoxicity[170-173]. Aluminum complexes of Aβ oligomers hold NMDA ion channels open longer than just Aβ oligomers. This allows even more calcium ions into the neuron resulting in neuronal death[16]. Memantine, a drug for moderate to severe AD approved by the FDA, blocks NMDA receptor channels and prevents excitotoxicity in AD patients[174,175]. Taurine also decreases excitotoxicity by modulating $GABA_A$ inhibitory receptors to produce IPSP's that filter out EPSPs [176,177].

Neurochemistry of Memory Impairment by Aluminum

Cognition and memory are due to long-term potentiation (LTP) that is created by spike-timing dependent-plasticity (STDP). Split second timing of neuronal synapses causes small amounts of extracellular calcium ions to diffuse into the neuron through NMDA and AMPA receptor ion channels. These ions create a mechanism for maintaining LTP. This maintenance involves three calcium ions complexing with each molecule of calmodulin. Too little calcium cancels LTP and results in long term depression (LTD) and too much calcium results in neuronal death.

Aluminum ions bind to calmodulin inhibiting calcium modulation and enzyme activation[123]. The calcium/calmodulin complex normally modulates calcium in the neuron and activates four enzymes (PKII, PKIV, PP2B, PDE4A) all of which are involved in LTP and cognition:

1) *The calcium/calmodulin complex activates a protein kinase (a.k.a. PKII or CaMKII) that is both required for long-term potentiation (LTP) and has been observed in post synaptic dendrites after LTP induction. CaMKII activity is involved in moving the location of AMPA neuroreceptors to synapses and thereby increasing the postsynaptic response to the presynaptic potential, resulting in late phase LTP[178]. CaMKII also phosphorylates AMPA receptors increasing calcium channel conductance and making the AMPA receptors more sensitive than normal during LTP. This provides even more synaptic strength[178]. Aluminum ions complex with calmodulin changing its confirmation and inhibiting its activation of CaMKII and thereby preventing LTP[101,102,123,127].*

2) *The calcium/calmodulin complex also activates a protein kinase (PKIV or CaMKIV) that phosphorylates CREB[179,180]. CREB is a cAMP response element-binding protein that binds to certain DNA sequences. When CREB is phosphorylated it increases the transcription of certain genes, including the gene for brain derived neurotropic factor (BDNF) production. CREB has been shown to be required for long term memory, brain plasticity, and learning. Low levels of CREB impair the maintenance of long term memory but not short term memory[181,182]. Aluminum chloride in the diet of neonatal and postnatal rats inhibits the phosphorylation of CREB and thereby lowers hippocampal expression of BDNF. This results in impairment of both long term memory and spatial learning[101,102].*

3) *In early phase LTP, calcium ions, that diffuse through an activated NMDA receptor, complex with calmodulin and activate PP2B (a.k.a. calcineurin). When activated by the calcium/calmodulin complex, PP2B normally activates $GABA_A$ inhibitory receptors by catalyzing the removal of a phosphate group from each $GABA_A$ inhibitory receptor. Aluminum ions complex with the calcium/calmodulin complex inhibiting PP2B and preventing both phosphate removal and $GABA_A$ inhibitory receptors from acting as*

voltage filters for unsynchronized EPSPs[128]. This results in LTD and short term memory impairment.

In late phase LTP the calcium/calmodulin complex normally increases the density of $GABA_A$ receptors at the synapse moving the location of $GABA_A$ inhibitory receptors into the synapse to act as filters for unsynchronized EPSPs[168]. Aluminum ions complex with the calcium/calmodulin complex, block the movement of $GABA_A$ receptors, and result in LTD and long term memory impairment[129].

4) *The calcium/ calmodulin complex also increases the activity of cAMP-phosphodiesterase (PDE4A) that normally lowers the concentration of cAMP in the prefrontal cortex. It has been shown that as the brain ages cAMP concentration in the prefrontal cortex rises. This keeps HCN channels open lowering synaptic efficiency by allowing potassium diffusion, reducing neuronal firing, and impairing cognition[102,183]. The reason for this is likely due to the slow accumulation of aluminum in the brain. Aluminum inhibits the effect of the calcium/calmodulin complex on PDE4[123] allowing the concentration of cAMP to rise. That keeps the HCN channels open and thereby impairs cognition. High levels of cAMP have also been shown to encourage the phosphorylation of tau protein leading to NFTs that are a characteristic of AD [184,185]. Therefore aluminum promotes both impaired frontal lobe cognition and NFT production by increasing cAMP levels.*

Chapter 2 – Stroke and Vascular Dementia

"Hippocrates, the father of medicine, first recognized stroke over 2400 years ago." History of Stroke – John Hopkins Medical Health Library

Stroke is an old disease that is currently the second most common cause of death in the world with the most common being ischemic heart disease. The World Health Organization estimates that 6.7 million people died of stroke in 2012 as compared with 5.7 million in 2000[186]. This is a 17% increase in stroke deaths worldwide in 12 years. The primary reasons for the increase are that people are living longer and accumulating more aluminum. Worldwide the number of people over 60 grew by approximately 50% during this 12 year period. Strokes can result in either death or damage to the brain called vascular dementia. Currently an estimated 6.8 million Americans are living after having a stroke[187]. But 40% of those who have a stroke have serious long-term disability requiring special care and 15% die shortly after having the stroke[188].

One reason I decided to write this book is an acquaintance had a stroke that had devastating consequences. Every year around Christmas my wife and I enjoyed the company of a small group of friends that included Dick and his wife. Dick was in his early sixties, enjoyed kayaking, and was looking forward to retiring. Unfortunately he had a stroke before retiring. In order to dissolve the clot he was treated within 3 hours with tissue plasminogen activator (tPA)[189]. But in spite of fantastic medical care, he was left with the inability to speak his thoughts and walking was difficult. After partial recovery it was all he could do to make it to and from the mailbox at the end of his driveway. Dick died within 15 months of having the stroke. This made stroke a painful reality for me. After attending Dick's funeral I began researching the causes of stroke.

A stroke occurs when a region of the brain has insufficient blood flow resulting in cell death. The brain, like a muscle, needs oxygen and nutrients in order to allow organelles inside neurons called mitochondria to make energy in the form of adenosine triphosphate (ATP). In the brain ATP powers the neurotransmissions involved in cognition, while in muscle ATP powers the contractions involved in movement. Like muscle, the brain without oxygen or nutrients weakens the mitochondria and ultimately some of the brain's neurons and their mitochondria die.

Symptoms of a stroke include feeling like the world is spinning and difficulty doing any of the following:

- Understanding
- Speaking
- Moving
- Feeling one side of the body

The symptoms of stroke are variable because a stroke can occur in different parts of the brain. There are three types of strokes and a related condition called white matter disease:

- **Ischemic strokes** involve a blood clot that obstructs blood flow to a portion of the brain. Ischemic strokes account for 87% of all stroke cases and, if treated within 4.5 hours with tissue plasminogen activator (tPA)[189], the blood clot can be dissolved, minimizing damage to the brain.
- **Transient ischemic strokes**, called mini-strokes, silent strokes, or TIAs, involve a temporary blood clot inside a blood vessel that obstructs oxygen and nutrient flow to a portion of the brain. These strokes can be a warning sign of a pending ischemic stroke and they can cause mild cognitive impairment (MCI).
- **Hemorrhagic strokes** involve rupture of a blood vessel due to high blood pressure or amyloid plaque on the walls of blood vessels (cerebral amyloid angiopathy). These strokes can occur within a week of tPA administration[189].
- **Leukoaraiosis (a.k.a. white matter disease)** involves partial obstruction of blood flow to small regions of the brain[190]. These regions appear on CT or MRI scans as bright white spots scattered through the white matter regions of the brain[191]. These white spots have been found in 40-50% of people over 50 years of age[191,192]. This damage can result in impairment of executive brain functions such as memory processing, decision-making, and priority-setting, as well as more basic functions such as balance, gait, and motor coordination[193].

Both strokes and ischemic heart disease are caused by a process called atherogenesis (a.k.a. calcification or hardening of the arteries) that results in weakened blood vessels and calcified arteries and heart valves. Factors such as aluminum accumulation, age, smoking, diet, and lipid metabolism have been linked to stroke. Unlike Alzheimer's, stroke is an old disease recognized over 2400 years ago. Since exposure to increased levels of aluminum has only occurred during the last century, it is not surprising that there are other causes of stroke with a longer history. Figure 2 is a flow diagram of atherogenesis showing the process by which aluminum and other factors cause ischemic and hemorrhagic strokes. The steps of atherogenesis are as follows:

- Aluminum impacts lipid metabolism by causing low density lipoprotein (LDL), cholesterol, and triglycerides to rise and the level of L-carnitine to fall.
- Aluminum accumulation, genetics, vitamin deficiency, chronic moderate alcohol consumption, animal-protein diet, caffeine, and nicotine can all individually cause levels of serum homocysteine to rise.
- Elevated levels of homocysteine weaken the ultra-thin smooth inner lining of arteries, called the endothelium[194,195].
- Particles of LDL penetrate the weakened endothelium.
- The LDL in the endothelium becomes oxidized.
- White blood cells stream in to digest the oxidized LDL[196].
- Foam cells form a plaque on the inside wall of the weakened endothelium.
- The plaque serves as nucleation sites for calcium and phosphate in the blood to crystallize as a solid on the plaque resulting in atherosclerosis.

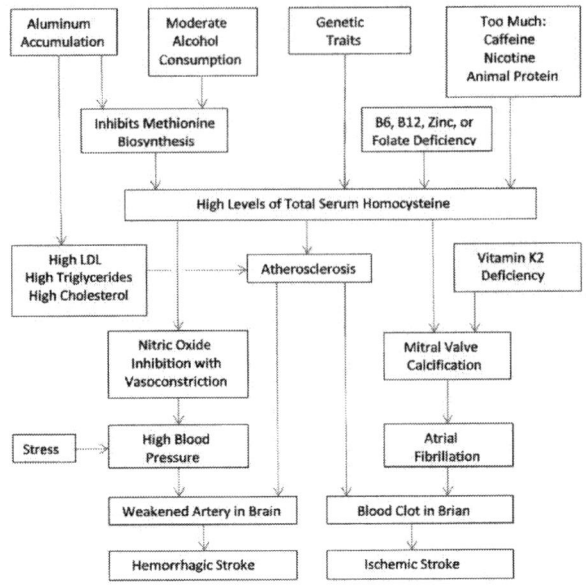

Figure 2 – Atherogenesis and aluminum's role as a cause of stroke

Aluminum a Causal Factor for Stroke

Atherogenesis can be caused by aluminum increasing the concentrations of homocysteine, low density lipoproteins (LDL), cholesterol, and triglycerides and decreasing concentrations of L-carnitine. The connection between strokes and aluminum was shown in 2013 by an occupational toxicology study of aluminum workers:

Forty workers exposed to aluminum while working in an aluminum factory were compared with 40 non-exposed subjects of comparable age who worked in administration at the same factory. The age range of the subjects was 18 to 62. The workers had been chronically exposed to aluminum dust levels of 0.33 to 3.4mg per cubic meter of air without any protective equipment. The study included a clinical examination of medical records of the subjects as well as blood tests for aluminum. Aluminum blood levels of the exposed group were on average nearly 10 times higher than the control group (24mcg/L versus 2.6mcg/L). The results of the clinical examination revealed a higher frequency of stroke, high blood pressure, and ischemic heart disease in the exposed group. In fact 5 of the 40 exposed workers had a stroke and 14 of the 40 had ischemic heart disease. This compared with 2 cases of stroke and 4 cases of ischemic heart disease in the control group. The exposed group also had higher levels of LDL, triglycerides, and cholesterol and lower levels of L-carnitine than the control group[197].

Aluminum accumulation causes elevated homocysteine levels[194,195] and elevated homocysteine levels can lead to stroke[198-203]. Homocysteine and its' methylated relative methionine are essential amino acids found in the proteins of our body and our diet. They are essential because our bodies can't make them from other biochemicals. When we digest proteins, homocysteine and methionine are set free from protein. Free homocysteine is toxic to our arteries and must be either converted to methionine or further metabolized in order to lower its toxicity.

In addition to elevating homocysteine levels, aluminum also promotes atherogenesis by increasing LDL, triglycerides, and cholesterol and decreasing L-carnitine in the blood[197]. Aluminum's ability to disrupt mitochondrial energy production, as discussed in Chapter 1, results in higher levels of LDL and triglycerides in the blood[204]. This is not only due to aluminum's inhibition of the Krebs (a.k.a. TCA) cycle, but also its inhibition of fatty acid transfer into the mitochondria by L-carnitine[204].

Do you diet and not lose weight? The reason may be accumulated aluminum in your body inhibiting the production of L-carnitine and the oxidation of fatty acids. L-carnitine acts as a chaperone that facilitates the transfer of large fatty acids into the mitochondria so they can be oxidized and metabolized for energy production. Aluminum lowers L-carnitine levels by inhibiting two enzymes involved in the biosynthesis of L-carnitine[205] and inhibiting the activation of an enzyme (e.g. MS) involved in the biosynthesis of a precursor of L-carnitine (e.g. methionine)[206,207]. Therefore aluminum impairs the body's ability to use stored fatty acids as an energy source by lowering L-carnitine levels in the blood and thereby reducing the effect of dieting for fat loss. Also since fatty acids are a component of triglycerides, it is not surprising that aluminum accumulation results in both low L-carnitine and high triglyceride levels in the blood[197]. Therefore aluminum promotes atherogenesis and increases the risk of stroke and ischemic heart disease by several mechanisms as diagrammed in Figure 2.

Obesity resulting from impaired stored fat utilization can be a symptom of aluminum accumulation. Since aluminum is a casual factor for stroke and Alzheimer's disease, obesity resulting from impaired stored fat utilization is correlated with a person's increased risk of stroke and Alzheimer's disease. Using body mass index (BMI=weight in kilograms divided by height in meters squared) as a measure of obesity:

- For each unit of BMI over 25 there is a 6% increased risk of stroke for men[208].
- Each unit of BMI at midlife predicts earlier onset of AD by 6.7 months[209].

Lifestyle choices leading to obesity may enhance aluminum accumulation and the impact of aluminum on brain health (see chapter 6). So does aluminum accumulation cause obesity or does obesity result in enhanced aluminum accumulation? This is a perfect example of how causes and symptoms can be difficult to untangle.

Homocysteine Metabolism

Normal blood oxygen levels stimulate an enzymatic pathway that safely and reversibly stores homocysteine as methionine. Under low blood oxygen levels our bodies been have evolved to use the metabolites of methionine and homocysteine for neuroprotection. Low blood oxygen levels can occur due to a stroke or from strenuous exercise. As a species we evolved to run down large game until it collapsed due to heat exhaustion[210]. This required anaerobic exercise that lowered our blood oxygen to harmful levels for the brain. These low blood oxygen levels stimulate an enzymatic pathway that metabolizes both methionine and homocysteine to produce the metabolites taurine and glutathione that protect the brain during and immediately after either anaerobic exercise or a stroke. As a highly adaptable species we have even evolved a third metabolic pathway as a backup to keep homocysteine levels safely under control.

Three pathways used by our bodies to metabolize homocysteine are diagrammed in Figure 3. Two of these three pathways are inhibited by aluminum and the third pathway can be made more efficient when supplemental betaine (a.k.a. TMG) is routinely taken orally. Inhibition of two pathways by aluminum accumulation increases total serum homocysteine levels in the blood. Highly elevated levels of total serum homocysteine (greater than 60μM/L), called hyperhomocysteinemia (HHC), and more commonly slightly elevated levels of total serum homocysteine (12-60μM/L) are correlated with increased risk of stroke[198-201].

Figure 3 diagrams the two methylation pathways that convert homocysteine to methionine and one transsulfuration pathway that converts homocysteine to taurine and glutathione (GSH)[195].

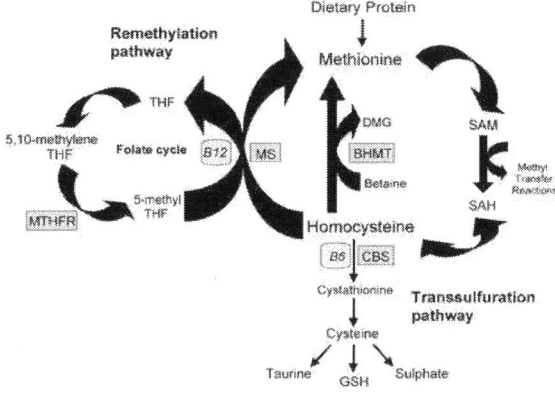

Figure 3 – Metabolism of homocysteine

Three Pathways of Homocysteine Metabolism

- *In one of three pathways of homocysteine metabolism the enzyme MS catalyzes the conversion of homocysteine to methionine and SAM. This pathway works under conditions of normal blood oxygenation keeping levels of homocysteine low. However aluminum inhibits activation of the enzyme MS[206,207]. Therefore aluminum blocks this pathway resulting in rising levels of homocysteine and declining levels of SAM.*
- *In the transsulfuration pathway the enzyme CBS is activated by either SAM or low blood oxygenation. With normal blood oxygenation and declining levels of SAM, due to aluminum, CBS activity is lowered adding to rising homocysteine levels. This is the "perfect storm" for creating high levels of homocysteine in the brain[207,211].*
- *When aluminum accumulation has blocked the other two pathways, only the pathway that uses betaine (a.k.a. TMG) to methylate homocysteine is available to lower homocysteine levels. Since the availability of TMG in the brain can be limited, TMG supplementation is a way to compensate for aluminum accumulation in the brain. TMG has been linked to heart disease in patients with diabetes and is not recommended for those patients[212].*

Additional Factors Linked to Elevated Total Serum Homocysteine

Aluminum is not the only factor that increases total serum homocysteine. The following additional factors have been linked to elevated levels of total serum homocysteine:

- Genetics
- Vitamin B6, B12, Zinc, and Folate Deficiency
- Chronic Moderate Alcohol Consumption
- Animal Protein
- Caffeine
- Smoking

Genetics Can Increase Homocysteine: Studying children with the rare genetic condition called homocystinuria revealed that elevated levels of homocysteine are a risk factor for atherosclerosis and stroke. People with homocystinuria develop atherosclerosis and have strokes much earlier than normal. This genetic condition occurs because of an enzymatic deficiency that causes high levels of total serum homocysteine. Homocystinuria affects 1 in 200,000 people.

A much more common genetic variant found in 48% of the population impairs the ability of the enzyme MTHFR to convert folic acid (THF) to 5-methlyl THF in the folate cycle (see Figure 3)[10,213]. 5-methyl THF is required for the conversion of homocysteine to methionine. This defective MTHFR gene leads to elevated levels of plasma homocysteine in those people who inherit this gene from both parents.

Vitamin B6, B12, Zinc and Folate Deficiency Increases Homocysteine: Homocysteine is metabolized by enzymes requiring vitamins B6, B12, zinc, and folic acid, a deficiency of any one of these chemicals can cause elevated homocysteine. B12 deficiency (<0.24ng/L) occurs in 3% to 4% of the general population[214], 15% of the over 65 population[215] and 29% of dementia patients[216]. Levels of both B12 and folic acid have been shown to decrease in cerebral spinal fluid with advancing age[218].

In order for folic acid to be used to lower homocysteine levels it must first be converted in the body to 5-MTHF (a.k.a. levomefolic acid, 5-methyltetrahydrofolate, methyl folate). In North American 48% of the population have genotypes that may increase the risk of an enzyme deficiency preventing the conversion of folic acid to 5-MTHF[213]. In order to circumvent this enzyme deficiency, taking 5-MTHF as a supplement instead of folic acid is recommended[219,220].

Since levels of both B12 and folic acid have been shown to decrease in cerebral spinal fluid with advancing age[218] both folic acid as 5-MTHF and vitamin B12 supplementation is recommended as you get older. The metabolism of homocysteine to taurine and glutathione requires vitamin B6. Therefore a B vitamin complex, including both vitamin B6, and B12 is recommended as a supplement to lower homocysteine and the risk of stroke[199,121,222].

Another pathway of homocysteine metabolism involves methylation of homocysteine using TMG (a.k.a. betaine, trimethylglycine)[223]. TMG supplementation (500mg/day) can lower homocysteine[221]. Advantages of this pathway are that B12 and the enzyme MS are not required and aluminum has not been shown to be an inhibitor. TMG supplementation is recommended for those people over 60 who have high homocysteine levels as they are more likely to also have high aluminum levels. TMG is not recommended for patients with diabetes as it has been linked to heart disease in those patients[212].

Caffeine and Smoking Increases Homocysteine: The caffeine induced neurotransmitters epinephrine and norepinephrine (a.k.a. noradrenaline) and the tobacco ingredient nicotine are metabolized via processes that use folic acid, diverting it from being used for homocysteine metabolism. Therefore it is not surprising that caffeine consumption and smoking are each correlated with a rise of approximately 1μM/L of homocysteine in the blood[224].

High Animal-protein Diet Increases Homocysteine: A study of how protein in the diet impacts total serum homocysteine levels was performed with 1,015 patients 40 to 85 years old who underwent coronary angiography. Based upon food-frequency questionnaires the patients were divided into four groups: those consuming low and high levels of animal protein and those consuming low and high levels of plant protein in their diets. The amount of protein consumed in the high animal-protein diet (protein greater than 8.4% of total energy intake) was positively correlated with high total serum homocysteine. Surprisingly the amount of protein consumed in the high plant-protein diet (also protein greater than 8.4% of total energy intake) was inversely correlated with total serum homocysteine[225]. This is because unlike animal-protein diets, vegetarian diets are normally high in folic acid. As long as there is sufficient vitamin B12 in the vegetarian's diet, their total serum homocysteine will decrease as they consume more plant-protein with folic acid. However vitamin B12 is not found in plants.

Therefore vegetarians must supplement their diets with vitamin B12, by eating fortified food or supplements. If they do not, their vitamin B12 levels will decline and their total serum homocysteine levels will become elevated to levels higher than omnivores. In 1999 there was a study of vegans who supplemented their diet with an average of 5.6mcg/day of vitamin B12. They were found to have total serum homocysteine levels averaging 7.96μM/L, only slightly lower than omnivores with an average animal-protein diet[226].

Because high animal-protein diets are low in folic acid, folic acid supplementation as 5-MTHF and TMG is recommended for those on such diets in order to lower homocysteine levels.

Chronic Moderate Alcohol Consumption Increases Homocysteine: The ethanol in alcoholic beverages is enzymatically oxidized in the body to acetaldehyde and acetate. Acetaldehyde inhibits the conversion of homocysteine to methionine by the enzyme MS. This inhibition was found to become irreversible with chronic exposure of MS to acetaldehyde[227]. MS is the same enzyme inhibited by aluminum. Therefore as in the case of aluminum inhibition, an above normal level of total serum homocysteine is expected with alcohol consumption.

A study of chronic moderate alcohol consumption and homocysteine levels was conducted with 60 healthy males aged 28 to 44. The subjects were divided into four groups of 15 based upon their alcohol consumption during the prior year. A control group, who were abstinent during the prior year, received no alcoholic beverage during the study. The other three groups got a daily alcoholic drink of either beer, red wine, or spirits depending upon the subject's preferred source of alcohol. The volume consumed of each of these three drinks was equivalent to 30 grams (38cc, 1.3 ounces) of pure alcohol. The study lasted 6 weeks. The data in the table shows that chronic moderate alcohol drinking during the 6 week study caused elevated total serum homocysteine. In addition, periodic alcohol consumption prior to the 6 week study had also caused elevated total serum homocysteine in the drinkers who had periodically drunk beer, wine, and spirits[228].

Group	% Ethanol	Ounces of Drink**	Initial tHcy*	Final tHcy*
Control			9	8.5
Beer	5	26	11.7	14.6
Wine	12	11	12.7	15.6
Spirits	40	3.2	13.8	16.2

*Average tHcy levels are µM/L of homocysteine in the blood.
**Ounces of drink that contain 30 grams of ethanol.

Additional Causes of Stroke

There are other causal factors of stroke in addition to the previously described factors that increase homocysteine. These additional causal factors for stroke include:

- High Blood Pressure – symptom of high serum homocysteine
- High Serum Levels of LDL Particles – can be caused by high aluminum levels
- High Serum Levels of Triglycerides – can be caused by high aluminum levels
- Amyloid plaque on blood vessels – can be caused by high aluminum levels
- Atrial Fibrillation – symptom of high serum homocysteine & low vitamin K2–MK-4

High Blood Pressure as a Causal Factor for Stroke: High blood pressure (a.k.a. hypertension) causes both hemorrhagic strokes, by bursting blood vessels in the brain, and white matter disease[229,230]. High blood pressure is caused by both stress and elevated total serum homocysteine levels[231]. Elevated total serum homocysteine levels can also cause atherosclerosis resulting in prehypertension and hypertension[232]. Prehypertension (i.e. blood pressure greater than 120/80 mm and less than 140/90 mmHg) has been shown to increase the risk of stroke by 66%[217]. Hypertension (e.g. blood pressure 140/90 mmHg or higher) is also known to increase the risk of stroke. Stroke patients with elevated total serum homocysteine are four times more likely to have hypertension and a recurrent stroke[233].

Elevated levels of total serum homocysteine increase blood pressure. Vasoconstriction of blood vessels causes high blood pressure by decreasing the diameter of blood vessels. Vasodilation lowers blood pressure by expanding the diameter of blood vessels. Nitric oxide (NO) is a vasodilator produced by the enzymatic conversion of the amino acid arginine to NO. Homocysteine acts to increase production of an inhibitor of this enzymatic conversion. Thereby elevated levels of total serum homocysteine act as a vasoconstrictor and cause high blood pressure by inhibiting the formation of NO[231].

Low Density Lipoprotein as a Causal Factor for Stroke: If atherogenesis were a drama, your brain would be the stage and aluminum, homocysteine, and low density lipoprotein (LDL) would be the main characters in a life and death or dementia struggle. Aluminum accumulation increases both homocysteine and LDL in the blood. Therefore lowering your aluminum accumulation will help to prevent stroke by lowering both your homocysteine and LDL.

There is a correlation between LDL and stroke risk. An updated meta-analysis of 165,792 patients in 24 randomized clinical trials showed that for every 39mg/dL decrease in serum LDL there is a 21% decrease in ischemic stroke risk[234]. The SPARCL and HPS clinical trials, that were part of this meta-analysis, did reveal a significantly increased hemorrhagic stroke risk in people taking statins, if they had a prior hemorrhagic stroke. This makes a recommendation to take statins controversial for these people. Statins taken before and after an ischemic stroke have been shown to result in significantly lower post-stroke mortality and lower risk of a worsening condition during hospitalization[235,236]. In general statins are recommended to lower the endogenous (i.e. internal) production of both LDL and cholesterol. Particles of LDL contain cholesterol however there is no conclusive correlation between high cholesterol and stroke risk.

Currently millions of people take statins to lower LDL. Statins inhibit a coenzyme involved in cholesterol's biosynthetic pathway. This in turn inhibits the internal production of cholesterol and formation of LDL. The absorption of dietary cholesterol can also be inhibited by drugs[237,238]. Note that vitamin D3 made in your skin requires both sunlight (UVB radiation) and a precursor of cholesterol that is made only by the internal production of cholesterol. Therefore statins could lower the production of vitamin D3 in the skin[239]. But a recent study indicates that 12 weeks of daily use of statins (e.g. Rosuvastatin: 10mg/day, or Atorvastatin: 20mg/day) had no significant effect on vitamin D3 levels[240]. Another study involving 77 participants revealed that one year of daily use of Simvastatin also had no effect on vitamin D3 levels[241].

A study of 700,000 people 65 and older suffering from cardiovascular disease clearly demonstrated that Simvastatin lowered the risk of dementia, including AD, by approximately 50%, while Atorvastatin and Lovastatin had no effect on the risk of dementia[242]. This has led people to suspect that Simvastatin's lipid lowering efficacy prevents both vascular dementia and sporadic AD caused by ischemic events[9]. The reason for the efficacy of Simvastatin versus the other two statins is currently unknown but Simvastatin's fat solubility (i.e. lipophilicity) may be an important factor[242,243].

Statins are not the only chemicals known to lower LDL. For instance in two separate studies it was observed that atherosclerosis was most prevalent in people with plasma chromium levels lower than 0.006mcg/L[244,245]. Chromium picolinate taken as a 200mcg/day supplement increases plasma chromium levels and has been shown to lower LDL by 11% over a 6 week period[246]. This was a study of only 28 subjects who had an average total cholesterol level of 276mg/dL and an average LDL level of 200mg/dL (dL is one tenth of a liter). There was no significant change in triglycerides and HDL with this dose of chromium picolinate.

Niacin (a.k.a. vitamin B3, nicotinic acid) is recommended in small doses (i.e. 20-35mg/day) to prevent pellagra (see Appendix II on metabolic dementia). But the use of large doses of niacin (i.e. 500-3000mg/day) to lower LDL while simultaneously raising HDL has become controversial[247]. This is because niacin only has a big impact on your LDL level, if you are not taking statins[248]. Also there has been no proven benefit of increasing HDL and there is an increased risk of disease when taking large doses of niacin[247].

High Plasma Triglycerides as a Causal Factor for Stroke: Elevated triglyceride levels in the blood have been correlated with increased risk of recurrent ischemic stroke[249]. The efficacy of the drug Gemfibrozil, that lowers triglycerides, was evaluated in a 5 year study of 2,531 men with coronary heart disease. The study showed that Gemfibrozil reduced the risk of initial ischemic strokes by 31%[250]. Therefore lowering triglyceride levels reduces the risk of stroke.

Non-drug approaches to reducing triglycerides include vitamin D3 supplementation lowering triglyceride levels in postmenopausal women[241,251]. In one study those with vitamin D levels greater than 32ng/ml have 23% lower serum triglycerides than those with vitamin D levels below 32ng/ml[241]. Also each gram of the omega-3 fatty acids DHA and EPA taken daily has been shown to reduce triglycerides by 5 to 10%[252]. Taking less than a quarter gram of the omega-7 fatty acid palmitoleic acid (PA) daily reduces triglycerides by 15% and LDL by 8%[253]. EPA supplementation does not increase LDL levels significantly while DHA supplementation increases LDL levels by 4.5mg/dL[254]. Therefore EPA and PA supplementation is recommended if both your serum triglycerides and LDL are too high. Before starting EPA, PA, or EPA + DHA supplementation in order to lower your triglyceride level, read the section on DHA in Chapter 3.

Amyloid Plaque on Blood Vessels as a Causal Factor for Stroke: Called cerebral amyloid angiopathy, the build-up of amyloid deposits on the walls of blood vessels of the central nervous system can cause hemorrhagic stroke. This build-up may be due to aluminum cross-linking amyloid protein thereby preventing amyloid from being cleared from the brain[255].

Atrial fibrillation as a Causal Factor for Stroke: Using data from the Framingham Study of 5,209 men and women who were examined for cardiovascular disease every 2 years for 34 years, it was discovered that both 50-59 and 80-89 year old individuals with atrial fibrillation (a.k.a. aFib) are 4-4.5 times more likely to have a stroke than those in these age groups without aFib[256]. Those individuals with aFib between 59 and 80 are 2.6-3.3 times more likely to have a stroke than those in this age group without aFib. aFib is believed to cause strokes because blood is incompletely pumped from the aorta causing blood stasis (i.e. slower fluid flow) resulting in atrial clots that can be pumped to the brain[256].

Because aFib can be a random event, it may not be detected in the doctor's office by an ECG (a.k.a. EKG). In order to detect aFib continuous monitoring for 24-48 hours by a Holter monitor or for several weeks with an event monitor may be required. Continuous event monitoring for aFib has recently been made possible by a paperclip sized heart monitor inserted under the skin of the chest. This monitor is battery powered and the batteries last for 3 years. The information is stored in the device and transmitted wirelessly to a patient's doctor who can be alerted even in the middle of the night to any problems. The device is the Reveal LINQ that was developed by Medtronic.

Atrial fibrillation is correlated with both high levels of total serum homocysteine and a vitamin K2 deficiency (see Chapter 3 for information on vitamin K2 supplementation).

Visiting my Doctor

Recently I looked at the results of my blood work for my last physical examination only to find that serum homocysteine had not been analyzed. My doctor of 25 years, who specialized in cardiology, had retired and a younger doctor who specializes in gastroenterology took over his caseload. During my next annual physical visit with my new doctor I requested a homocysteine analysis. The blood work came back showing I have elevated total serum homocysteine with 15μM/L of homocysteine. I asked my doctor for his advice on how to lower this elevated homocysteine level. In order to give me this advice he first had to ask my former, and now retired doctor, what he might advise. The answer was a daily supplement of folic acid (1mg = 1,000mcg). This is the correct answer although more information would have been useful. For starters folic acid and folate are not the same. Folic acid is a synthetic mono-glutamate of folic acid while dietary folate is a natural product containing polyglutamates of folic acid that are quickly converted to 5-MTHF (a.k.a. methyl folate, levomefolic acid) in your body[222].

A more complete answer would also have mentioned that 400mcg/day is the normal recommended daily supplemental dose of folic acid and that there can be side-effects of higher doses of folic acid. These side-effects can include abdominal cramps, diarrhea, rash, sleep disorders, irritability, confusion, nausea, stomach upset, behavior changes, skin reactions, seizures, gas, excitability, and a tendency toward anxiety. Also 1mg of folic acid taken daily as a supplement has been linked to an increased risk of prostate cancer while dietary folate is linked to a slightly decreased risk of prostate cancer[257].

If your doctor recommends taking supplemental folic acid for high homocysteine levels, first check the label on your B vitamin complex. You may be already taking 400mcg of folic acid a day as part of your daily B vitamin complex. 5-MTHF (a.k.a. methyl folate, levomefolic acid) is more effective than folic acid at lowering homocysteine[220]. Also taking 5-MTHF is essential for those people with the MTHFR gene who have an impaired ability to use folic acid. Folic acid and 5-MTHF have the same side-effects. If taking other drugs, check 5-MTHF on the internet for drug interactions.

This experience shows that you may have to ask your doctor for a homocysteine analysis of your blood. Once the results are back the amount of advice you get as what to do about high levels may depend upon your doctor's specialty. High homocysteine levels can be treated with the low cost non-patented non-prescription folic acid or 5-MTHF and, if you are not diabetic, TMG.

Biochemical Mechanism of Supplements to Lower Homocysteine

Methylation is a process wherein a CH_3 group is added to a molecule. Methylation lowers the homocysteine concentration in the blood and brain as shown in Figure 3. Vitamin B12 and the enzyme methionine synthase (MS) catalyze the methylation of homocysteine to methionine in the folate cycle. Folic acid (a.k.a. folate, vitamin M, vitamin B9) enters the remethylation pathway as tetrahydrofolate (THF) and is converted to 5-MTHF (a.k.a. levomefolic acid, methyl folate, (6S)-5-methylTHF, 5-methyltetrahydrofolate, (6S)-5-methyltetrahydrofolate) that methylates vitamin B12. Folic acid supplementation (1mg/day) lowers plasma homocysteine levels and 5-MTHF taken as a supplement (1mg/day) has been shown to be more effective than folic acid for lowering plasma homocysteine levels[220]. Aluminum inhibits the activation of MS and slows the methylation of homocysteine to methionine[206,207].

Homocysteine can also be methylated to methionine catalyzed by the enzyme betaine homocysteine methyltransferase (BHMT) that uses betaine (a.k.a. trimethylglycine, TMG) as a source of methyl groups while demethylating TMG to dimethylglycine (DMG)[223]. Aluminum has not been shown to inhibit BHMT. A study of 3,042 people showed that those who consumed >360 mg/day of TMG had on average 10% lower homocysteine than those who consumed <260 mg/day[221]. TMG has been linked to heart disease in patients with diabetes and is not recommended for those patients[212]. TMG has been found to be most effective for lowering homocysteine in people with a B12 or folate deficiency[258] or in those with inhibited MS catalyzed methylation of homocysteine[259]. This inhibition can be due to aluminum inhibition of MS activation or chronic alcohol consumption leading to acetaldehyde inhibition of MS.

Another way to lower the concentration of homocysteine is the transsulfuration pathway that converts it to cysteine with catalysis by two enzymes (cystathionine beta synthase CBS and cystathionine gamma-lyase CGL)) and the help of vitamin B6 and zinc. Cysteine can be further metabolized to sulfate, that is excreted, and to taurine, and glutathione (GSH), both of which are protective to neurons before, during, and after a stroke. This pathway is sped up in the brain by a lack of oxygen created by anaerobic exercise or stroke.

Conclusion of Stroke and Vascular Dementia

Strokes resulting in death or vascular dementia can occur due to the following factors:

- Aluminum accumulation in the brain
- Low levels of B6, B12, folic acid, and/or zinc
- Increased homocysteine in the blood
- High blood pressure due to homocysteine, stress and/or atherosclerosis
- High levels of LDL in the blood
- High levels of triglycerides in the blood
- Atrial fibrillation due to vitamin K2 deficiency and elevated homocysteine
- Chronic moderate alcohol consumption
- Smoking and nicotine
- Stress
- Caffeine ingestion

This chapter has discussed how aluminum accumulation increases the concentration of homocysteine, LDL, triglycerides, and cholesterol in the blood that initiates the process of atherogenesis (a.k.a. hardening of the arteries). This can end badly with a stroke, vascular dementia, or death. A high homocysteine level in the blood weakens the smooth inner lining of arteries and is correlated with an increased risk of strokes.

The following steps are recommended to lower your homocysteine level and the risk of stroke:

- Lower your aluminum ingestion and accumulation as described in Chapters 4 and 5.
- Get your serum B12, homocysteine, LDL, and triglyceride levels tested.
- If your homocysteine level is too high, take supplemental vitamin B12 (100mcg/day), B6 (100mg/day), and take folic acid (400-1000mcg/day) or 5-MTHF (400-1000mcg/day).
- If your homocysteine level remains high, try less caffeine, less nicotine, less stress, and less alcohol and take trimethylglycine (TMG 500mg/day). TMG should only be used if you are not diabetic.
- If your B12 level is low and your homocysteine is very high, B12 injections will quickly increase your B12 and lower your homocysteine levels. Ten injections will lower homocysteine levels from $50\mu M$/liter to $10\mu M$/liter in 10 days.
- If your LDL level is too high, take a statin, unless you have had a hemorrhagic stroke. Otherwise take chromium picolinate (200mcg/day).
- If your triglyceride level is too high, try a diet high in omega-3 fatty acids, as described in the section on DHA in Chapter 3, and take a quarter gram per day of the omega-7 palmitoleic acid, or take Gemfibrozil by prescription.
- If both your LDL levels and serum triglyceride levels are too high take 1 – 2 grams per day of the omega-3 fatty acid EPA and a quarter gram per day of the omega-7 palmitoleic acid.
- In order to lower the risk of atrial fibrillation causing a stroke, lower your total serum homocysteine and take a vitamin K2 supplement as described in Chapter 3.
- In order to lower the risk of a recurrent stroke, after the first stroke take aspirin daily (100mg/day).

Chapter 3 – Preventing and Possibly Reversing Dementia with 7 Supplements

"I believe that you can, by taking some simple measures, lead a longer life and extend your years of well-being" Linus Pauling

This chapter describes "The 7 Samurai Warriors" for brain protection. These 7 supplements can reverse brain ageing and keep your brain youthful while preventing Alzheimer's, autism (chapter 9), and stroke. A friend describes these supplements as a 401K plan for his brain that requires a small investment every year that pays dividends in brain health both before and after you retire.

| **Seven Supplements to Reverse Brain and Heart Ageing and Provide Brain Protection** ||
Supplement	**Benefits of Supplements**
PQQ	Reverses Brain Ageing – Prevents Dementia and Possibly Autism
CoQ10	Provides More Brain Energy – Counters Mitochondrial Disease
Vitamin D	Prevents Aluminum Absorption and Possibly Autism
Taurine	Reverses Brain Ageing - Prevents Damage due to Stroke & Metals
Vitamin K2-MK-4	Reverses Heart Ageing – Prevents Stroke
Vitamin B100 Complex	Prevents Hardening of Arteries – Lowers Homocysteine Levels
5-MTHF	Prevents Hardening of Arteries – Lowers Homocysteine Levels

PQQ as an Oral Supplement to Prevent Dementia and Possibly Autism

PQQ (a.k.a. pyrroloquinoline quinone) is a molecular super-hero for the body. PQQ is found in mother's milk at concentrations five times higher than any food. Its' presence in mother's milk is no evolutionary accident. PQQ promotes generation of both new mitochondria for brain energy and new neurites for memory storage. PQQ is a heavyweight antioxidant that can deliver 20,000 knockout punches to oxidants compared to only 4 delivered by a lightweight antioxidant like vitamin C.

PQQ was first isolated in 1979, but only a few milligrams could be obtained from natural sources. This low availability prevented PQQ's chemistry and mode of action from being defined. In order to obtain larger quantities of PQQ a total organic synthesis from readily available chemicals became a vital part of improving our understanding. My former doctoral thesis advisor, Professor E. J. Corey was awarded a noble prize for developing a logical "retro-synthetic" method of designing synthetic routes to complex molecules. Corey and Alfonso Tramontano performed the first total synthesis of PQQ at Harvard in 1981[260]. This synthesis made large amounts of PQQ available for research and has opened our eyes to PQQ's remarkable properties. PQQ has been claimed to be a vitamin. This claim is controversial as PQQ is produced by our bodies, so for now we will call PQQ a cofactor or coenzyme.

There are six reasons to take PQQ:

- PQQ protects mitochondria from oxidative stress due to nitric oxide (NO) produced by the brain's glial cells in response to aluminum. PQQ lowers NO production by inhibiting the expression of genes responsible for the production of inducible nitric oxide synthase (iNOS)[121,261-263]. With the help of glutathione PQQ also acts as a stable antioxidant[264,265].
- PQQ promotes the generation of new mitochondria, called mitochondrial biogenesis[266] that increases energy efficiency of mitochondria[267].
- PQQ increases production of nerve growth factor (NGF) in the mitochondria[268] that results in increased neurite growth and improved memory[269,270].
- PQQ when taken before and after a stroke can help to avoid vascular dementia by reducing memory impairment due to lack of oxygen[271,272]. Since we don't know when a stroke might occur, taking PQQ daily is advised.
- PQQ partially inhibits Aβ oligomer formation from Aβ peptides, one of the hallmarks of AD[273].
- PQQ binds to α-synuclein preventing formation of aggegates[274]. Formation of α-synuclein aggregates is believed to be the first step in Lewy body formation leading to Lewy body dementia (see Appendix I).

PQQ as an Antioxidant: Too much or too little oxygen or some metal ions act as physiological stressors in the brain by stimulating brain cells to produce oxidizing chemicals (a.k.a. ROS)[121,122]. The metal ions stimulate inducible nitric oxide synthase (iNOS) in microglial and astroglial cells of the brain to produce nitric oxide (NO) that reacts to produce ROS. This ROS can damage and kill neurons creating inflammation in the brain. Aluminum tops the list of metal ions as a generator of ROS by the brain's glial cells[58].

PQQ inhibits genetic expression of iNOS and thereby inhibits ROS formation in the brain[263]. Also oxidized PQQ and reduced PQQ (a.k.a. $PQQH_2$) both exist in the brain as a highly stable redox cycle that protects the brain. The redox cycle works by glutathione first reducing PQQ to $PQQH_2$ and then by $PQQH_2$ reducing ROS and regenerating PQQ[264,265]. PQQ's high stability allows this redox cycle to be repeated 20,000 times before PQQ becomes degraded as opposed to only four cycles for vitamin C^{264}. The PQQ redox cycle protects the mitochondria, from oxidative stress due to too much or too little oxygen or toxic metals[122].

Safety of PQQ Supplementation: There have been no toxicological signs or symptoms reported as a result of daily PQQ supplementation given orally to humans at a dose of 20mg (milligrams, thousandths of a gram) per day[264,270]. In a 13 week study of PQQ given orally to rats a no-observed-adverse-effect-level (NOAEL) of 100mg per kilogram body weight per day was observed[275]. Experiments with mice showed no interaction with DNA (i.e. genotoxicity)[276]. High daily doses of PPQ in excess of 60mg/day should be avoided due to the potential of kidney damage as observed in rats exposed to high doses of PQQ[264].

PQQ Bioavailability and Sources: PQQ is biosynthesized by the human body at a rate of 100-400 ng/day (100-400 billionths of a gram per day) with an estimated tissue concentration of 1-3 ng/gr of body weight (5-15nM)[269]. Oral supplementation of 20 mg of PQQ in humans resulted in a PQQ serum peak of 9nM after each dose in 2-3 hours and a half-life in the serum of 3-5 hours[269]. Ingested PQQ is both metabolized and reacts with proteins in humans resulting in only 0.1% being eliminated in the urine as PQQ. PQQ is a natural product found in human breastmilk and some foods[277-279].

Dietary Sources of PQQ[277-279]	
Food	**Nanograms PQQ per gram**
Human Breastmilk	160*
Parsley	34
Kiwi Fruit	30
Papaya	30
Green Peppers	28
Tofu	24
Spinach	22
Celery	6

*Note: Currently PQQ is not listed as an ingredient in any baby formula

PQQ and Autism: Biochemical characteristics of autism include activation of iNOS in glial brain cells with increased ROS production[280]. This is a neuro-inflammatory process leading to local cell damage, synapse destruction, and brain under-connectivity[280]. PQQ prevents this situation by both decreasing the expression of iNOS and chemically reducing ROS. PQQ also prevents brain under-connectivity by enhancing nerve growth factor (NGF) production that in turn stimulates the growth of neuronal connections. It is therefore not surprising that PQQ is found in mother's milk at a concentration 5 times higher than found in any other food[279]. However PQQ is not found as an ingredient in any currently available baby formula. Since an amount of PQQ equivalent to 160 nanograms per gram of mother's milk is inexpensive, there is no reason to continue the practice of not adding it to baby formula.

PQQ as an Oral Supplement for Reversing Brain Ageing

PQQ stimulates neurite growth in the ageing brain. A neurite is a projection grown from the cell body of a neuron resulting in an axion or dendrite that can extend a considerable distance in the brain in order to make a synaptic contact with another neuron's neurite. The process of neurite growth involves each neuron growing hundreds of neurites resulting in a complex neural network that allows the brain to store and process memory. Neurite growth is stimulated by neural growth factor (NGF), a protein made in the brain. NGF induces tau and MAP protein production that promotes microtubule assembly during neurite growth. When NGF is removed from neurons, neurites disappear, microtubule mass decreases, and tau and MAP proteins decline to lower levels[281]. Neurite growth is important for short to long term memory conversion, brain plasticity, and for damage repair due to stroke.

PQQ stimulates both neurite growth and mitochondrial biogenesis. CoQ10 improves the energy efficiency of mitochondria. PQQ taken together with CoQ10 improves cognition in the ageing brain. A study of how oral supplements of PQQ and CoQ10 enhance cognition involving 75 people who were 53 years old was recently conducted and published in Japan[270]. In the 12 week study 1/3 of the group were given 20mg/day of PQQ at breakfast, 1/3 were given 20mg/day of PQQ and 300mg/day of CoQ10 at breakfast, and 1/3 were a control given a placebo. People taking just PQQ and PQQ plus CoQ10 significantly out-performed the control group on the CogHealth test. The group on PQQ plus CoQ10 significantly out-performed both the PQQ and control groups on the Stroop test.

Biochemistry of PQQ Stimulating NGF Production

PQQ administered to mouse astroglial cells induces the production of NGF by the astroglial cell[282]. Astroglial cells are star shaped and are located at synapses. Astroglial cells produce extracellular signaling chemicals that remove excess potassium ions, and control the flow of chemicals from the blood to the brain. Astroglial cells form a membrane called the glial limitans that regulates the movement of molecules, such as PQQ, from the blood into the brain. This membrane forms what is called the blood-brain barrier. Like PQQ the methyl ester of PQQ (2-carbomethoxy-pyrroloquinoline quinone) induces NGF production in cells from the CA1 region of the hippocampus[283]. This methyl ester of PQQ has low toxicity and is believed to more readily cross the blood-brain barrier than PQQ. Unlike PQQ, the methyl ester of PQQ is not yet commercially available or approved as an oral supplement.

CoQ10 as an Oral Supplement for Brain Energy

The brain needs oxygen, nutrients, cofactors, and coenzymes (i.e. CoQ10) in order to allow mitochondria, organelles inside neurons, to make energy in the form of adenosine triphosphate (ATP). In the brain ATP powers the neurotransmissions involved in memory and cognition. Too much or too little oxygen or too much toxic metal can disrupt the biosynthesis of ATP. This is called oxidative stress and results in damage to the mitochondria during and after a stroke and after exposure to some metal ions, such as aluminum. There are five reasons to take CoQ10:

- CoQ10 protects mitochondria from oxidative stress and improves energy efficiency.
- CoQ10 protects the brain by improving cerebral metabolism during and after a stroke[284]. Since we don't know when a stroke might occur, taking CoQ10 daily is advised.
- CoQ10 decreases Aβ plaque in brain tissue and improves cognitive performance[285].
- The amount of CoQ10 biosynthesized by humans declines with age. At 80 the concentration in some tissues is only half of what it was at age 20[286].
- The biosynthesis of CoQ10 is inhibited by statins prescribed for LDL and cholesterol reduction[287].

Therefore supplemental CoQ10 is recommended especially for the elderly and those taking statins. CoQ10 has two forms: ubiquinone and ubiquinol. Ubiquinol is more water soluble, more bioavailable, and more expensive than ubiquinone. So although ubiquinol results in 60% higher serum levels as compared with ubiquinone after a single 100mg. dose[288], currently it is three times less expensive to take 200mg of ubiquinone rather that 100mg of ubiquinol.

Vitamin D3 as an Oral Supplement

Vitamin D3 supplementation has been shown to provide the following benefits in **infants and children:**

- Lowers serum and tissue aluminum levels and strengthens bones[289]
- Lowers the risk of autism[290]
- Lowers the risk of developing ADHD-like symptoms in the offspring of mothers taking a vitamin D supplement during pregnancy[291]

Vitamin D3 supplementation has been shown to provide the following benefits in **adults:**

- Lowers the risk of Alzheimer's disease[292]
- Slows the rate of decline of episodic memory and executive function[293]
- Lowers the risk of stroke by lowering triglyceride levels[294]
- Minimizes stroke severity and functional impairment due to stroke[295]
- Increases glutathione levels in the brain[296]
- Improves muscle strength and balance in older adults[297]

Vitamin D deficiency has been found to correlate with AD[292,294], autism[290,298], and stroke[294] risk. In a longitudinal study of 1,658 elderly ambulatory adults it was found that the occurrence of Alzheimer's disease markedly increased below a vitamin D2 threshold serum level of 20ng/ml[292]. In a similar longitudinal study of 382 participants the rate of decline in episodic memory and executive function also increased below a vitamin D2 threshold serum level of 20ng/ml or 50nmole/liter[293]. In a study of sibling pairs, siblings with autism spectrum disorder (ASD) had lower vitamin D2 levels after birth than did their paired non-ASD siblings[290]. In a cross-sectional study of 318 elderly participants receiving home care from 2003 to 2007 it was found that vitamin D deficiency is associated with Alzheimer's disease and stroke with or without vascular dementia symptoms[294]. Vitamin D's ability to prevent AD, autism, and stroke suggests a common causal factor for these three diseases. As we know from Chapters 1 and 2 aluminum is a causal factor of AD and stroke. Therefore vitamin D's unique ability to prevent all three diseases suggests that aluminum may also be a causal factor for autism. See Chapter 9 for a complete discussion of aluminum as a causal factor for autism.

The active form of vitamin D (a.k.a. calcitriol, 1,25-dihydroxycholcalciferol) was discovered in an effort to find the dietary substance lacking in rickets, the childhood form of osteomalacia. Rickets causes soft or easily broken bones in children. The active form of vitamin D increases the level of calcium in the blood by increasing the absorption of calcium from the gut to the blood and possibly increasing the release of calcium from the bone to the blood[299].

The active form of vitamin D does not meet the definition of a true vitamin as it can be made by our bodies in three steps from 7-dehydrocholesterol (see following diagram). Vitamin D3 (a.k.a. cholecalciferol) is either made in the skin by sunlight (e.g. UVB) induced photochemical conversion from 7-dehydrocholesterol or ingested in food or vitamin D3 supplements. Vitamin D3 is first converted in the liver to vitamin D2 (a.k.a. calcidiol, ergocalciferol) and then vitamin D2 is converted to the active form of vitamin D in the kidney. Vitamin D2 is circulated in the blood and its level is used as an indicator of active vitamin D excess or deficiency. Osteomalacia can occur because enhanced aluminum levels inhibit the production of the active form of vitamin D from vitamin D2 in the kidney[300,301].

7-Dehydrocholesterol	→	Vitamin D3	→	Vitamin D2	→	Vitamin D
Produced by:		Skin + UVB		Liver		Kidney
Inhibited by:		Lack of Sunlight				Aluminum

The prevalence of vitamin D deficiency is dramatically rising in the U.S. A study published in 2009 compared the mean serum vitamin D2 levels of 18,883 participants measured from 1988 to 1994 with the mean serum vitamin D2 level of 13,369 participants measured from 2001 to 2004. The mean level of serum vitamin D2 in the U.S. during the decade between 1994 and 2004 fell 18.6%[302]. By measuring vitamin D2 instead of D, could the prevalence of vitamin D deficiency be even worse due to an increased incidence of aluminum inhibition of vitamin D biosynthesis in the kidney? It is possible because demand for aluminum has increased 30-fold since 1950 and is estimated to increase by 3-fold current levels by 2050[119]. Based upon this data on aluminum demand, it is estimated that human exposure to and absorption of aluminum has and will continue to increase at a rate of 65% per decade during the 100 year period from 1950 to 2050[39].

Lower Aluminum Accumulation with Vitamin D Supplementation

Vitamin D supplementation has been found to lower serum aluminum levels in people with higher than normal levels of aluminum. For instance, people with kidney disease (KD) have more aluminum in their brains and kidneys and are more susceptible to softening of bones (osteomalacia). Enhanced aluminum levels in the blood of KD patients result in 70% higher than normal aluminum burdens in their brains[303].

During 2009, 10 pediatric patients with KD and 20 healthy controls were studied. With 4 weeks of active vitamin D supplementation at a level of 15-45 ng/kg/day = 0.27-0.82 IU/lb/day (dosed according to parathyroid hormone levels) serum aluminum concentration declined from a median level of 27.2ng/ml to 3.8ng/ml compared with a median level of 2.5ng/ml for healthy controls[289]. There was no significant change in serum and tissue aluminum levels in KD patients not supplemented with active vitamin D. Since aluminum absorption is a function of parathyroid hormone levels in rats[304,305], it must be noted that the parathyroid hormone levels remained unchanged in the group with KD given active vitamin D supplementation.

Animals with and without KD whose diets are supplemented with vitamin D have lower aluminum levels in their bones and organs. Active vitamin D supplementation lowers aluminum levels in the brain, bone, and liver of rats with KD dosed with aluminum containing food[306]. Dogs with normal kidney function when orally exposed to aluminum and supplemented with 2,200IU/kg of vitamin D3 have dramatically less aluminum accumulation in their bones as compared with vitamin D deficient dogs[307]. Rats with normal kidney function when orally exposed to aluminum and supplemented with active vitamin D had two-fold less aluminum accumulation in their liver as compared with un-supplemented rats[308]. From these studies it can be concluded that vitamin D supplementation lowers aluminum levels in the bones and organs of animals with and without KD. This decrease in aluminum levels is in spite of active vitamin D-enhanced absorption of aluminum from the gut to the blood, particularly in animals with low calcium diets[309-311]. The reason for the decrease in aluminum levels in bones and organs may be due to vitamin D-enhanced aluminum absorption from the gut being coupled with vitamin D-enhanced aluminum excretion by the kidneys in humans[289].

It has been reported that in 2003-2005 six infants from First Nation communities located north of Manitoba at 54 degrees latitude had been diagnosed with vitamin D deficiency, even though they were being fed cow's milk formula containing vitamin D3 at 400 IU/liter[312]. These cases highlight the following factors that may require greater vitamin D3 supplementation:

- High latitudes have less UVB solar radiation and therefore breastmilk has less vitamin D
- American Academy of Pediatrics recommends babies under 6 months get no sun
- Infants may consume less than 1 liter of formula per day
- High levels of aluminum can decrease the effectiveness of vitamin D3 supplementation

Several levels (e.g. 400, 800, 1200, and 1600 IU/day) of D3 supplementation of infants have been tested in double-blind randomized clinical trial of 132 breastfed 1 month old infants living in Montreal Quebec[313]. Of the infants who receiving vitamin D3 supplementation at 400 to 1200 IU/day, 97% had acceptable vitamin D2 plasma levels of 50nmol/liter or greater at 3 months of age. Supplementation at 1600 IU/day resulted in some infants having D2 levels associated with hypercalcemia (see Appendix II on metabolic dementia). Bone growth and mineral content of the bones of all infants tested did not change based upon their dose of supplemental D3[313]. So a supplemental vitamin D3 daily dose of 400IU is recommended for infants.

The Vitamin D Council, the Endocrine Society, and the American Academy of Pediatrics[314] all recommend that babies get daily intake of 400 – 800 IU of vitamin D3 from formula and/or breastmilk. In order to give their children breastmilk with this level of vitamin D3 requires the mothers take a vitamin D3 supplement. Researchers at the Medical University of South Carolina found that mothers who took a 6,400 IU vitamin D3 supplement every day gave their babies on average 800 IU per liter of vitamin D3 in their breastmilk[315]. With this high level of vitamin D3 supplementation a calcium supplement is also recommended for mothers in order to improve bone health and decrease aluminum absorption.

There is controversy regarding recommended daily intake of vitamin D3 for pregnant women[316]:

- Vitamin D Council recommends 4,000 to 6,000 IU/day
- Endocrine Society recommends 1,500 to 2,000 IU/day
- Food and Nutrition Board recommends 600 IU/day[317]

Researchers at the Medical University of South Carolina found in a study of 350 pregnant mothers that taking vitamin D3 supplement of 2,000 to 4,000 IU per day was optimal for achieving a concentration of vitamin D2 greater than 80nmole/liter in the neonate[316]. Since there was no adverse event attributed to the supplementation, the authors recommended supplementation at 4,000 IU per day of vitamin D3 for pregnant mothers[316]. With this high level of vitamin D3 supplementation a calcium supplement is also recommended for pregnant mothers to improve bone health and decrease aluminum absorption.

Reduce Stroke Severity and Functional Impairment with Vitamin D3 Supplementation

During 2010, 386 stroke patients admitted to the Department of Neurology in Dijon France were evaluated during admittance for both vitamin D2 levels in their blood and their stroke severity and were reevaluated at the time of discharge for functional impairment. There was a significant positive correlation found between vitamin D2 levels in the blood and both minimal stroke severity and minimal functional impairment at the time of discharge[295]. Those who do not take a vitamin D3 supplement typically have D2 levels under 20ng/ml. Those who properly supplement have D2 levels above 50ng/ml. It has been shown that each 10ng/ml decrement in D2 level doubles the odds of a poor 90-day post stroke functional outcome[318,319].

Ischemia-reperfusion injury occurs with the sudden return of blood containing nutrients and oxygen to the region(s) of the brain deprived of blood during a stroke. This sudden return of blood to the brain causes mitochondria to generate reactive oxygen species (ROS) that result in mitochondrial dysfunction and damage[320]. Also following a stroke reactive nitrogen species (RNS), enzymatically produced by inducible nitric oxide synthase, causes stress on the neurons and long-term neurological damage[321]. Both vitamin D and PQQ inhibit the production and activity of nitric oxide synthase thereby inhibiting the production of RNS in humans[263,265]. Unlike the observed beneficial effects of acute PQQ administration both before and after a stroke, vitamin D3 administered acutely after a stroke didn't reduce functional impairment[322]. This may be due to slow multi-day biosynthesis of vitamin D from D3.

Recommendations for Vitamin D3 Supplementation

A combination of increased aluminum accumulation, air pollution, and usage of UVB sunscreen and sunblock have made most of the U.S. population deficient in active vitamin D[302]. Elderly people living in developed countries at high latitudes, institutionalized elderly, and geriatric patients have also been found to be deficient in vitamin D[323]. Also children in general are spending more time indoors. So vitamin D3 supplementation is recommended for everyone.

Infants should take a daily supplement of 400 IU of vitamin D3[313,324]. Children and adolescents should get a total of at least 800 IU per day of vitamin D3. This vitamin D3 should come from their diet, exposure to sunlight when possible, and an added 600 IU per day of supplementation. Healthy levels of active vitamin D can be maintained prior to age 71 by taking a daily 600 IU vitamin D3 supplement as suggested in 2010 by the Food and Nutrition Board of the Institute of Medicine[317]. I recommend 2,000 IU of supplemental D3 be taken daily by those 71 and over, in light of the fact that aluminum absorption by the brain increases in your seventies. The recent scientific literature presented in this section recommends that mothers should take 4,000 IU/day while pregnant and 6,000 IU/day of vitamin D3 while breastfeeding. With these high levels of vitamin D3 supplementation a calcium supplement is also recommended to improve bone health and decrease aluminum absorption.

Vitamin D2 supplementation is not recommended[325]. Vitamin D2 taken orally as a supplement is not as effective as vitamin D3 at raising serum levels of vitamin D2. This may be due to vitamin D2 having a different range of metabolites than vitamin D3 when taken orally. Also vitamin D2 has a shorter shelf-life than vitamin D3.

Vitamin D3 Toxicity

Vitamin D3 has extremely low toxicity[326]. In 2010 the Institute of Medicine's Food and Nutrition Board set the following upper daily limits for vitamin D3 supplementation for adults and children without the safety of doctor supervised periodic blood tests for vitamin D2[326].

- Children ages 1 through 3: 2,500 IU
- Children ages 2 through 8: 3,000 IU
- Adults and Children ages 9 through 18: 4,000 IU

Adults and children over 1 year of age should also be exposed to sunlight for short periods of time without sunscreen protection. For instance 20 minutes of exposure to full body midday summer sun for light-skinned adults results in 10,000 IU of vitamin D3[326]. For a child this same amount of exposure to sun will result in approximately 5,000 IU of vitamin D3[326]. The rate of vitamin D3 production depends on skin coloration – darker skin produces vitamin D3 slower[326].

Active vitamin D causes both enhanced absorption of calcium and aluminum in the gut[654]. This is a competitive process dependent upon the relative concentration ratio of aluminum to calcium. Therefore maintaining sufficient calcium in your diet will lower aluminum absorption[310]. However, too much active vitamin D and calcium will result in too much calcium in the blood (a.k.a. hypercalcemia – see Appendix II). This can promote calcification of the arteries and heart valves and lead to stroke[327]. Therefore, as with everything in life - moderation is the best policy. As you get older do not take supplements greater than 2000IU of vitamin D3 continuously and supplement your calcium intake with 500mg per day of calcium as calcium citrate. Also drinking water with more than 80mg/L of calcium is recommended.

Dietary Sources of Vitamin D

Vitamin D is naturally present in some common foods. The highest levels are found in oily fish. The following table lists the common dietary sources naturally containing vitamin D:

Dietary Sources of Vitamin D	
Food and Serving Size	**IU of Vitamin D per Serving**
Cod Liver Oil (1 Tbsp.)	1,360
Salmon – cooked (3.5 oz.)	360
Mackerel – cooked (3.5 oz.)	345
Sardines – canned in oil & drained (1.75 oz.)	250
Tuna Fish – canned in oil & drained (1.75 oz.)	200
Egg (1 – vitamin D is found in the yolk)	20
Beef Liver – cooked (3.5oz.)	15
Swiss Cheese (1 oz.)	12

Source: National Institutes of Health Office of Dietary Supplements

Vitamin D Increases Glutathione

Glutathione and PQQ protect the brain from oxidative damage after a stroke. Supplemental glutathione is not recommended, as it is not well absorbed by the body. But vitamin D taken prior to a stroke has been found to significantly increase glutathione in the brain[296]. Ischemia-reperfusion injury after a stroke results from the generation of free-radicals in the brain that react to produce the oxidants ROS and RNS. Antioxidants, such as $PQQH_2$ and glutathione, are free-radical scavengers that prevent ROS and RNS production. NADH made in the Krebs cycle (a.k.a. TCA cycle) reduces glutathione. Reduced glutathione in turn reduces PQQ to $PQQH_2$ at the pH of the brain[265]. Glutathione is found in concentrations more than 300 times greater than PQQ in the human brain[328,329]. Therefore NADH and glutathione keep PQQ in the reduced form in the brain. That allows $PQQH_2$ to act as a free-radical scavenger protecting the brain from ROS and RNS after a stroke[330,331].

Taurine Improves and Protects the Ageing Brain

Taurine is an amino acid that is biosynthesized from methionine, homocysteine, and cysteine in the brain, liver, and kidney and is also sourced from our diet in foods such as meat and seafood. Taurine has a sulfonic acid and lacks a carboxylic acid making it unusable as a protein building block. Taurine crosses the blood-brain barrier with the help of a specific amino acid transporter[332]. Taurine is 3-4 times more abundant in the developing brain as compared with the mature brain[333] and its concentration in the brain decreases with ageing[334].

Taurine supplementation does the following things for an ageing brain:
- Reverses brain ageing by increasing hippocampal neurogenesis
- Lowers the risk of a stroke and prevents stroke damage
- Ameliorates metal toxicity

Taurine Reverses Brain Ageing by Increasing Hippocampal Neurogenesis

The creation of new neurons from stem cells (a.k.a. neurogenesis) persists during adulthood in the dentate gyrus region of the hippocampus of our brains. These new neurons allow the brain to rewire broken synaptic connections and make new synaptic connections allowing the brain to maintain old memories and create new memories in a dynamic process called plasticity. Neurogenesis declines with age leading to age-related cognitive impairment. Taurine increases stem cell proliferation and increases the survival of new neurons, resulting in an increase in adult neurogenesis. Taurine supplementation reverses brain ageing by increasing hippocampal neurogenesis and ameliorating age-related cognitive impairment[335].

Taurine Lowers the Risk of Stroke and Prevents Stroke Damage

It has been shown experimentally and epidemiologically that taurine consumption in food and/or supplementation can lower blood pressure and the risk of stroke in humans and other animals[336]. Also taurine prevents three harmful mechanisms involved in killing neurons during and immediately after an ischemic stroke[337,338]:

- **Glutamate excitotoxicity** is prevented by taurine activating inhibitory receptors on neurons that decrease calcium diffusion into the neurons and prevent neuronal death[176,177].
- **Calcium imbalance** is corrected when taurine decreases calcium levels in sensitive portions of the neuron by increasing calcium levels in the neuron's mitochondria thereby preventing neuronal death[339].
- **Oxidative stress** is reduced in the brain by taurine. When taurine is present both before and during a stroke it reduces reactive oxygen species generated by the mitochondria as a result of oxygenated blood returning to those portions of the brain starved for oxygen and nutrients by the stroke[340].

Taurine Ameliorates Metal Toxicity

Without complexing with metals taurine ameliorates the toxic effects of aluminum and other metals in the body[341-344]. Taurine's mechanism of action is a mystery – See "Mystery of How Taurine Protects Against Metal Toxicity" on the next page.

Taurine Supplementation

Taurine supplementation is recommended in order to promote new brain cell formation and provide brain cell protection both before and after a stroke. Supplementation is particularity important as we age due to taurine levels declining with age. Also low levels of taurine have been observed in Parkinson's disease patients (see Appendix I). Long term supplementation of taurine at a dose of 500mg/day in "energy" drinks or pill form is considered safe. This level of supplementation can be compared to 400mg/day as the highest estimated dietary intake from natural sources[345]. Optionally a blood check can be performed prior to supplementation to verify a need for supplementation. The normal range of whole-blood taurine levels is 164-318 micromoles/L[346]. Taurine is stored in blood cells and therefore your whole-blood and not plasma taurine level should be measured[346].

Dietary sources of taurine are limited to cheese, meats, seafood, eggs, and milk[347]:

Dietary Sources of Taurine[348]	
Food	Grams Taurine per 100 grams food
Oysters	1.19
Scallop	0.93
Cheese	0.85
Eggs (2 medium)	0.70
Chicken Liver	0.68
Mackerel	0.65
Pork	0.46
Salmon	0.44
Lamb	0.37
Whole Milk and Yogurt	0.17
Chicken	0.16
Beef	0.02

Mystery of How Taurine Protects Against Metal Toxicity

Taurine combined with a metal chelator (e.g. monoisoamyl DMSA) improves the protection of rats from arsenic induced oxidative injury[341]. In addition combined administration of taurine and a chelator (e.g. mseo-2,3-dimercaptosuccinic acid) improves the treatment of chronic lead intoxication of rats[342]. Taurine lowers the concentration of lead ions in the blood, brain, and liver to levels below those achieved by using just the metal chelator[342]. In addition, taurine has prophylactic and therapeutic effects against aluminum induced acute liver toxicity[349].

Taurine does not complex with metal ions. So the mystery lies in the mechanism whereby taurine causes these beneficial effects. Are taurine's beneficial effects another example of its ability to lower oxidative stress caused by these metals? If so, what effect does taurine have on protecting the brain from aluminum damage? For instance does taurine protect enzymes in the brain from aluminum toxicity?

Vitamin K2-MK-4 for Preventing Stroke and Possibly Reversing aFib

There are a number of types of atrial fibrillation (a.k.a. aFib):

- **Paroxysmal aFib** – faulty internal electrical stimulation of the heart causes sudden rapid heart rate that usually slows to normal within 24 hours to one week.
- **Persistent aFib** – abnormal heart rate continues for more than a week and may stop spontaneously or with treatment.
- **Permanent aFib** – normal heart rate can't be restored with treatment. Over time both paroxysmal and persistent aFib can become permanent.

One type of permanent aFib is caused by aortic mitral valve annulus calcification (MAC). The Boston Area Anticoagulation Trial of warfarin and a placebo revealed that the sole statistically significant clinical characteristic of the stroke group of patients versus those who remained free of stroke was the presence of MAC as determined by echocardiography[256]. MAC results in the mitral valve closing only partially and the orifice narrowing (stenosis) leading to a pocket of slow blood flow (stasis) in the aorta. This local slowing of blood flow in turn causes an increased incidence of arterial clot formation resulting in stroke. The prevalence of MAC increases with age as described in the Cardiovascular Health Study (CHS) of 3,929 elderly individuals who had a 46% prevalence of MAC and a mean age of 76[350]. Those over 85 years old in the CHS had a 60% prevalence of MAC.

Causes of MAC include a high plasma homocysteine level as shown by a study of 76 patients with a mean age of 66. They underwent cardiac surgery at the Cleveland Clinic Foundation. An echocardiography was used to screen for MAC. A high correlation was found between the degree of MAC and plasma homocysteine concentration. Those without MAC had plasma homocysteine levels of 8.5-12.9µM/L (avg. 10.4µM/L) versus levels of 12.7-17.8µM/L (avg. 16.6µM/L) for those with MAC[351]. The homocysteine level in blood can be elevated with aluminum accumulation, moderate alcohol consumption, genetic traits, smoking, too much caffeine, too much animal protein, and vitamin B deficiency (see Chapter 2 for details).

Causes of MAC also include a low level of vitamin K2-MK-4 (a.k.a. menaquinone and menatetranone) as shown by a study of 387 patients with a mean age of 56.8 who were on hemodialysis for greater than one year. A three year observational study was carried out on this population to study the correlation between aortic calcification and vitamin K deficiency[352]. A correlation was found between MAC and vitamin K2-MK-4 deficiency and no correlation was found between MAC and vitamin K1 (a.k.a. phylloquinone) or vitamin K2-MK-7 deficiency. The ten year Rotterdam Study of 4,807 subjects with no history of myocardial infarction also found that lower than normal levels of vitamin K2-MK-4 intake was related to an increased incidence of MAC and coronary artery calcification, while vitamin K1 intake was unrelated to MAC[353].

Vitamin K Supplementation Reverses Arterial and Aortic Calcification

It has recently been shown in humans and rats that arterial and aortic calcification can be reversed by vitamin K supplementation[354,355]. In humans the arterial wall produces a protein (e.g. MGP) that, when activated, complexes with calcium preventing arterial and aortic calcification. Usually MGP is 30% inactive. This percentage of inactivity rises as we age and can be lowered with vitamin K2-MK-4 and K2-MK-7 supplementation that may reverse MAC and decrease the risk of vascular dementia. Therefore it can be considered preventative to take a vitamin K2 supplement as we age[356]. Since the primary source of vitamin K2 in our diets is meats and cheeses[353], vegetarians and vegans should consider supplementation. Vascular calcification is also associated with chronic kidney disease and vitamin K2 supplementation is recommended as a preventative[357].

Vitamin K2-MK-4 only lasts in the serum for 8 hours while vitamin K2-MK-7 last three times longer. When vitamin K2-MK-7 was compared with other K2 vitamins, it has been shown to have the most beneficial effects on cardiovascular disease[358]. Large doses of these vitamins taken over a several year period by thousands of people have not been found to lead to an increased risk of thrombosis and are considered safe[358]. There is one exception to this and that is those people taking oral anticoagulants, like warfarin (a.k.a. Coumadin), that are vitamin K antagonists. Therefore it is recommended that these people do not take vitamin K2 supplements.

Maxx Labs currently makes a combination K2-MK-4 (500mcg) and K2-MK-7 (100mcg) supplement.

Vitamin K2-MK-4 Prevents Osteoporosis

What is the impact of long-term vitamin K2-MK-4 supplementation on bone health? High serum concentrations of undercarboxylated osteocalcin are known to decrease bone mineral density (BMD) and high serum concentrations of pentosidine have been identified as an increased risk factor for bone fracture in older adults. A group of 48 women 50-60 years of age was divided into two sub-groups. One sub-group took a 1.5 mg K2-MK-4 supplement daily for 12 months and the other sub-group took a placebo. After 12 months the BMD of the forearm was significantly lower in the control sub-group while the K2-MK-4 sub-group had no change. Also there was an observed decrease in both pentosidine and undercarboxylated osteocalcin serum concentration in the K2-MK-4 sub-group[359]. A pharmacological dose of 45mg/day of vitamin K2-MK-4 has been used in Japan for the treatment of osteoporosis[359]. Carlson currently distributes gel caps containing 5mg of K2-MK-4 (Menatetrenone). These gel caps are available from online vendors.

Vitamin K2-MK-4 Activates Proteins to Prevent MAC

Vitamin K is required for activating the carboxylation of Gla proteins (MGP) and Gla rich proteins (GRP) catalyzed by the enzyme gama-carboxylase. When either MGP or GRP proteins are carboxylated, they can complex with calcium in the blood which prevents arterial and aortic calcification and MAC[360-362]. The MK-4 species of vitamin K2 has the highest efficacy of all K vitamins for preventing MAC. This is possibly because it is the only K2 vitamin that is both water and fat soluble[358].

Vitamin B12 and B6 as a B100 Supplement to Keep Homocysteine Levels Low

Vitamin B12 is the largest and most structurally complex of all vitamins. Only bacteria and single-celled microorganisms have the enzymes necessary to produce vitamin B12. B12 has a key role in the functioning of the brain and nervous system as a catalyst for methylation. We have already discussed in Chapter 2 vitamin B12's vital role in methylating homocysteine. Robert Burns Woodward (Nobel Prize in Chemistry 1965) and his group at Harvard were the first to perform a total synthesis of Vitamin B12. They worked on the 100 step total-synthesis from the early 1960's until it was published in 1973. Like no other synthesis before or after, it marked a landmark in organic chemistry. In 1973 I attended Woodward's concluding talk on this synthesis and will never forget his detailed multicolored chalk diagrams brilliantly standing out on those blackboards. It was beautiful organic chemistry described by a great chemist.

Both Vitamin B12 and B6 are required to keep serum homocysteine levels low. High levels of homocysteine increase the risk of vascular dementia and AD. The level of B12 declines with age unless B12 supplements are taken daily. B12 deficiency (<0.24ng/L) occurs in 3% to 4% of the general population[214], 15% of the over 65 population[215] and 29% of dementia patients[216,217]. Levels of B12 have been shown to decrease in cerebral spinal fluid with advancing age[218].

The results of a vitamin B6 (pyridoxal-5-phosphate - P5P) deficiency are the same as B12 malabsorption - elevated levels of homocysteine and increased risk of vascular dementia and AD. A vitamin B6 deficiency in the venous blood and elevated homocysteine levels in the cerebrospinal fluid have both been correlated with chronic fatigue syndrome (CFS)[363].

Chronic malabsorption of vitamin B12 and/or B6 in the small intestine will result in low levels of these vitamins and high levels of homocysteine in the blood and neurological tissue. Also chronic malabsorption of vitamin B12 can result in a neurological syndrome commonly characterized by neuropathy and occasionally by cognitive disturbance. Vitamin B12 taken into the stomach as food must first be released with stomach acid and then must bind to intrinsic factor (IF) prior to absorption. IF is produced in the parietal cells of the stomach. Malabsorption of vitamin B12 occurs when there is insufficient IF being produced by the parietal cells[364].

Autoimmune diseases are an abnormal immune response of the body against substances and tissues normally present in the body. Pernicious anemia is an autoimmune disease that destroys parietal cells in the stomach thereby stopping IF production and preventing B12 absorption by the small intestine. It is theorized that something, perhaps a virus, triggers the immune system to make antibodies that attack not only the virus but also the parietal cells. Once engaged, the immune system continues to attack the parietal cells resulting in chronic malabsorption of B12.

Other diseases or conditions that result in chronic gastrointestinal malabsorption of B12 include:

- Surgery to remove the stomach or end of the small intestine.
- Stomach conditions such as atrophic gastritis that may affect the production of IF.
- Diseases such as Crohn's that affect the small intestine where vitamin B12 is absorbed.
- Drugs such as metformin that are commonly used in the treatment of diabetes may affect the absorption of B12. Other drugs that result in B12 malabsorption include colchicine, neomycin, and some anticonvulsants used to treat epilepsy.
- Because stomach acid is needed to release B12 bound to proteins in food, long term use of drugs that affect stomach acid production, such as H_2 antagonists or H_2 blockers (i.e. Zantac and Tagamet), or proton pump inhibitors (i.e. Nexium and Prilosec) can result in B12 malabsorption. Chronic use of proton pump inhibitors by people 75 years of age and older has been shown to result in a 44% higher risk of dementia[365] and also B12 malabsorption of both B12 bound to proteins and oral B12 supplements[366].

A supplemental daily time-release B-100 complex taken orally is recommended, if gastrointestinal absorption of vitamin B12 is not a problem. This will provide 100mg of vitamin B6, 100mcg of vitamin B12, and 400mcg of folic acid. Also included is 100mg of niacin, vitamin B1, and B2. If gastrointestinal malabsorption of vitamin B12 is diagnosed or suspected take a daily sublingual (i.e. under the tongue) B12, B6, folic acid, and biotin tablet (Wonder Laboratories), the methyl form of B12, B12 nasal spray, or B12 injections. Also take 15mg of chelated zinc every day in order to help vitamin B6 lower levels of homocysteine.

There are three forms of vitamin B12 (a.k.a. cobalamin) available as supplements: cyano, hydroxy, and methyl. The **cyano form** is the least expensive and is converted in the body with the help of glutathione to the two active forms of vitamin B12: methyl and adenosyl[367]. For these reasons the cyano form is usually recommended. The **hydroxyl form** of vitamin B12 (a.k.a. hydroxycobalamin) is converted in the body to the two active forms without using glutathione[368]. The **methyl form** of vitamin B12 (a.k.a. methylcobalamin) taken orally is more bioavailable than cyanocabalamin, since it does not require either intrinsic factor for absorption[369] or glutathione for activation, but it is more expensive as a supplement[367].

5-MTHF Supplement as Insurance to Keep Homocysteine Levels Low

Levels of folic acid have been shown to decrease in cerebral spinal fluid with advancing age[218]. In order for folic acid to be used as a methylation agent it must first be converted to 5-MTHF (a.k.a. methyl folate, levomefolic acid, 5-methyltetrahydrofolate) in the folate cycle (see Figure 3). Approximately 48% of the North American population have MTHFR genotypes that increase the risk of an enzymatic deficiency preventing the conversion of folic acid to 5-MTHF[213]. It is possible to test for the MTHFR mutation, but taking 5-MTHF is not expensive and can be viewed as low cost insurance in case you have the mutation.

In order to circumvent both the decline of folic acid with old age and this enzymatic deficiency, taking 5-MTHF as a supplement (400mcg/day), in addition to the folic acid (400mcg/day) in the B-100 supplement, is recommended[219,220].

There can be side-effects of folic acid and 5-MTHF supplementation. These side-effects can include abdominal cramps, diarrhea, rash, sleep disorders, irritability, confusion, nausea, stomach upset, behavior changes, skin reactions, seizures, gas, excitability, and a tendency toward anxiety. This list of side-effects underscores why I recommend testing for high levels of homocysteine before taking a 5-MTHF supplement.

DHA in a Healthy Diet for Memory Improvement

DHA (a.k.a. docosahexaenoic acid) is an omega-3 fatty acid and a structural component of the human brain. DHA is the most abundant omega-3 fatty acid in the brain accounting for 40% of the brain's polyunsaturated fatty acids[370]. Fifty percent of the weight of a neuron's cell membrane is DHA[370]. DHA modulates the transport of choline, glycine and taurine in the brain[371].

Due to its prevalence in the brain it is not surprising that a DHA deficiency is associated with cognitive decline in healthy adults. In 2010 485 people 55 and older with age-related memory impairment found that DHA supplementation (900mg/day) for six months improved memory and learning ability[372]. A study with 37 Alzheimer's and 17 control subjects showed only a weak statistical correlation with AD being associated with deficits of brain DHA levels. The region of the brain where the DHA deficit was most statistically significant was the cerebellum, a region of the brain regarded as less vulnerable to Alzheimer's pathology[373]. Currently there is no evidence that low levels of DHA can cause AD.

DHA supplementation has been shown to improve memory and slow AD progression in mice genetically modified to model AD symptoms. Also there is an observed correlation between the decreased biosynthesis of DHA and cognitive impairment in AD[373]. However results published in 2010 involving elderly human patients with AD show that DHA supplementation does not slow their rate of declining mental function. This test was conducted with 402 people with an average age of 76 who had mild to moderate AD. These people were divided into two groups: one group taking a DHA supplement (2gr/day) and the other group taking a placebo for 18 months. Although DHA supplementation appeared to increase brain levels of DHA, there was no change in mental function, dementia severity, activities of daily living, or behavior[374].

DHA is both found in our diet and biosynthesized in our bodies from α-linolenic acid, a shorter essential omega-3 fatty acid found in only in plants and not biosynthesized in our bodies. DHA is found at high concentrations in cold-water oceanic and fresh-water fishes. Therefore, assuming you are eating a balanced diet and have no age-related memory impairment, there is no need for

DHA supplementation. Otherwise DHA supplementation of one gram per day might help improve your memory. DHA is usually found with EPA (a.k.a. eicosapentaenoic acid) in fish and fish oils. EPA, like α-linolenic acid, is a precursor of DHA[373].

Dietary Sources of DHA[375]	
Dietary Source	**% DHA + EPA**
Salmon	2.1%
Herring	2.0%
Anchovies	1.5%
Sardine	1.0%
Trout	0.9%
Sea Bass	0.8%
Shark	0.8%
Swordfish	0.8%
Mussels	0.8%
Carp	0.5%
Flounder	0.5%
Halibut	0.5%
Lobster	0.5%
Pollack	0.5%
Sole	0.5%
Crab	0.4%
Oyster	0.4%
Clam	0.3%
Perch	0.3%
Shrimp	0.3%
Snapper	0.3%
Tuna	0.3%
Haddock	0.2%

Dietary Sources of α-Linolenic Acid[375-377]	
Dietary Source	**% α-Linolenic Acid**
Kiwifruit seeds	62%
Flax (a.k.a. linseed)	55%
Lingonberry (a.k.a. cowberry)	49%
Hemp (a.k.a. cannabis)	20%
Walnut (a.k.a. English walnut, Persian walnut)	11.4%
Rapeseed (a.k.a. canola)	10%
Butternuts	8.7%
Soybean (a.k.a. Soya)	8%
Beechnuts	1.7%
Filberts	1%
Pecans	0.7%
Wheat Germ	0.7%
Radish Microgreens	0.7%
Tofu	0.6%
Pine Nuts	0.5%
Macadamias	0.3%
Almonds	0.2%

Try the following recipe in order to taste an example of delicious brain-food. Based upon the information in the previous two tables a single 4 ounce portion of this salmon dish contains 1.6 grams of α-linolenic acid and 2.4 grams of DHA/EPA. This recipe proves that a good diet is tastier than taking supplements.

Pecan Encrusted Salmon

- 32 ounces of salmon (32 oz. containing 19 grams DHA/EPA)
- 2 cups of pecans (7.2 oz. containing 1.4 grams α-linolenic acid)
- 1 tbsp. minced garlic
- ½ tsp. salt
- 1/8 tsp. cayenne
- ½ cup canola oil (4 oz. containing 11.3 grams of α-linolenic acid)

Cut the salmon into eight equal 4 ounce portions. Chop the pecans to a coarse meal. Add together and mix the ground pecans, minced garlic, salt, and cayenne. Dip the salmon fillets in canola oil. Then roll the salmon in pecan crumble mixture covering both sides. Heat a large non-aluminum fry pan and lightly sauté the salmon only on one side. Flip the salmon sautéed side up onto a non-aluminum sheet pan. Bake the fish at 450°F in an oven for approximately 10 minutes or until done to taste.

Conclusion of Preventing and Possibly Reversing Dementia with 7 Supplements

As a species we evolved to fill the niche of persistence hunting during the heat of midday when our prey was most vulnerable to heat exhaustion[210]. We are unlike our ancestors in that we do not routinely aerobically and anaerobically exercise for hours each day in the midday sun. Thus we have less taurine, less glutathione for PQQ reduction, and less vitamin D. Also we did not evolve to live any older than the age required for reproduction and child rearing. Longer life results in the levels of some of our enzymes such as MS, cofactors such as B12/folic acid, and coenzymes such as CoQ10, declining past age 50. Because of these biochemical and cultural changes, and in order to prevent Alzheimer's, autism, and stroke, seven daily supplements are recommended.

Seven Supplements:

- **PQQ:** Protect your brain during and after a stroke, increase the energy available in your brain, and enhance your memory and keep your brain young with more neurites by taking a PQQ supplement (20mg/day).

- **CoQ10:** Protect your brain during and after a stroke and increase its energy efficiency by taking a CoQ10 supplement (ubiquinone 200mg/day).

- **Vitamin D3:** Lower your aluminum absorption and risk of Alzheimer's, autism, and stroke with a vitamin D3 supplement. Prior to age 71 take a daily 600 IU of supplemental vitamin D3 and at age 71 start taking a daily 2,000 IU's of supplemental D3. Mothers should take daily 4,000 IU while pregnant and 6,000 IU each day of vitamin D3 while breastfeeding. Also infants should get 400 IU per day. Children and adolescents should get a total of at least 800 IU per day of vitamin D3. This 800 IU vitamin D3 should come from a combination of diet, exposure to sunlight, and an added 600 IU per day of supplementation.

- **Taurine:** Protect your brain during and after a stroke and lower the risk of stroke with a taurine supplement (500mg/day)

- **Vitamin K2-MK-4:** Prevent and possibly reverse aortic mitral valve calcification. Take a daily supplement of vitamin K2-MK-4 (500mcg/day) and K2-MK-7 (100mcg/day). For osteoporosis take K2-MK-4 (5mg/day). Do not take these supplements if you are taking oral anticoagulants, like warfarin (a.k.a. Coumadin), that are vitamin K antagonists.

- **B100 Supplement:** Keep your homocysteine levels low - take 100mg/day of vitamin B6, 100mcg/day of vitamin B12, and 400mcg of folic acid. These are all found in a time-release B100 complex. In the case of vitamin B12 malabsorption, use sublingual absorption tablets containing B12, B6, folic acid and biotin from Wonder Laboratory or get B12 injections from a doctor.

- **5-MTHF (Methyl Folate):** Keep your homocysteine levels low even if you have the MTHFR gene that prevents your body from converting folic acid to methyl folate. Take 400mcg of 5-MTHF per day.

Biosynthesis of Taurine and Glutathione

Both taurine and glutathione, two primary neuroprotectors, are biosynthesized from cysteine as shown in Figure 3. Cysteine is toxic to neurons and its concentration in the brain is kept low by the enzyme CDO that oxidizes cysteine to cysteine sulfinic acid. CDO is found in astroglial cells (astrocytes) in the brain and is activated by cysteine, keeping cysteine levels low in the brain[378]. Cysteine sulfinic acid is converted to hypotaurine by the enzyme CSD that is also found in astroglial cells. Both hypotaurine and taurine can cross the blood-brain barrier and hypotaurine acts as an antioxidant as it is oxidized to taurine in the brain by either oxygen or reactive oxygen species (ROS). Glutathione is biosynthesized in the astroglial cells by combining cysteine with both glutamate and glycine[378].

Cysteine is biosynthesized by transsulfuration from homocysteine catalyzed by the enzyme CBS as shown in Figure 3. CBS is not activated by homocysteine, and thus high homocysteine levels can occur. Instead CBS is activated either by SAM (see Figure 3), a methionine derivative, or low oxygen levels[379]. When there is sufficient oxygen in the blood, resulting in normal redox levels in the brain, and sufficient folic acid, B12, and B6, homocysteine is methylated to methionine by the enzyme MS (see Figure 3). This results in the equilibrium of high levels of methionine with low levels of homocysteine. But under conditions of low oxygen, such as a stroke or anaerobic exercise, CBS is activated to convert homocysteine to cysteine resulting in a biosynthetic cascade of methionine conversion to homocysteine that is in turn converted to cysteine and then taurine and glutathione as shown in Figure 3 [379,380]. This biosynthetic cascade results in a 3 fold increase in taurine levels during a stroke[381].

The biosynthesis of taurine and glutathione is an example of how evolution has shaped our biochemistry to keep our brains self-medicated under adverse conditions such as a stroke or anaerobic exercise. Whenever low oxygen levels are sensed these two neuroprotective chemicals are synthesized in larger than normal amounts and used by the brain to protect its normal functioning. As we will see later in this book the brain also needs both aerobic exercise to cleanse the brain and increase neurite connections and sleep to also cleanse the brain of Aβ peptides.

Chapter 4 - Controlling Aluminum Ingestion

"The positive relationship between aluminum in drinking-water and Alzheimer's disease ... cannot be totally dismissed." World Health Organization 1998 and 2003

"...the MWRA does not routinely analyze for aluminum as it is not on our list of toxic metals." F. Laskey – Executive Director Massachusetts Water Resources Authority - 2013

Aluminum as an ionic salt is a neurotoxin that is a causative factor in Alzheimer's, autism, and stroke. Aluminum is also the third most common element in the earth's crust and it is one of the most remarkable elements in the periodic table. Things made from aluminum metal are strong, light-weight, durable, and electrically conductive. Aluminum's melting point is low enough that it can be readily recycled. As a consequence of its availability and unique properties, aluminum, as an ionic salt and a metal, is found in a variety of things that add to our body's accumulation (i.e. body-burden) of aluminum as estimated in the following table:

Estimates of Daily Intake of Aluminum in Humans		
Major Sources of Aluminum	**Daily Aluminum Intake (mg/day)**	**Amount Delivered Daily into Systemic Circulation (mcg/day)**
Natural Food[130]	0.7 – 11.5	1.4 – 23 [A]
Pharmaceuticals[382]	126 - 5000	315 – 12,500 [A]
Vaccines[383]	0.25 – 0.75 [E]	250 – 750 [C]
Formula (U.K. Data)[384,385]	0.06-0.7	0.015-1.75 [A]
Antiperspirants[386]	0.32	0.4 [B]
Aluminum Cookware[387]	0 - 500	0 – 1,250 [A]
Drinking Water[68]	0.03 – 0.600 [D]	0.09 – 1.8 [A]
Beverages – Tea[388-390]	0.75 [F]	1.9 [A]

A) Average absorption 0.2%[131]; B) Single use per day with average absorption 0.012%[391]; C) Absorption 100%[391] but the rate of absorption is unknown; D) Average drinking water absorption 0.3%[391] and intake 3liters/day with aluminum concentration of 10 to 200mcg/liter; E) 1 to 3 vaccines per day; F) Equivalent to 3 cups of green or black tea per day.

The percentages of aluminum ion absorbed into systemic circulation (i.e. bioavailable aluminum) are averages. Among individuals there is at least a 3 fold variation in these percentages of aluminum bioavailablity[51]. The data in the table shows that chronic use of aluminum containing pharmaceuticals and aluminum cookware can be the largest sources of bioavailable aluminum. The largest acute source of bioavailable aluminum is from the adjuvant in vaccines.

Aluminum in Food

Analysis of 451 foodstuffs revealed that aluminum content of unprocessed plant derived foods is significant and that processed foods contained even more aluminum than unprocessed foods. Most unprocessed foods, with the exception of certain herbs, tea leaves, and coco, contain low (less than 2mg/lb.) levels of aluminum. Because of aluminum's neurotoxicity this amount should be minimized as much as possible. This table is a result of 1,431 food samples analysed for aluminum[392].

Aluminum Content of Food[392]	
Food Product	**Mean Aluminum Concentration**
Flour	2 mg/lb
Baking Premixes	3 mg/lb
Bread and Pastry	1 mg/lb
Herb Tea	250 mg/lb (1-6% eluted into hot water)
Green and Black Tea[388-390]	272 mg/lb (25% eluted into hot water)
Coffee	7 mg/lb (3% eluted into hot water)
Cheese[131]	450-900 mg/lb
Confectioneries (i.e. candy)	25 mg/lb
Chocolate and Coco Powder	83 mg/lb
Beer (no difference between bottles and cans)	0.5 mg/qt
Wine and Fruit Juice	2 mg/qt
Mineral Water	<0.2 mg/qt
Human Breastmilk[393]	15-30 mcg/qt
Food sold in Aluminum Packaging	1 mg/lb

The data in this table came from data on aluminum ingestion published by the U.S. Food and Drug Administration's Center for Food Safety and Applied Nutrition. The aluminum content of the core foods of the FDA Total Diet Study were determined by analyses, recipe calculation, and literature values. Estimates of aluminum intake ranged from 0.7mg/day for 6 to11 month infants, 11.5mg/day for 14 to 16 year old males, and 7 to 9mg/day for adult men and women[130].

High levels of aluminum in some foods is due to plants growing in high aluminum soils, including soybeans, tea, and cocoa trees producing cocoa beans used to make chocolate. So aluminum ingestion can be reduced by avoiding these foods.

SALPs and Alumsb as Major Sources of Aluminum in Food

Acidic SALPs (a.k.a. sodium aluminum phosphates) and alums (a.k.a. aluminum sulfates) are FDA-approved food additives generally recognized as safe. SALPs and alums contribute the greatest amount of aluminum to our diet. In his book "Practical Dietetics" written in 1897 N.Y. University Professor of Clinical Medicine, W. Gilman Thompson, M.D. stated: "Baking powder ... should be free from alum ...". His words of wisdom have been ignored as today aluminum due to acidic SALP and alum can be been found in many popular food products including: waffle and pancake mixes and ready-to-eat waffles and pancakes. For example a daily diet of pancakes, waffles, muffins, and biscuits made with SALP or alum increases the risk of AD by 8.6 fold[65].

Friends were cleaning out their kitchen cabinets and came upon a can of leavening agent "for better baking". The ingredients were phosphoric acid salts and the recipes on the can called for mixing the leavening agent with baking soda (a.k.a. sodium bicarbonate) as an alternative for baking powder. Acidic SALP (a.k.a. food additive E541) and alum are the most common acidic salts used in baking. Upon heating, acidic SALP or alum reacts with baking soda to form carbon dioxide gas. It has been found that 0.1% of the aluminum in a biscuit leavened with acidic SALP or alum and baking soda is absorbed by the body after ingestion[394]. I recommended in the future my friends avoid aluminum ingestion by making baking powder with cream of tartar as the acid (see page 146 of this book for a baking powder recipe).

Basic SALP (a.k.a. basic sodium aluminum phosphate) is one of many emulsifying agents used to process cheese and cheese spread. The basic SALP reacts with and changes the protein in the cheese producing a film around fat droplets preventing them from separating from the cheese. This results in a low melting cheese with a soft texture and easy slicing properties. Up to 3% basic SALP is permitted by the FDA in pasteurized process cheeses, cheese foods, and cheese spreads. If cheese contains 1.5% to 3% basic SALP, the percentage of aluminum orally absorbed from ingestion of 1 gram of cheese is 0.1% to 0.3%. The resulting maximum serum aluminum concentration occurs 8 to 9 hours after ingestion[131]. Cheeses containing SALP are currently not sold by certain grocery chains, such as Whole Foods.

Alum as a Source of Aluminum in Food

Growing up in Iowa I enjoyed going to my grandparents for holiday meals because I loved grandma's homemade bread and butter pickles. They had such a memorably crunchy texture that I decided to get the recipe. Needless to say I was shocked to see that one teaspoon of alum (a.k.a. aluminum sulfate) was used in each pint of pickles for crunchiness. This sparked my interest in finding if alum is still used in commercial pickles. I was again surprised to find that alum was listed as an ingredient on a bottle of commercially available gherkins that I had in the refrigerator. I threw out the bottle of pickles and vowed to always read labels in the future.

In order to lower the level of aluminum in foods we should stop the practice of using alums in our food and fertilizer. Alums are aluminum containing salts. When just "alum" is listed as an ingredient on food or fertilizer it is sodium or potassium aluminum sulfate. Otherwise it will be listed with the cation or cations specified, for example ammonium alum (a.k.a. ammonium aluminum sulfate).

Aluminum in Pharmaceuticals

Many pharmaceuticals contain aluminum compounds as both active and non-active ingredients for anticaking and compounding. For example, aluminum trisilicate is used in buffered aspirin. Aluminum is also present in certain antacids, pain-killers, and anti-diarrhea medicines. Styptic pencils contain alum (a.k.a. aluminum sulfate) as the active ingredient. Ammonium alum (a.k.a. ammonium aluminum sulfate) is used for treating canker sores. Some aluminum containing pharmaceutical additives (i.e. aluminum trisilicate, aluminum hydroxide) have very low solubility in neutral water solutions unlike some of the halide salts of aluminum (i.e. aluminum chloride). But acidification in the stomach results in even insoluble aluminum containing pharmaceutical additives being solubilized and made more bioavailable[391,395].

Colorants for Food, Drugs, and Cosmetics that Contain Aluminum

Although some food, pharmaceutical, and cosmetic color dyes and artificial food colors (AFCs) are aluminum free, some synthetic color dyes contain the aluminum salt of the colorant and in some cases colorants are combined with alumina (a.k.a. aluminum oxide). Manufacturers of foods, pharmaceuticals, and cosmetics (FD&C) containing colorants must list these inactive ingredients on product labels. Aluminum salts of colorants are listed as "Aluminum Lake". The name of the aluminum lake is defined in the U.S. Code of Federal Regulations as being made up of the name of the colorant followed by "Aluminum Lake"[396]. Aluminum Lakes have low water soluble but are used to color food because they tint by dispersion. These foods include: icings, candies, fats, gums, waxes, and oils[397,398]. Aluminum Lakes are also used to color fruit drinks prepared from a powder mix but not ready-to-drink beverages[398].

Usually the colorant is combined with an extender, particularly in pill coatings, that prevents the colorant from migrating out of the coating. If "FD&C" appears as a prefix on the listed colorant name, alumina is likely used as an extender. When "D&C" appears as a prefix on the listed name, the colorant can only be used for drugs and cosmetics and alumina is not used as an extender. However when the aluminum salt of a D&C colorant is used, the colorant is listed as an "Aluminum Lake"[396].

The total amount of AFC's added to food per person in the U.S. rose 5-fold from 1950 (12mg/person/day) to 2012 (62mg/person/day)[397]. This does not include AFC's added to drugs and cosmetics. Not all AFC's contain aluminum. AFC's that do contain aluminum are on average 10% aluminum with a range of 6 to 15%. The most common Aluminum Lakes by their U.S. FD&C name and their European (E) Number are: FD&C Blue No. 1 (E133), FD&C Blue No. 2 (E132), FD&C Yellow No. 5 (E102), Yellow No. 6 (E110, Banned in Norway), FD&C Red No. 3 (E127), FD&C Red No. 40 (E129, Banned in Switzerland), and FD&C Green No. 3 (E143, Banned in the E.U.).

Aluminum in Vaccines

Aluminum hydroxide, aluminum phosphate, and alum are used as adjuvants in human vaccines because they potentiate the response of our bodies to the vaccine. The mechanism for this potentiation is not fully understood. As early as 1995 R.K. Gupta pointed out that calcium phosphate, which has adjuvant properties similar to aluminum hydroxide, also has the advantage of being a natural component of the body[399]. The use of aluminum containing vaccines is most concerning for infants and young children whose brains are developing. For instance at birth and at 2 and 6 months of ages infants are vaccinated for hepatitis B with 250mcg of aluminum per dose. Between birth and 18 months of age children are dosed with 16 vaccines, many on the same day, totaling 3.45mg of aluminum[383]. When there is an alternative available, like calcium phosphate, there should be no reason to continue administration of neurotoxic aluminum containing vaccines to children or adults[399-401].

Aluminum hydroxide and aluminum phosphate were injected into rabbit's muscle tissue simulating a vaccination. In all cases aluminum was found in blood samples one hour after the intramuscular injection. Aluminum remains in the blood for 28 days after the injection and its level slowly declines. A portion of the injected aluminum was found in the rabbit's brains[402].

Aluminum in Infant Formula

Fifteen to twenty brands of infant formula in the U.K. and Canada were analyzed for aluminum and the results were published in 2010[384], 2011[403], and 2013[385]. Using the manufacture's guidelines of formula consumption the average daily ingestion of aluminum from infant formulas for a child of 6 months varied from 53 to 725mcg. The concentration in ready-made milk varied from 176 to 700mcg /liter. The 700mcg /liter milk was for preterm infants. This is 3 times higher than the World Health's Organization's (WHO's) maximum limit on aluminum in drinking water[83].

Generally the aluminum consumption was higher from powdered than ready-made formulas. Also two soy-based formulas have the highest levels of aluminum corresponding to an ingestion rate for a 6 month old child of 627 – 725mcg/day[385,404]. These high levels in soy-based formulas either reflect prior aluminum accumulation in the soybean plant or aluminum added during processing.

The papers published in 2010, 2011, and 2013 warning of high aluminum levels found in infant formula were not the first publications warning of high aluminum levels in infant formula. N.M. Hawkins, et al. reported in 1994 that infant formula was the cause of aluminum toxicity in infants[405].

Recent data on aluminum in baby formula made in the U.S. could not be found. But Nestles manufactures and sells both the Sma brand of formula in the U.K. and the Gerber brand of formula in the U.S. The Sma brand was tested and found to vary from 65-116mcg/day for Sma First Infant and 354-627mcg/day for Sma Wysoy Infant formula for birth to 6 months[406].

Absorption of Aluminum in Antiperspirants and Astringents

Alum, aluminum chloride, aluminum chlorohydrate, and aluminum-zirconium compounds are the most widely used active ingredients in antiperspirants. Application of aluminum chloride to the skin of mice resulted in aluminum accumulation in the hippocampal region of their brains[407]. Aluminum chlorohydrate applied to human underarms was shown to be absorbed at a rate of 4mcg aluminum per single-use[386]. A five year study of 130 matched pairs of humans showed antiperspirant use slightly increases the risk of AD and this risk increases with frequency of use[408].

Aluminum acetate is found in some astringent solutions for minor skin irritations. These solutions should be avoided because the aluminum acetate is as absorbable through the skin as aluminum chloride. Epsom salts that contain magnesium, instead of aluminum salts, are a safe substitute for minor skin irritations.

Aluminum in Beverages

Alum Fertilizer as a Source of Aluminum in Beverages

Alum (a.k.a. aluminum sulfate) used as a fertilizer increases root growth in tea plants and makes tea grow quicker. For this reason alum is used for tea fertilization. However this practice has enhanced the aluminum concentration in tea leaves. Aluminum in a 1.5 gram tea bag varies with the type of tea and is approximately 0.8-1.0mg. in both green and black tea[388]. Approximately 25% of this aluminum dissolves in hot water resulting in a cup of tea with an aluminum concentration of 700mcg/liter[389,390]. Less aluminum dissolves from herbal teas and coffee, with coffee also containing much less aluminum than teas.

Alum is popular as a soil-acidifier because it works quickly as opposed to pure sulfur containing soil-acidifiers. However, ammonium sulfate containing fertilizers work just as quickly as alum. Also ammonium sulfate fertilizers are recommended instead of alum because aluminum is toxic to some plants[409]. It is disturbing to see alum advertised as a fertilizer for plants that need acidic soils, such as blueberries. Ammonium sulfate is a much safer alternative. The amount of aluminum in alum fertilized blueberries has not been reported.

Aluminum Beverage Cans as a Source of Aluminum in Beverages

There are 180 billion aluminum beverage cans produced annually and beverages of various kinds are packed and sold all over the world in these cans[410]. These beverages include:

- Water
- Carbonated soda
- Carbonated beer
- Wine
- Tea
- Energy drinks
- Fruit juice and concentrate

These beverages can all cause aluminum corrosion. The rate of this corrosion is dependent upon the acidity of the beverage, the ions in the beverage, and the storage temperature of the canned beverage. In order to slow the rate of corrosion, manufacturers line the inside of aluminum cans with a thin layer of polymer or copolymer (a.k.a. epoxy, lacquer). The exact chemical composition of the liner is proprietary and varies depending upon the beverage[410].

In spite of can liners some of the beverage diffuses through the lining or imperfections in the lining. This results in corrosion with the conversion of aluminum metal to aluminum ions. The aluminum ions then migrate through the lining and into the beverage. The rate of aluminum ions being added to the beverage by corrosion has been shown to increase with the acidity of the beverage. When a beverage is carbonated, carbonic acid is formed. Fruit juices contain citric acid and teas contain tannic acid and are therefore naturally acidic. Additional acids are added to beverages as ingredients, preservatives, or for taste. These acids include:

- Amino acids (i.e. taurine)
- Salts of organic acids (i.e. sodium benzoate)
- Salts of inorganic acids (i.e. phosphoric acid)

One study found that after seven months of storage at room temperature in aluminum cans, beer's aluminum concentration had increased by 140mcg/liter and tea's aluminum concentration had increased by 600mcg/liter[411]. In a second study by a different group of researchers 273 samples of 7 different varieties of soft drinks in both aluminum cans and glass bottles were stored for one year at room temperature. The aluminum concentration in the beginning of the test was 39-55mcg/liter and after one year in aluminum cans it had increased to 188-848mcg/liter[412]. There was no significant change in beverages stored in glass bottles[412,413]. After seven months of storage at room temperature in dented aluminum cans, beer had increased its aluminum concentration by 9,600mcg/liter[411]. Since the World Health Organization (WHO) recommends a limit of 100mcg/liter of aluminum in drinking water, these stored beverages were too toxic to drink[68].

Juice boxes and juice and snack packs are lined with a metallized aluminum film. Metallized films are plastics containing a thin layer of aluminum metal. The migration rate of corroded metallized aluminum into juice and snacks needs to be studied.

Recommendations based upon these results are:

- When given a choice, purchase beverages in glass
- When purchasing a beverage in an aluminum can, drink it and do not store it
- Do not purchase beverages in dented aluminum cans
- Check the canned food you plan to purchase with a magnet – aluminum is nonmagnetic

Aluminum in Drinking Water

It is not surprising that aluminum is in drinking water as it comprises 8% of the earth's crust. Also 0.3% of the aluminum ingested in drinking water is absorbed[131]. The 1998 and 2003 documents published by WHO on aluminum in drinking-water concluded[83]:

> *"The positive relationship between aluminum in drinking-water and AD ... cannot be totally dismissed."*

In these documents WHO recommends a limit of 100mcg/liter of aluminum in drinking water, but in 2010 WHO allowed 200mcg/liter at small water treatment facilities[68].

WHO concluded that there is a positive correlation between high levels of aluminum in drinking water and the occurrence of dementia among those who had drank the water. This conclusion was based upon a number of epidemiological studies. In 1989 a high incidence of AD was reported in areas with a high level of aluminum in the drinking water in England and Wales[80]. In 1991 high levels of aluminum in drinking water were linked with high dementia mortality in an area of Norway[81]. In 1991 and 1996 a positive relationship between aluminum in drinking water and AD risk was identified in Canada[75,82]. In 2000 high levels of aluminum in drinking water were correlated with increased risk of dementia or cognitive decline in a 15-year study of 1,700 people in France[414].

In 1988 an accidental contamination of aluminum ions in drinking water occurred in the Camelford area of the UK. Over 20,000 people were exposed to high levels of aluminum. Hundreds of residents exposed to the aluminum exhibited various symptoms related to cerebral impairments, such as loss of both concentration and short term memory, as reported in a 10-year follow-up study. Incidence of these cerebral impairments was significantly higher in the group exposed to aluminum than in the unexposed population. A 58 year old woman living in the Camelford area in 1988 at the time of the contamination died 15 years later due to a rapidly progressive, fatal dementing illness. An autopsy showed AD-like neurodegeneration and very high levels of aluminum in affected brain regions[415].

The water in Quabbin Reservoir, located in central Massachusetts, is the drinking water source for most of the communities inside of the Route 95 inner beltway around Boston. Water taken directly from the Quabbin Reservoir contains of 10mcg/liter aluminum[416]. However Quabbin water delivered by the Massachusetts Water Resources Authority (MWRA) and town water pipes to a tap in Somerville, Massachusetts contained 18.6mcg/liter aluminum[416].

Melrose, Massachusetts tap water was filtered through a Brita pour-through pitcher system with a mixed activated carbon and ion exchange resin filter (filter #OB03). The Brita filter lowered aluminum from 17mcg/liter to zero mcg/liter[417]. This Brita filter reduces 100mcg/liter of labile neurotoxic aluminum in water to less than 2.5mcg/liter[417]. Since activated carbon has a small capacity for aluminum ions it can be assumed that the ion exchange resin is primarily responsible for aluminum removal by the Brita filter[418]. In spite of the filter's proven performance, Brita's product literature does not mention aluminum removal as a benefit of this filter. Brita, like the MWRA, may not have aluminum on their list of toxic metals. Some water filtration systems have been found to add aluminum to tap water[416].

Cement as a Source of Aluminum in Drinking Water

The added 8.6mcg/liter of aluminum found in Somerville tap water[416] equals over 14 pounds/day of aluminum being added to Metropolitan Boston's drinking water. That water is consumed at the rate of 200 million gallons/day. So who is adding this aluminum to the drinking water?

To answer this question I had to become a private detective, ask some questions, and make some observations. My first opportunity to ask questions came when the MWRA gave a tour of a partially built 20 million gallon buffer-reservoir for drinking water. This reservoir is being constructed on the side of a hill near my neighborhood. Mr. Frederick A. Laskey, Executive Director of the MWRA, gave the tour along with the chief engineer for the project. During the tour I told Mr. Laskey about the added aluminum reaching our taps and asked him if he knew where it was coming from. Mr. Laskey said

> "... the MWRA does not add aluminum to Quabbin water"

He admitted he did not know where the aluminum was coming from. I also asked Mr. Laskey why the aluminum concentration of our drinking water is not analyzed and reported annually as are other toxic trace metals. His response was

> "... the MWRA does not routinely analyze for aluminum as it is not on our list of toxic metals."

The first clue came while standing in the middle of the partially constructed 20 million gallon reservoir that looked like a concrete bathtub with 50 foot high sides. I asked the chief engineer if she knew how long the reservoir would last. She said it would only last 50 years because drinking water leaches minerals out of concrete thereby weakening the concrete.

The second clue came from an observation in my front yard. The town hired a contractor to replace the water pipe on my street and during the project I noticed a section of the old pipe had been dug up, thrown in my yard, and had been killing the grass. After inspecting this piece of pipe I was shocked to find that it had been killing more than my grass. It had been killing my neurons and those of my family and neighbors for a long time. The steel pipe was internally lined with two inches of mortar that had become highly porous and crumbled due to mineral leaching. That was the "straw that broke the camel's back". I purchased a Brita water filter with an OB03 filter and have used it regularly ever since.

After this initial detective work to find who added the aluminum, I found no one person was the culprit. Instead I found that Portland cement mixed with sand and water to form mortar is the predominant water pipe lining used for public water supply to homes in the U.S and homes around the world. Also Portland cement mixed with sand, gravel, and water to form concrete is the predominant lining of water storage basins. Leaching of aluminum ions from mortar lined pipes and concrete lined storage reservoirs used to supply drinking water is a common source of aluminum in drinking water. The aluminum content in Portland cement varies from 5% to 36% and one of the predominant crystalline phases in cement is celite (a.k.a. tricalcium aluminate), that leaches from mortar and concrete dissolving in water as follows[419]:

$$Ca_3Al_2O_6 + 6H_2O \rightarrow 3Ca^{2+} + 2Al^{3+} + 12OH \quad \text{Tricalcium Aluminate Dissolution Reaction}$$

The rate of aluminum (Al^{3+}) leaching from mortar into drinking water was studied by analyzing aluminum in desalinated and fluoridated water flowing through 7,200 feet of freshly mortar lined pipe. With an average water residence time in the pipe of 2.3 days, over the course of the first two months aluminum levels went from 5mcg/liter in the intake water to 690mcg/liter in the outflow water. Even after two years of using the pipe the outflow water had levels of aluminum greater than 100mcg/liter[420].

From my investigation I have concluded that aluminum leaching from the mortar lined pipes and concrete lined storage reservoirs used by the MWRA to transport and store water in the Boston area adds 8.6mcg/liter of aluminum to drinking water going from Quabbin to Somerville, MA. This represents 14.4 pounds of aluminum being added per day, since the MWRA supplies 200 million gallons of water per day to the Boston area. This also corresponds to tricalcium aluminate leaching rate of 72 pounds per day or 650 tons in 50 years. This accounts for MWRA's 50 year lifetime estimate for concrete structures exposed to drinking water.

Alum Pretreatment as a Source of Aluminum in Drinking Water

Aluminum sulfate (a.k.a. alum), with a water solubility of 320 grams/liter, is added by many public water departments as a drinking water pretreatment. By adjusting the water's pH from 6.5 to 8.5 the soluble aluminum sulfate is converted to insoluble aluminum hydroxide while impurities are coagulated and removed. However, if the precipitated aluminum hydroxide is not removed or if the water's pH is improperly adjusted, the insoluble coagulate may again dissolve increasing the level of aluminum in drinking water[421-423]. A survey of 380 U.S. community water supplies has shown that alum treated water contains residual aluminum in the range 3 to 1,600mcg/L with a mean of 179mcg/L[424].

Studies indicate that raw drinking waters generally have aluminum predominantly in particulate form (e.g. complexed with silicic acid as hydroxyaluminum silicates, HAS) that is non-bioavailable[425-428]. Whereas in the alum treated water the aluminum exists as soluble chemically labile neurotoxic forms (i.e. ionic aluminum), that are much more bioavailable[424,429].

Alum has been applied over the last 40 years to hundreds of nutrient rich lakes and storm water retention ponds in the U.S. to lower the phosphate level of the water and prevent harmful algae blooms. When added to water at a basic pH, alum complexes with the phosphate and precipitates lowering the phosphate level of the water. But as shown in a recent study the result of these alum treatments is not effective at lowering phosphate due to the lack of pH control. In addition these treatments have resulted in both high levels of dissolved aluminum and nitrous oxide in surface and subsurface waters[430]. Adding alum to our surface waters should be made illegal. It is contaminating our drinking water and harming microbial and invertebrate communities in these lakes that play a role in nutrient recycling and sediment transport.

Defluoridation as a Source of Aluminum in Drinking Water

Alum and activated alumina are both used for defluoridation of water high in fluoride in order to render the water potable. Drinking water resulting from both of these processes results in levels of residual aluminum that are higher than 200mcg/liter[431-433]. Therefore only use water filters that claim to remove fluoride by anion exchange as they will not add aluminum to the water.

Enhancement of Aluminum Corrosion by Fluoride

Aluminum metal in contact with drinking water at a pH near neutral forms a transparent layer of aluminum oxide on the metal's surface. This layer of aluminum oxide can slow down the dissolution of aluminum. The following factors may affect the stability of the aluminum oxide and thereby cause faster corrosion and dissolution of aluminum cookware adding aluminum ions to cooking water:

- The oxide is not stable in acidic (pH < 4) or alkaline (pH > 9) environments
- Aggressive ions, such as fluoride, may attack the oxide forming pits in the aluminum

Two events occurred in 1901 that have resulted in enhanced aluminum in our diet today:

1) At the 1901 Pan-American Exposition in Buffalo, New York, aluminum cookware was first introduced to housewives, who wisely viewed it with suspicion because of concerns about the quality of the cookware and the toxicity of aluminum. It would take about 50 years before aluminum pots and pans gained acceptance.

2) In 1901 a young dental school graduate named Frederick McKay left the East Coast to open a dental practice in Colorado Springs, Colorado. When he arrived, McKay was astounded to find scores of people with brown stains on their teeth. He also found that teeth afflicted with these stains were surprisingly and inexplicably resistant to decay. It took McKay 30 years to find that fluoride in the drinking water was responsible.

The CDC recommended in 2011 that drinking water be fluoridated to a level of 0.7 ppm instead of then current 1 ppm level introduced to help prevent tooth decay[434]. This lower 0.7 ppm level was recommended because in a 1999-2004 study it was found that 41% of those between 12 -15 years of age had fluorosis[435]. Fluorosis is streaking or spottiness of teeth due to too much fluoride. The percentage in this age group with mild to severe dental fluorosis had doubled since a 1986-1987 study[435].

Community fluoridation was shown to reduce the risk of dental caries by 27% in 5 studies of older adults (total of 2,530 participants) published after 1979[436]. But self-applied fluoride from either tooth paste or mouth rinse was shown to reduce the risk of dental caries by 25% in 4 studies of older adults published after 1979[436] and in studies of children and adolescents using toothpastes[437] and mouth rinses[438]. Since there is no proven significant difference in risk reduction of dental caries between community and self-applied fluoride, the wisdom of community fluoridation of drinking water should be questioned[439].

Toothpaste with an active ingredient usually contains 1,500ppm fluoride and is usually sold in aluminum lined tubes. The aluminum lining on some brands, including Colgate and Crest, have a layer of clear plastic separating the aluminum from the toothpaste to prevent corrosion.

In 1987, experiments showed that water used for cooking in aluminum cookware containing fluoride ion at 1ppm, resulted in water with an aluminum ion concentration of as much as 600 mg/liter (3,000 times WHO's drinking water limit). Neutral water without fluoride used in an identical manner did not add aluminum ions to the water[440]. Almost all stainless steels alloys contain no aluminum. Only stainless steel 405 contains 0.1 - 0.3% aluminum.

Other factors that speed up corrosion and dissolution of aluminum include acidic foods, such as tomato sauces and citrus juices[387]. Cooking temperature in aluminum cookware is also a factor as the higher the cooking temperature the faster the aluminum corrodes, particularly in the presence of fluoride ions and/or acidic foods[387]. For instance cooking meat for three people in aluminum foil at 350 °F increased its aluminum concentration to 500mg/person intake levels[387].

This is a quote from the USDA website in response to the question: "If aluminum foil pits, is food endangered?"

"No. Pinholes in foil or a blue liquid that may form on the food that has come in contact with the foil are not harmful. These reactions can occur when salt, vinegar, highly acidic or highly spicy foods come in contact with aluminum foil. The product is a harmless aluminum salt and presents no safety problem if consumed." USDA website under meat and poultry packing materials 2015

This quote is disturbing in that the USDA is the food product watchdog for the U.S. Based upon the information in Chapter 1 of this book we now know that aluminum salts dissolve in water to form neurotoxic aluminum ions that are absorbed and accumulated by our brains. Also from Chapter 1 and 2 we know that aluminum ingestion causes Alzheimer's and stroke.

The problem of aluminum corrosion during cooking is underscored by this recipe for soup.

Beef and Aluminum Soup

Place an aluminum foil baking pan in a porcelain-lined Dutch oven and add:

- 0.6 cup of tap water
- 0.4 cup of beef broth
- 1 cup of tomato juice
- 2 tablespoons of apple cider vinegar

Put the lid on the Dutch oven and place it in a 350°F oven for one hour.

Remove from the oven and discard the aluminum foil baking pan.

Finally discard the soup because it contains an extremely high level of aluminum ions equal to more than 10 times WHO's recommended maximum aluminum in drinking water[387].

I recently attended a children's birthday party for my great niece and became sick to my stomach when the catered food arrived in six big disposable aluminum foil pans containing various Italian pastas in meat and tomato sauce. There was no protective liner between the food and the aluminum. I could not bear to watch children ingesting all that aluminum.

Testing pots and pans to see if they are made of aluminum is easy due to aluminum being a soft metal that is easily scratched. Test pots and pans for scratch resistance using a metal key. The metal used to make keys is harder than aluminum. If a scratch mark is easily made with the key, the pot or pan is aluminum and it should be discarded. Note that some stainless steels can be scratched with a key by applying sufficient pressure.

Fluoride Increases Aluminum Absorption

Fluoride ions form an ionic bond with aluminum. This ionic bond is stronger than 60 other metal fluorides[441]. The aluminum-fluoride ionic bond is highly stable *in vivo*[442]. After a year of adding either fluoride or aluminum trifluoride to the drinking water of rats at a level of 2.1 ppm, the amount of aluminum in their brains was nearly double that of a control group of rats who had no added fluoride in their drinking water. The aluminum concentration of their rat chow was at least 150ppm[443]. It is hypothesized that when fluoride and aluminum are both present they form fluoroaluminum complexes in the stomach that exhibit both increased absorption into the blood and transport across the blood-brain-barrier into the brain. An epidemiology study in China has shown that both high aluminum and fluoride in drinking water coincides with a lower IQ in children aged 8 to 12[444,445].

The conversion of aluminum cations to aluminum trifluoride is favored by levels of fluoride with at least a 3 to 1 ratio of F to Al. The level of fluoride in drinking water recommended by the Center for Disease Control and Prevention (CDC) has recently been lowered from 1.0ppm to 0.7ppm (700mcg/L)[446]. This is 3.5 times higher than WHO's 200mcg/liter maximum aluminum concentration in drinking water and 37 times higher than the 18.6mcg/liter of aluminum contained in Quabbin tap water arriving in Somerville, MA. It is typical of most fluorinated drinking water that there is more than three times the level of fluoride to aluminum. Therefore there is sufficient fluoride added to drinking water to make aluminum trifluoride.

One-half of a gram (1cm from a tube of toothpaste) of fluoride containing toothpaste has approximately 750mcg of fluoride. The number of fluoride molecules in that amount of fluoride is equivalent to the number of aluminum molecules in 40 liters of Quabbin tap water. Therefore if swallowed that amount of fluoride is sufficient to form aluminum trifluoride. But a study with rats showed that only 7% of the fluoride taken orally can be absorbed in the oral cavity even if left in the mouth over a 2.5 hour period[447]. Therefore, if not swallowed and if tooth brushing requires less than 1 minute, fluoride containing toothpaste or mouth rinse is not a major source of absorbed fluoride (approximately 0.35mcg per brushing).

Coffee Percolators and Tea Warmers as an Aluminum Source

Every day I pour fluorinated tap water in my coffee percolator to make coffee in the morning and tea in the evening. My wife read on the internet that inside these plastic and glass devices there can be a tube of aluminum with an attached heating element. All the water flows through this tube and is heated to near the boiling point. In the process of heating the water, fluoride pits the aluminum surface corroding the metal and polluting my coffee and tea with aluminum.

I disassembled my coffee and tea maker and found an aluminum tube with an attached ceramic heating element. One pass of tap water through this device increased the aluminum level four fold. There are coffee percolators and tea makers safe to use that are all glass and stainless steel. Beware as there are also stainless steel clad percolators and tea makers with a heated aluminum bottom plate in contact with the water. You can use the key scratch test to verify the type of metal used internally in these stainless steel coffee percolators and tea makers (see Avoid Aluminum Ingestion in Chapter 6 of this book for recommendations).

Conclusion of Controlling Your Aluminum Ingestion

Aluminum ingestion can be controlled by being selective in how you cook and what you ingest:

- Read labels on food products and drugs
- Avoid alum and SALP containing products
- Don't buy or store beverages in aluminum cans
- Filter water to remove aluminum
- Avoid foods, pharmaceuticals, and cosmetics that contain high levels of aluminum
- Avoid foods, pharmaceuticals and cosmetics colored with aluminum lakes
- Get one vaccine at a time
- Use an antiperspirant without aluminum
- Don't cook in aluminum cookware or aluminum foil
- Don't use a water filter that filters fluoride out of drinking water as it will add aluminum to the water.

Aluminum ingestion can also be controlled at a government level by:

- Requiring the labeling of all food and pharmaceutical products that contain aluminum as food additive, inactive ingredient, or active ingredient. The warning label should both state that the product contains aluminum and that aluminum is a known neurotoxin causing Alzheimer's, autism, and stroke.

- Require the labeling of all food, including baby formula, with the amount of aluminum per serving. This will allow producers of baby formula with low aluminum levels to differentiate their formula from other brands with higher aluminum levels.

- Recommending that water departments cease adding fluoride to drinking water. This will decrease aluminum corrosion while cooking in aluminum cookware and will decrease the absorption of aluminum by the brains of those who drink the water.

Chapter 5 – Controlling Your Aluminum Retention with a Dissolved Mineral

In "One Hundred Years of Solitude" the Colombian author Gabriel Garcia Marquez describes a mythical village of Macondo where the villagers have acquired a disease that causes them to lose their memories and "the name and notion of things and finally the identity of people." The disease persists until a travelling gypsy visits Macondo and introduces the villagers to a drink "of a gentle color" that restores their memory and identity. Is this fiction or could it be a portent of things to come?

Aluminum is the third most common element in the earth's crust so why, given aluminum's cellular toxicity, is there life on earth? The answer is the ability of the second most common element in the earth's crust, silicon, to form silica that complexes with aluminum rendering it harmless. This fact and three questions open our eyes to a remarkably simple way to decrease our aluminum retention and increase our aluminum excretion with orthosilicic acid (OSA):

1) **What does social drinking have to do with AD?** A 2011 review of the literature found that moderate drinking correlates with a lower risk of memory problems and dementia, including AD[448]. The authors of the review analyzed results of 143 studies, dating back to 1977 that included 365,000 participants in 19 countries. The studies compared drinkers with non-drinkers. Moderate drinkers were 23% less likely than teetotalers to develop signs of memory problems or AD. Moderate drinking was defined as one drink per day for women and two drinks per day for men where one drink was defined at 1.5oz of sprits, 5 oz. of wine, or 12 oz. of beer.

2) **What does the dissolved mineral orthosilicic acid (OSA – a.k.a. dissolved silica, silicon hydroxide, silicic acid) have to do with AD?** In 2009 the results of a 15 year study of 1,900 people was published[76]. It found that cognitive decline with time was greater in people with a higher daily intake of aluminum from drinking water. The study also found that there is a lower frequency of AD when OSA intake is at a level of ≥ 11.25mg of dissolved silica a day (equivalent to ≥ 3.3mg silicon/day since 29% of silica is silicon). The lower frequency of AD is theorized to be due to OSA binding with aluminum in the body and facilitating the excretion of the aluminum[76].

3) **Is there a connection between why both social drinking and OSA lower the frequency of AD?** OSA is present in beer, wine, and some sprits due to the use of silicic acid as a clarifying agent to remove colloidal hazes from these beverages. Also the grain used for brewing may add dissolved silica to beer during preparation. The mean silicon level of 76 different beers has been found to be 19.2mg/liter[449]. Therefore one drink, or 12 oz. of beer, corresponds to ingesting approximately 7mg of silicon in 24mg of OSA.

Dietary and Supplementary Silica Decreasing Aluminum Retention

There are three forms of aluminum that are ingested:

- Labile aluminum – absorbable and bioavailable
- Non-labile aluminum – non-absorbable and non-bioavailable
- Particulate aluminum – non-absorbable and non-bioavailable

Labile aluminum is in the form of trivalent aluminum ions (Al^{3+}) complexed with molecules of water. Because of the acidity of the human gut (e.g. pH 4 $\pm$2) some of the non-labile aluminum we ingest, such as aluminum silicates, hydroxides, and fluorides, are converted to labile aluminum in the gut[450]. Labile aluminum competes with calcium for absorption from the gut to the blood and is excreted in the urine[451]. Both non-labile and particulate aluminum that are stable at the pH of the human gut are not absorbed and are excreted in the feces.

There are two ways that dissolved silica as OSA and oligomers and nanoparticles of OSA in the diet or as a supplement can regulate the amount of ingested aluminum reaching the brain:

- Monomeric OSA increases aluminum excretion in the urine
- Oligomers and nanoparticles of OSA increases fecal excretion of aluminum

OSA when taken orally is readably absorbed and therefore bioavailable. OSA is a nearly neutral acid (pKa 9.84) that complexes with labile aluminum in the blood and kidneys (pH 6.5-8) increasing the urinary excretion of aluminum[36,37,452]. Oligomers of OSA (i.e. short ultra-filterable polymers) are not absorbed and therefore non-bioavailable[452]. These oligomers of OSA can form nanoparticles of silica that have a high affinity for aluminum and are also non-bioavailable[452,453]. Both oligomers and nanoparticles of OSA bind to aluminum in the gut and intestine making particulate aluminum. This decreases gastrointestinal absorption and facilitates increased fecal excretion of aluminum[51,452,454].

Studies on the bioavailability of OSA indicated that after OSA ingestion there is a significant increase in urinary excretion of aluminum as compared with no OSA ingestion[36,452]. Also 56% of the silicon ingested as OSA is excreted in the urine within 8 hours of ingestion[36]. After OSA ingestion excretion of aluminum reaches a maximum and then declines, consistent with depletion of aluminum in the blood and kidneys[36]. A low serum but high urine concentration of silicon suggests that when aluminum and OSA interact to form a chemical complex they do so mostly in the kidney lumen[36]. Also OSA limits the reabsorption of aluminum from the kidney lumen back into the blood without disturbing iron levels[37].

The chemical affinity of both OSA and oligomers of OSA for aluminum has been shown to reduce levels of aluminum in blood plasma by 85% in human studies (see Figure 4)[51,452]. Also OSA in drinking water lowers the amount of aluminum accumulated in ageing rat brains[454,455].

Dietary and Supplementary Silica Improving Cognition in AD Patients

In a 2013 British study 15 AD patients and their caregivers, 15 men and 15 women, drank one liter of Spritzer water every day for 13 weeks. The Spritzer water contains approximately 35mg/liter of silicon as 121mg/liter of dissolved silica and is bottled in Malaysia. Comparison of the participant's serum aluminum levels at the beginning and end of the study revealed declines as large as 50% to 70%. The AD patients' cognition at the beginning and end of the study was assessed using the ADAS-Cog (e.g. Alzheimer Disease Assessment Scale-Cognitive) test. After 13 weeks eight of the AD patients had no further cognitive deterioration during the study and three of the AD patients had significantly improved cognition[456]. This result is encouraging but tests with more patients for longer periods of time are needed for confirmation.

Content of Silicon and Aluminum in Drinking Water[416,417,456]					
Drinking Water	**Location of Source**	**pH**	**TDS[A] 25°C**	**Silicon[B] (mg/liter)**	**Aluminum[B] (mcg/liter)**
AquaFina	Ayer, MA, USA	5.8	22	~0 (0.5)	5 (18.4)
Dansi	Atlanta, GA, USA	5.7	45	~0 (1.0)	~0 (0)
Eska	St. Mathieu, Quebec	4.5	80	7	5
Evian	Evian-Les-Bains, France	7.3	278	10 (14.6)	7 (0)
Fiji	Fiji Islands	7.1	153	36 (27.1)	~0 (0)
Perrier	Vergeze, France	5.4	342	6	13
Poland Spring	Maine, USA	6.5	48	10 (10.2)	~0 (0)
Pure Life – Nestle's	Breinigsville, PA, USA Allentown, PA, USA	6.7	50	~0 (0)	~0
San Pellagrino	Bergamo, Italy	5.0	420	5	23
Silicade+Ca[C]	Quabbin Reservoir, MA, USA	6.6	450	36	~0
Smart Water	?	7.3	45	~0	~0
Starkey Water	Fruitvale, ID, USA	9.1	270	28.5	~0
Volvic	Volvic, France	7.2	96	15	~0

A) TDS = level of total dissolved solids the most common of which are calcium and magnesium.

B) Data is from a 2016 analysis[417] and data in parenthesis is from a 2007 analysis[416]. The "~" means approximately as the limit of detection is 2 ppm/L of silicon and 2 mcg/L of aluminum.

C) Silicade plus Ca is tap water, originating from Quabbin, acidified to pH 4.0 – 5.0 and filtered through a Brita OB03 filter lowers aluminum by 98.5%[417] but does not decrease silicon levels[417].

The amounts of both labile aluminum (e.g. aluminum extracted at pH3.3) and OSA as silicon in drinking have been measured and are summarized in the table[416,456]. Note that silicon is 29% of OSA (i.e. dissolved silica) the rest being oxygen and hydrogen. The amount of OSA in bottled water depends on both what the source water has been in contact with underground and the length of time it has been underground. Quartz is the mineral silicon dioxide and in water it slowly hydrates to form water soluble OSA at a rate dependent upon its crystalline structure. Geochemically over time quartz is made from opal deposits that consist of the skeletons of siliceous marine organisms. Water in contact with opal deposits leaches out dissolved OSA.

Diatoms as a Source of Silica in Drinking Water

Marine diatoms transport silicon as part of their skeleton and the concentration of OSA in deep (i.e. 1,000m) ocean water increases as the water travels along ocean currents (e.g. the global ocean conveyor belt)[457,458]. The global ocean conveyor belt flows deeply from the Atlantic, partly between Australia and Antarctica, and north through the Pacific. The current upwells in the middle of the Pacific and changes direction. Some of this current then flows Northwestward through the Malacca Strait into the Indian Ocean. Areas along the Malacca Strait and islands in the pacific are on the receiving end of this OSA transport and are composed of high levels of OSA rich subsurface deposits. Both Malaysia and Singapore are located on the Malacca Strait. Singapore has levels of silica in their drinking water averaging 4.0 to 7.7 mg/liter.

Life Expectancy and AD Death Rate by Country		
Country	**Life Expectancy (yrs.)***	**AD Death Rate (per 100,000)****
Iceland	83.3	34.1
United States	79.8	45.6
Malaysia	75.7	0.7
Singapore	84	0.2

*Life expectancy data from WHO 2014, **AD death rate data 2016 worldlifeexpectancy.com

The death rate from AD in the U.S. is one of the highest in the world while Singapore and Malaysia are near zero ranking them at the bottom of the list of 192 countries[459]. Singapore and Malaysia's comparable life expectancy with the U.S. and a significantly lowered death rate for AD may be due to high silica levels in Malaysia's and Singapore's drinking water. The high death rate from AD in Iceland may be due to high levels of aluminum in their surface waters due to extensive bauxite deposits that are rich in aluminum but poor in silicon[460].

Preparation of Silicade

Making silicon rich water weekly at home is easy and much less expensive and more sustainable than purchasing water bottled in Fiji or Malaysia. I call this water "Silicade". Silicade provides dissolved silica to keep your body-burden of aluminum under control. Silicade preparation requires only two ingredients and a set of small measuring spoons that are all easy to purchase online and have shipped to your home. Silicade can be stored indefinitely in the dark like Fiji water. The chemicals to make Silicade store well and should be kept out of children's reach:

- **Low Alkalinity Sodium Silicate:** a hydrous powder available from Chemical Store Online. The powder is safer and easier to measure than the liquid form and has a purity of 99.5% with a ratio of SiO_2 to Na_2O of 3.22 (Na_2O=19.2%, SiO_2=61.8%) and a water of hydration to SiO_2 ratio of 1.0. **Only order "sodium silicate – low alkalinity". Do not order "sodium silicate – alkaline" from the Chemical Store.**
- **Sodium Bisulfate:** a white powder 99.5% pure of micro-prills (i.e. very small pellets) from Professor Fullwood of LoudWolf Ltd. is available from Amazon. Note that both optional calcium chloride and magnesium sulfate are available from the same source.
- **Mini Measuring Spoon Set:** Norpro 3061D from Dine Company Online. Currently priced under $4 without shipping. Three measuring spoons come attached to a single ring. Only the dash and smidgen are used for Silicade preparation. In order to avoid accidental use of the wrong measuring spoon, remove the pinch from the ring.
- **Spatula:** Any small spatula with a straight-edge works to level the contents of the measuring spoons prior to addition.

By following these instructions you can easily prepare a gallon of Silicade:

1) A level dash and two level smidgens (3/16 of a teaspoon, 600mg. with 597mg as $SiO_2[NaO_2]_{1/3.22}$ H_2O (mw 88.66) of hydrous powdered sodium silicate is placed in a Pyrex glass measuring cup, suspended in 1/8 cup of tap water, brought to boiling in the microwave or on the stove, and boiled for 30sec. The powder contains 99.5% water soluble sodium silicate and 0.5% max. of water insoluble materials as required by the American Waterworks Standard B104-98 for adding sodium silicate to drinking water.

2) The hot water with dissolved sodium silicate is immediately diluted to one gallon (3.785 liters) with cold tap water resulting in a 1.29 mM/liter (124ppm) solution of pH 9.8 OSA.

3) One level dash (1/8 of a teaspoon, 0.83 gr, 6.9 mM) of sodium bisulfate is added to the solution of OSA and dissolved with stirring in order to acidify the solution to pH 4.0 to 5.0. **Optionally**, if tap water is more basic than pH 8.5, use a pH meter while slowly adding a little more sodium bisulfate in order to lower the pH to 4.0-5.0. Etekcity pH pen meter PH-2011 is a temperature compensated low cost pH meter available online. A pH 7.0 standard solution is recommended for periodic calibration of the pH meter.

4) The clear colorless acidic solution of OSA is further purified by filtering through a Brita pitcher style filter (i.e. OB03) resulting in OSA at a pH of 4.4.

5) Two level smidgens of sodium bicarbonate (a.k.a. baking soda) are added and dissolved with stirring in the gallon of filtered OSA, resulting in Silicade with a pH of 6.5, a TDS of 285 at 25°C, and less than 2mcg/L labile aluminum. Each quart of Silicade contains 34mg of dissolved silicon as 117.3mg of monomeric (OSA).

6) **Optionally make Silicade Plus Calcium,** if tap water is low in calcium, add two level dashes of calcium chloride flakes or prills (840mg 36% calcium) 99% pure from Loudwolf/Amazon. This will increase the calcium level by 80mg per liter, the TDS to 450 at 25°C, and the pH to 6.6 in a gallon of Silicade + Ca. Labile aluminum in calcium enriched Silicade is less than 2mcg/L. It has been found that calcium at concentrations greater than or equal to 75mg/L have a significant protective effect on cognition[461]. Optionally add a heaping dash of magnesium sulfate to increase magnesium by 20mg/L.

7) **Optionally make Sparkling Silicade** - Carbonate Silicade resulting in pH 4.5 beverages.

Drink 3 to 4 cups of Silicade a day around meal times in order to provide a total of 25.5 to 34mg of silicon as monomeric OSA. This is 7.7 to 10.3 times the 3.3mg of silicon that when consumed as OSA per day was observed to lower the frequency of AD[76]. In the U.S. 160mg per liter of OSA (i.e. 100mg per liter of SiO_2) is generally recognized as safe in drinking water[462].

Why This Recipe Works

The goal of this recipe for orthosilicic acid (OSA) in drinking water is to use an easily measured solid silica powder and an acidic microprill that are commercially available online and shipped to anyone, not just chemical laboratories. Both of these chemicals are high purity (e.g. 99.5%).

- **Solubilize and hydrolyze sodium silicate to OSA:** Boiling powdered sodium silicate for 30 seconds in an eighth of a cup of tap water keeps the pH high enough (e.g. pH = 13) to solubilize and hydrolyze 99.5% to monomeric OSA and short silica polymers[463-465].
- **Neutralize and prevent re-polymerization of OSA:** In order to prevent OSA re-polymerization, immediately dilute the basic (e.g. pH=13) OSA solution to a gallon with tap water. **To render the solution non-hazardous**, acidify the solution to pH 4.0 to 5.0 with the solid acid sodium bisulfate. A 1.29mM OSA solution is well below OSA's saturation level in water (e.g. 2-3mM) but requires 7 days to fully stabilize rising from 108ppm immediately after preparation to 124ppm[417]. Polymerization of OSA has been observed at neutral pH only well above OSA's saturation level (i.e. 42mM)[453,464,465].
- **Remove Aluminum:** For optimal aluminum removal acidify the OSA solution to pH 4.0 to 5.0 and then filter through a Brita pitcher style filter (OB03)[417]. A significant portion (e.g. 98.5%) of the labile aluminum introduced in tap water is removed[416,417]. This Brita filter is a combined activated carbon and cation exchange resin that removes cations like aluminum but does not remove OSA[417]. If the tap water used for Silicade is between pH 6.5 to 8.5, as per EPA's secondary drinking water standard, then after acidification, filtration, and bicarbonate addition Silicade will be pH 6.5.
- **Optionally add Calcium and/or Magnesium:** Have your tap water checked and if it is low in calcium and/or magnesium, add supplemental calcium and/or magnesium to Silicade. The Brita filter reduces calcium and magnesium in Quabbin tap water by one half[416]. Drinking water with calcium at levels of 80mg/L and magnesium at levels of 20mg/L has been found to be optimal for good health[466]. This may be due to calcium and magnesium competing with aluminum for absorption by the gut[451]. Calcium catalyzes the polymerization of OSA but only at pH greater than 8[467,468]. Silicade + Ca is pH 6.6 and at this pH OSA in Silicade + Ca is primarily a non-polymeric monomer[417].

Conclusion of Controlling Your Aluminum Excretion with a Dissolved Mineral

Silica supplementation is a proven and recommended way to increase aluminum excretion by your body. There are six silica supplements available:

- **High silica mineral water**, such as Fiji or Starkey water, taken as 3 to 4 cups per day will result in 25.5 to 34mg of silicon as OSA per day. This source of silica taken orally results in 43% of the OSA being absorbed and bioavailable[469].
- **High silica Silicade water** is prepared in your home by mixing powdered sodium silicate with powdered sodium bisulfate in tap water. Silicade taken as 3 to 4 cups per day will result in 25.5-34mg of silicon as OSA per day. Like high silica mineral water, this source of silica taken orally results in 43% of the OSA being absorbed and bioavailable[469].
- **Stabilized concentrated OSA**, such as Natural Factor's Biosil choline stabilized OSA[470], can be taken as 5 drops twice a day in a quarter cup of flavored liquid, as it has a slight taste, or as 2 veg caps a day. Note that low choline supplementation (200mg/day) may have benefits but there is a 70% greater risk of lethal prostate cancer with high (500mg/day) choline diets[471]. The European Food Safety Authority recommended that liquid choline stabilized OSA be taken at a maximum dose of 10 mg. of silicon with 200mg of choline per day[472,473]. Choline stabilized OSA taken orally results in 17% of the OSA being absorbed and bioavailable and 42% being oligomeric OSA[469].
- **Colloidal silica**, such as Eidon's Ionic Minerals Silica Concentrate, taken as 30 drops per day, or Saguna's Silicolgel Colloidal Silicic Acid, taken as 10cc per day equals 175mg or 163mg of silicon, respectively, per day. Only 0.25% or less of silicon in colloidal silica taken orally has been shown to be absorbed and bioavailable[417,469]. Also silica colloids made synthetically and sold commercially as nanoparticles have been tested *in vitro* on human cells and shown to have cytotoxicity[474].
- **Plant Extracts**, such as bamboo (33% silicon) and horsetail (3.3% silicon) as silica SiO_2
- **Diatomaceous Earth**, sold as food grade contains less than 0.46% silicon as silica SiO_2

Silica Supplements[417,469]

Supplement	Dose/Day	Silicon\Dose\Day	Bioavailable OSA	Cost/Day
Mineral Water[AK]	3 - 4 cups	25.5-34mg	11 – 14.7mg	$1.00 - $1.50
Silicade[BK]	3 - 4 cups	25.5-34mg	11 – 14.7mg	$0.04 - $0.05[C]
Choline Stab OSA[DK]	10 drops	10mg	1.7mg	$0.42
Choline Stab OSA[EK]	2 veg caps	10mg	1.7mg	$0.83
Colloidal Silica[F]	30 drops	175mg	0.15mg	$0.60
Colloidal Silica[G]	10cc	163mg	0.40mg	$0.59
Bamboo[H]	1cap(300mg)	99mg	0.29mg	$0.10
Horsetail[I]	1cap(500mg)	16.5mg	0.11mg	$0.04
Diatomaceous Earth[H]	625mg	<2.9mg	0.07mg	$0.01

A. Fiji and Starkey – Mineral Waters; B. Silicade - preparation Chapter 5; C. Excluding cost of tap water; D. Biosil Choline Stab. OSA; E. Biosil Veg Caps; F. Eidon – Ionic Minerals Silica Concentrate; G. Saguna – Silicolgel Colloidal OSA; H. Swanson; I. Swanson; J. Swanson K. Samples acidified to pH3.2 for 4 hours all other samples for 24 hours prior to testing for OSA

OSA in drinking water acts to lower the amount of soluble aluminum in the drinking water[426]. After examining 214 water supplies in northern England it was found that when drinking water contained greater than 3.5mg/liter of soluble silicon as OSA, the level of soluble aluminum was always below 20mcg/liter[426]. When drinking water contained less than 3.5mg/liter of soluble silicon as OSA, the level of aluminum ranged from 25 to 125mcg/liter. Communities and agencies responsible for drinking water should be adding OSA (i.e. soluble silica) to public drinking water to keep the level of soluble silicon at or above 50mg/liter. They should also refrain from adding fluoride to drinking water. In place of fluoride in drinking water the public should be encouraged to use tooth paste and/or mouthwash containing fluoride. These two actions could lower the amount of AD, autism, and stroke.

Chemistry of Orthosilicic Acid Complexation with Aluminum

As the pH rises, OSA will more completely complex with aluminum. The pH in the kidney lumen and blood, where this complexation can occur, is between 6.5 and 8.0. In the kidney lumen and blood 98-99% of the aluminum ion is complexed with OSA at pH 6.5 to pH 8.0..

As the pH falls, OSA will not completely complex with aluminum. The pH in the stomach, where this complexation can also occur, is between 1 and 5. It is calculated that at pH 4.5 only 12% of the aluminum ion is complexed with OSA in the stomach and at pH 4.0 only 1% of the aluminum ion is complexed with OSA in the stomach and upper GI track.

OSA (100 μM/L = 9.6mg/L) in 0.1 liter of orange juice laced with isotopic aluminum-26 lowers human plasma levels of aluminum-26 by 85% on average as compared with the same human volunteers drinking aluminum-26 laced orange juice without OSA (see Figure 4)[51]. From these data it can be concluded that OSA does complex with almost all free aluminum in both the blood and the kidney lumen and can lower plasma aluminum levels by 85%. It has been reported that OSA does not lower aluminum absorption in rats[475]. Therefore OSA may lower plasma aluminum levels not by decreasing absorption but by complexing with aluminum in the kidneys and preventing its reabsorption from the urine into the blood.

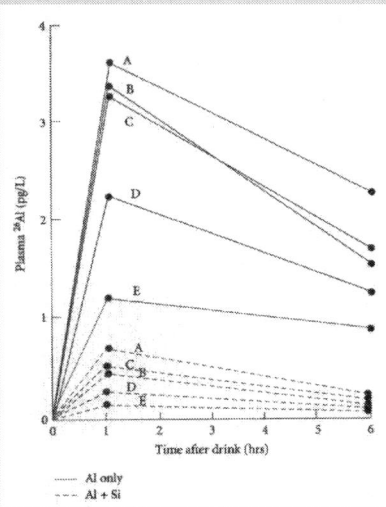

Figure 4 – Effect of OSA on aluminum in blood plasma
Five volunteers (A-D) drank orange juice first containing aluminum-26 without OSA and then drank orange juice with OSA. Conclusions: 1) some humans excrete 3 times more aluminum than others. 2) OSA at 100μM/L =2.8mg of silicon/liter lowers the amount of aluminum in the blood by approximately 10 fold[51].

Siliceous Organisms and their Contribution to OSA in Drinking Water

A group of small marine siliceous organisms (i.e. diatoms, radiolarians, silicoflagellates) have a silica skeleton. For these creatures OSA (a.k.a. dissolved silica) is an essential nutrient. On a global scale diatoms sustain more than 40% of the ocean's primary biological production[458]. When these organisms die their skeletons fall to the bottom of the ocean accumulating as opal (a.k.a. opaline siliceous ooz,, biogenetic silica). The opal undergoes partial dissolution as OSA back into the ocean sustaining the growth of more siliceous organisms. The rest of the opal becomes buried as ocean sediment and this opal is a precursor of quartz[458]. After the ocean conveyor belt upwells in the mid-pacific, opal sediments become concentrated along its path. A portion of the ocean conveyor belt flows northwest through the Malacca Strait between Sumatra and Malaysia. When ocean sediment becomes landmass due to geological processes, rainwater can dissolve OSA out of the opal and quartz. This results in OSA rich drinking water in regions of the world such as Malaysia, Singapore, and Fiji that have underground aquifers surrounded by opal and quartz deposits.

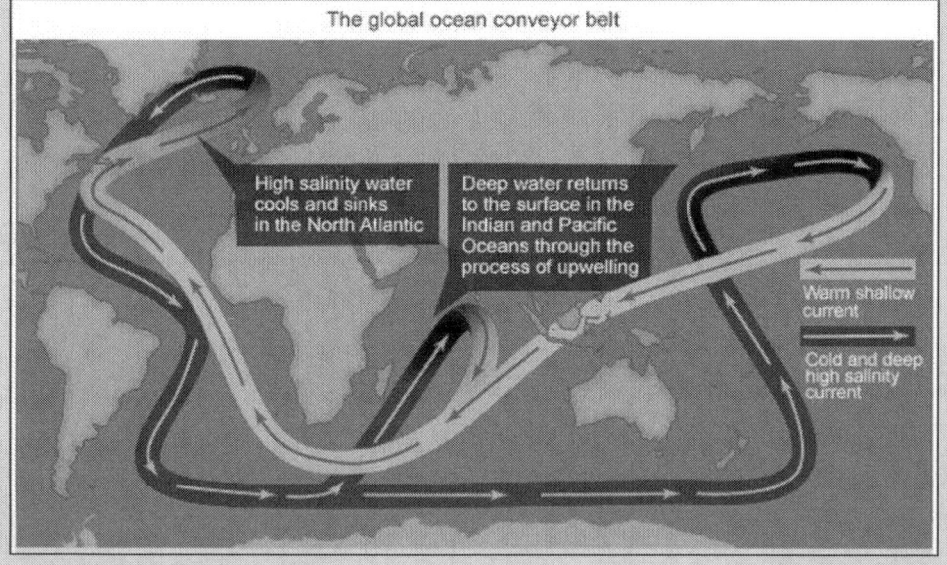

Figure 5 – Global ocean conveyor belt

Geologically the Malacca Strait belongs to the Sunda Shelf that was an extensive low-relief land surface formed at the beginning of Quarternary time about 2.6 million years ago. The Sunda Shelf has remained undisturbed by coastal movements for about the past 7 million years. The strait has attained its present configuration after having been inundated by the postglacial rise of sea level resulting from the melting of land-ice at higher latitudes after the last ice age. It is possible that opal was deposited on the current sites of Singapore and Taiping Malaysia during this period of inundation or prior inundations. At Taiping the deposited opal could have been covered by siltation from rivers that drain into the strait. Spritzer water is pumped from a 450 foot deep well near Taiping Malaysia that is near the coast on the Malacca Strait. Singapore is on the coast at the southern end of the Malacca Strait. The abundance of silica in drinking water accounts for why Malaysia and Singapore have the lowest rates of AD in the world.

Obtaining fresh water from underground opal or quartz deposits has the advantage of drinking water enriched in OSA and low in aluminum. The opposite situation exists in other parts of the world that have drinking water with low concentrations of OSA and high concentrations of aluminum. One example is Iceland where geothermal activity enriches surface waters with much more aluminum than silicon[460]. Icelandic surface waters that have gone through boiling before reaching the surface have a pH greater than 8 and an aluminum concentration of 21 to 1,510mcg/liter. Icelandic surface waters that have been mixed with condensed steam have a pH less than 4 and an aluminum concentration of 200 to 267,000mcg/liter. These high levels are due to heating and acidification causing the breakdown of Icelandic bauxite deposits that contain a high concentration of aluminum and only a few percent of silicon. These high surface levels of aluminum may account for why Iceland has the second highest rate of AD in the world.

Chapter 6 – Seven Lifestyle Choices to Prevent Alzheimer's, Autism, and Stroke

"Lack of activity destroys the good condition of every human being, while movement and methodical physical exercise save it and preserve it." Plato

This chapter discusses how some lifestyle choices can be modified to prevent Alzheimer's, autism, and stroke. The seven lifestyle choices discussed in this chapter are:

- Stop smoking
- Decrease alcohol consumption
- Avoid aluminum ingestion
- Increase dissolved silica in your diet
- Aerobically exercise
- Avoid lack of sleep
- Avoid head trauma

Stop Smoking

In 2010 the results of a long-term study of 21,123 members of one health care system in Finland were published. The results showed that smoking two packs of cigarettes a day between age 50-60 doubles the risk of stroke (416 cases) and AD (1,136 cases) two decades later between age 70-85. Those who smoked less than a half a pack per day did not show an increased risk of stroke. Smoking contributes to higher homocysteine levels and inflammation of blood vessels leading to decreased blood flow through the brain (e.g. leukoaraiosis and atherosclerosis) and increased risk of strokes. Also high homocysteine levels caused by smoking are correlated with an increased risk of AD. The correlations found in this study between smoking and dementia did not vary by race or sex[476].

In 2012 a study of 45 men and 29 women with an average age of 76 took place. All the participants showed signs of early memory loss. The participants were divided into two groups.

For six months one group wore a 15mg. nicotine patch while the other group was given a placebo. By the end of the study, the patients who had worn the nicotine patches were better able to pay attention and also demonstrated better long-term memory than patients who didn't use the nicotine patches[477].

Nicotine appears to enhance attention and long-term memory by binding to ganglion type nicotinic acetylcholine receptors in the adrenal medulla portion of the brain increasing the concentration of acetylcholine. Unfortunately, nicotine binding to this receptor also increases the concentration of dopamine providing the feelings of euphoria and relaxation that leads to addiction[478]. Nicotine can't be recommended in any dose because cigarette smoking is the single largest cause of premature death in the U.S., killing approximately 490,000 people a year[479].

There is aluminum in both tobacco and cannabis at concentrations that vary from 0.1 to 3.7 mg per gram[480]. Some of this aluminum is volatilized during smoking and is absorbed by the lungs during both active and passive smoking[480]. This may explain why smokers have a higher body burden of aluminum than nonsmokers[480]. In addition it may be the reason that smoking is related to an increased risk of stroke[224].

Therefore **stop smoking** as there are non-addictive ways to improve your memory and ability to concentrate. See Chapter 7 for a discussion of non-addictive cholinergic drugs for the treatment of the symptoms of dementia, such as memory loss.

Nicotine Patches: Beware that aluminum acetylacetonate is toxic but still used as an adhesive promoter and listed as an ingredient of some nicotine patches. This organometallic aluminum complex has been shown to facilitate aluminum accumulation in regions of the brain responsible for memory[42]. It is soluble in both fat and water and has been shown to gain entry to the body by inhalation[42] and likely absorption through the skin.

Decrease Daily Moderate Alcohol Consumption

As discussed in Chapter 2 an elevated level of plasma homocysteine is a causal factor for high blood pressure and stroke. Daily moderate drinking causes elevated levels of plasma homocysteine as shown by the following study:

A study of daily moderate alcohol consumption and homocysteine levels was conducted with 60 healthy males aged 28 to 44. The subjects were divided into four groups of 15 based upon their alcohol consumption during the prior year. A control group, who were abstinent during the prior year, received no alcoholic beverage during the study. The other three groups got a daily alcoholic drink of either beer, red wine, or spirits depending upon the subject's preferred source of alcohol. The volume of these drinks was equivalent to 30 grams (38cc, 1.3 ounces) of pure alcohol. The study lasted 6 weeks. The data in the table shows that daily moderate alcohol drinking during the 6 week study caused elevated levels of plasma homocysteine. In addition, periodic alcohol consumption prior to the 6 week study had also caused elevated levels of plasma homocysteine in two of the three groups of drinkers who periodically drank wine and spirits[228].

Group	% Ethanol	Ounces of Drink**	Initial tHcy*	Final tHcy*
Control	--	--	9	8.5
Beer	5	26	11.7	14.6
Wine	12	11	12.7	15.6
Spirits	40	3.2	13.8	16.2

*Average tHcy levels are μM/L of homocysteine in the blood.
**Ounces of drink that contain 30 grams of ethanol.
Note: Elevated total serum homocysteine level is 12-60μM/L

Therefore **decrease daily moderate alcohol consumption** to avoid high blood pressure and stroke.

Avoid Aluminum Ingestion

We ingest aluminum daily in our drinking water and food but how much aluminum can we safely ingest without increasing our risk of AD? Aluminum taken at daily doses ranging from 0.003 to 0.063 mg per liter (e.g.1.06 quart) in drinking water averaging 0.023 mg per liter has been linked to a higher risk of AD in a study of 1462 women over 75[531]. The World Health Organization (WHO) has put a 0.1 mg per liter limit on aluminum in drinking water due to concerns about the risk of AD[83]. The WHO has also attempted to lower the weekly limit on ingestion of aluminum in food to 1 mg per kilogram (e.g. 0.45mg per pound) of body weight[68].

Avoid aluminum containing pharmaceuticals – We consume more aluminum from ingestion of pharmaceuticals than any other source. The following table is an example of the amount of aluminum consumed per day by taking a maximum strength antacid at the full daily dose:

Aluminum in Antacids			
Antacid – Max Strength	**Max. Dose/Day**	**Antacid Compound**	**Max. Aluminum/Day**
CVS Natural Antacid (Peppermint Tablets)	3 tablets	Calcium Carbonate	0.09mg
Equate (Liquid)	12 teaspoons	Aluminum Hydroxide	1,660mg
Maalox (Liquid)	8 teaspoons	Aluminum Hydroxide	1,110mg
Mylanta (Adult)	12 tablets	Aluminum Hydroxide	830mg
Mylanta (Liquid)	60ml/day	Aluminum Hydroxide	2,080mg
Gelusil (Tablets)	12 tablets	Aluminum Hydroxide	830mg

Check labels and product literature of pharmaceuticals for aluminum compounds used as either active or inactive ingredients. Look for alternative pharmaceuticals without aluminum.

Avoid using aluminum containing baking powder – Baking powders contain sodium bicarbonate (a.k.a. baking soda), powdered acid, and corn starch for anti-caking. The powdered acid can be an aluminum salt, calcium phosphate, or potassium bitartrate (a.k.a. cream of tartar). Baking powders made with calcium phosphate are usually advertised as "aluminum free". This is an effort by the manufacturer to differentiate baking powders made with calcium phosphate from those made with an aluminum salt. In reality there is a large amount of aluminum impurity in baking powders made with calcium phosphate and of course even a larger amount of aluminum in baking powders made with aluminum salts as shown in the following table:

Aluminum in Baking Powders[417]		
Baking Powder	**Powdered Acid**	**Aluminum mg/tsp**
Homemade	Cream of Tartar	Less than 0.004
Rumford Aluminum Free	Monocalcium Phosphate	0.79
Market Pantry Aluminum Free	Monocalcium Phosphate	0.93
Trader Joe's Aluminum Free	Monocalcium Phosphate	Greater than 1.0
Whole Foods 365 Aluminum Free	Monocalcium Phosphate	Greater than 1.0
Davis	Sodium Aluminum Sulfate & Monocalcium Phosphate	48.6

From this table it is clear why some baked goods (i.e. bread, cake, pancakes, waffles) have high levels of aluminum (see Chapter 4). In order to bake aluminum free it is recommended that you make your own homemade baking powder with cream of tartar as the powdered acid according to the following recipe. The manufactures whose products were tested and found to have an undetectable amount (less than 0.004mg/tsp.) of aluminum are in parentesis[417]:

    2 Tbsp.   Cream of Tartar (McCormick and Signature Kitchens)

    1 Tbsp.   Baking Soda (Arm & Hammer and Davis)

    1 Tbsp.   Corn Starch (Davis)

Mix the ingredients together and put the mixture through a screen wire sieve. Place in a container with a snap on plastic lid for storage. Store the homemade baking powder in a cool dry place.

Avoid using aluminum cookware – Aluminum in contact with hot food is a source of high levels of aluminum in the food. Fluoride or mild acids in the water used for cooking enhances aluminum corrosion and makes the amount of aluminum in the food even higher. Therefore always use cookware that puts stainless steel, cast iron, or other non-aluminum surface in contact with hot food. For example to boil water many stainless steel and glass coffee makers heat an aluminum tube that comes in contact with the water. One pass of water through such a coffee maker (i.e. Black & Decker DLX1050) increased the aluminum level from 16 to 280mcg/liter[417]. The following coffee makers have been tested in the same way and found to add no aluminum to the coffee: Jura Capresso MG900, BUNN Speed Brew, Krups Moka Brew, Keurig K90, and Nespresso C110 coffee makers and Krups Glass Electronic Kettle (FL700) for tea. Silica water used to make coffee in drip coffee makers does lose approximately 7% OSA during brewing.

Note that the only known stainless steel that contains aluminum is 405 and it contains 0.1 - 0.3% of aluminum. Also, when purchasing aluminum foil, select the non-stick variety and always place food in contact with only the non-stick side of the foil. Alternatively place a layer of parchment paper or plastic wrap between food and the aluminum foil.

There are several low cost alternatives to cooking and serving food in aluminum or aluminum foil cookware. Disposable thin plastic liners for aluminum food containers heated by steam not only keep the hot food away from the aluminum but also make cleanup easier for reusable pans. These liners are made of PET (a.k.a. polyethylene terephthalate, PTL, PETE, CPET) that has a safe temperature range of -100 to +400°F. These liners can be used in microwaves or ovens. They are called "steam table pan liners" and are available from the "Webstaurant Store" in a variety of sizes for lining aluminum and aluminum foil cookware.

There are several nonmetallic disposable cookware alternatives to aluminum. The company "Go Solut!" manufactures disposable sheet cake pans and trays, baking cups, and pizza trays made of corrugated multi-ply paper coated with PET capable of being heated to 400°F. The company "CPT - Coextruded Plastic Technologies" manufactures disposable baking pans made of PET.

Testing pots and pans to see if they are made of aluminum is easy due to aluminum being a soft metal that is easily scratched. Test pots and pans for scratch resistance using a metal key. The metal used to make keys is harder than aluminum. If a scratch mark is easily made with the key, the pot or pan is aluminum and it should be discarded. Note that some stainless steels can be scratched with a key by applying sufficient pressure.

Filter your drinking water – Portland cement is used to make the mortar that lines most of the drinking water pipes in the U.S. Also alum is used to treat drinking water in many communities in the U.S. Both the mortar lining and alum treatment result in dissolved labile neurotoxic aluminum in the water. Therefore it is recommended to filter drinking water through a filter known to remove aluminum. There are three types of filters known to remove 80-100% of aluminum from drinking water: cation exchange resin, reverse osmosis, electrodialysis[424].

Filters made by Brita, PUR, and Zero Technologies remove aluminum from drinking water by cation exchange and are more affordable than reverse osmosis and electrodialysis filters. Brita makes a combination activated carbon (57gr/filter) and cation exchange resin (38gr/filter) filter[481] that has been found to remove more than 98.5% of labile neurotoxic aluminum and none of dissolved silica from water[417]. That filter is the Brita OB03 filter. It is replaceable, good for filtering 40 gallons of water, and compatible with the following Brita pitchers: Brita Aqualux SMART Pitcher, Brita Atlantis Pitcher, Brita Bella Pitcher, Brita Chrome SMART Pitcher, Brita Classic Pitcher, Brita Deluxe Pitcher, Brita Everyday Pitcher, Brita Fjord SMART Pitcher, Brita Grand SMART Pitcher, Brita Marina Pitcher, Brita Riviera SMART Pitcher, Brita Slim Pitcher, Vintage Pitcher, and Brita UltraMax SMART Dispenser.

The problem with filters made by Zero Technologies is they contain both a cation and anion exchange resin and they do not remove as much aluminum as the Brita OB03 filter. The anion exchange resin removes anions such as fluoride and silica. Removal of fluoride from drinking water is beneficial as fluoride facilitates aluminum absorption by the brain. But removal of silica from drinking water is detrimental as silica facilitates aluminum excretion and lowers aluminum absorption. Filters for Zero Technologies' Tumbler lower the total dissolved solids (a.k.a. TDS) in drinking water to near zero but only remove 80% of 100mcg/liter of labile aluminum in water as compared with greater than 98.5% removal by the Brita OB03 filter and PUR pitcher style filter[417]. PUR filters remove 8% of silica while Zero filters remove 96% of silica from water[417].

In order to avoid both cognitive impairment due to aluminum absorption and bone fractures due to impaired bone remodeling (a.k.a. skeletal ossification), both calcium and magnesium should be present in drinking water[310,461,466,482]. Brita filters lower the concentration of calcium and magnesium by half[483]. But Zero water filters remove almost all calcium and magnesium from drinking water, facilitating both the absorption of ingested aluminum and increasing the risk of bone fractures. Other filters that were tested and failed to absorb more than 50% of 100mcg/liter of labile aluminum included the Seychelles Radiologic, and Clearbrook Bottle Filter[417].

Aluminum and Silica Removal From Drinking Water[417]		
Filter	**Percent Aluminum Removed**	**Percent Silica Removed**
Brita Pitcher Style	98.5%	0%
Up&Up Replacement Filter	74%	0%
PUR Ultimate Pitcher Style	98.5%	8%
Zero Tech. Pitcher Style	98.5%	93%
Zero Technologies Tumbler	80%	96%
Seychelles Radiologic	49%	--
Clearbrook Bottle	0%	--

Drinking water filters have a limited life and must be replaced periodically. With water having total dissolved solids (TDS) of around 100, Brita filters need to be replaced every three months. Filter lifetime is shorter when there are higher levels of TDS in drinking water. In order to check the Brita filter's performance use an inexpensive handheld TDS meter (such as HM Digital TDS-EZ) to compare the TDS reading of drinking water just prior to and just after filtration. The TDS reading is temperature dependent and this procedure ensures the two measurements are made at approximately the same temperature. Normally a new Brita filter lowers the TDS by 30 to 45%. The Brita filter needs to be replaced when there is less than a 10% decrease in TDS by filtration.

Use aluminum free antiperspirants and astringents – Alum, aluminum chloride, aluminum chlorohydrate, and aluminum-zirconium compounds are the most widely used active ingredients in antiperspirants. Application of aluminum chloride to the skin of mice resulted in aluminum accumulation in the hippocampal region of the brain[407]. Aluminum chlorohydrate applied to human underarms was shown to be absorbed at a rate of 4μg aluminum per single-use[386]. A five year study of 130 matched pairs of humans showed antiperspirant use slightly increases the risk of AD and this risk increases with frequency of use[408].

Avoid deodorants containing aluminum compounds. Use either Arm & Hammer's "Essentials" or Tom's of Maine "Original" deodorants that are both aluminum free. **Avoid astringents containing aluminum salts.** Use Epsom salts for minor skin irritations.

Don't purchase and store beverages or food in aluminum containers – If possible, buy food and beverages in glass or plastic containers. Beverages or food purchased in aluminum containers should not be stored. The thin layer of corrosion protection applied to the aluminum surface exposed to the beverage or food has small holes that result in aluminum corrosion. This corrosion slowly adds aluminum to the beverage or food during storage[411,412]. Dented cans can have cracks in the protective layer resulting in even faster corrosion and higher levels of aluminum in the beverage or food[411]. Aluminum levels do not increase during storage in beverages stored in glass[412,413]. **Whenever possible you should purchase and store beverages and food in glass or plastic.**

Avoid using soy-based infant formula – Soybeans prefer acidic soil that makes aluminum more bioavailable to soybeans[405]. Therefore the soybeans accumulate high levels of aluminum during growth and this aluminum ends up in soy-based baby formula. Soy-based baby formula contains 600-700μg/liter of aluminum[385,402]. That level of aluminum corresponds to more than 3 times the World Health Organization's (WHO's) maximum aluminum in drinking water limit[68]. Even some non-soy based formula has been found in the U.K. to be higher than WHO's limit. **Avoid soy-based infant formula and any formula suspected of containing high levels of aluminum.**

Avoid using food, drugs and cosmetics containing aluminum lake colorants – Synthetic dyes containing the aluminum salt of colorants (a.k.a. Aluminum Lake) and possible alumina as an extender should be avoided when there is a choice. Daily use of the products that contain Aluminum Lakes results in regular aluminum accumulation[397,398].

Examples of the names of common food, drug, and cosmetic (FD&C) colorants for food, drugs, and cosmetics that likely are listed as containing an "Aluminum Lake" with alumina as an extender include: Blue No. 1 and 2, Green No. 3, Red No. 3 and 40, and Yellow No. 5, and 6[396].

Examples of the names of common drug and cosmetic (D&C) colorants for drugs and cosmetics that may be listed as containing an "Aluminum Lake" without alumina as an extender include: Blue No. 4, Green No. 5 and 6, Orange No. 4, 5, 6, 10, and 11, Red No. 6, 7, 17, 21, 22, 27, 28, 30, 31, 33, 34, and 36, Violet No. 2, Yellow No. 7, 8, and 10[396].

Aluminum Lakes in Levothyroxine Sodium Tablets	
Levothyroxine Sodium (mcg/pill)	**Aluminum Lake Colorants**
25	FD&C Yellow No. 6 Aluminum Lake
50	None
75	FD&C Red No. 40 + FD&C Blue No. 2 Aluminum Lakes
88	FD&C Blue No. 1 + FD&C Yellow No.6 + D&C Yellow No. 10 Aluminum Lakes
100	D&C Yellow No. 10 + FD&C Yellow No. 6 Aluminum Lakes
112	D&C Red No. 27 & 30 Aluminum Lakes
125	FD&C Blue No. 1 Aluminum Lake
137	FD&C Blue No 1 Aluminum Lake

In order to compensate for our thyroid gland producing insufficient T_4, some of us require a daily levothyroxine sodium (a.k.a. synthetic T_4, Synthroid^R) supplement. These supplements are formulated as tablets that are color-coded based upon the amount of levothyroxine sodium that they contain. As shown in the previous table provided by the manufacturer most of these tablets contain Aluminum Lakes. Since levothyroxine sodium tablets represent a daily intake of aluminum, requesting a prescription for 50mcg tablets containing no Aluminum Lake is recommended. Not all colored drugs contain Aluminum Lakes. For instance, Simvastatin tablets (10, 20, and 40mg) are colored with red iron oxide and a mixture of red and yellow iron oxide.

Since children prefer colorful food and sweets, manufactures have added FD&C dyes containing Aluminum Lakes to many foods and sweets[397]. Only a careful reading of the ingredients on the package will allow you to avoid these products, some of which are listed in the following table:

Foods and Sweets Containing Aluminum Lake as an AFC[397]		
Food or Sweet Colored with Aluminum Lake (Serving Size in Parentheses)	**AFC* per Serving (mg/Serv.)**	**Estimated** Amount of Aluminum per Serving (mcg/Serv.)**
Kellogg Frosted Cherry Poptart (1) – Red 40	10.1	1,110
Marsh Green Sprinkles Cookie (1) – Yellow 5, Blue 1	1.4	154
Hostess Orange Cupcake (1) – Yellow 5 & 6	3.5	470
Betty Crocker's Blue Cupcake (1) – Blue 1	1.2	84
Betty Crocker's Red Cupcake (1) – Red 40	34.7	3,470
Okedoke Cheesy Popcorn (1 cup) – Red 40	3.8	420
Combos (1/3 cup) – Yellow 5 & 6, Blue 1	3.2	350
Hamburger Helper (1 cup prepared) – Yellow 5 & 6	7.7	1040
Scalloped Potatoes (1/2 cup prepared) – Yellow 5 & 6	1.4	190
M&M Milk Chocolate (48 Pieces) – Blue 1 & 2, Yellow 5 & 6, Red 40	29.5	2,950
M&M Peanuts (15) – Blue 1 & 2, Yellow 5 & 6, Red 40	14.1	1,410
Skittles Original(61) –Blue 1 & 2, Yellow 5 & 6, Red 40	33.2	3,320
Reese's Pieces (51) – Blue 1, Yellow 5 & 6, Red 40	6.6	660
Rainbow Nerds (1 tablespoon) – Blue 1 & 2, Yellow 5 & 6, Red 40	3.7	370
Sprees (8 pieces) – Blue 2, Yellow 5, Red 40	1.9	230
Red Jawbreakers (3) – Red 40	1.2	130
Orange Jawbreakers (3) – Yellow 5 & 6, Red 40	0.4	50
Purple Jawbreakers (3) – Blue 1 & 2, Red 40	0.7	70
Green Jawbreakers (3) – Blue 1 & 2, Yellow 5 & 6	0.5	50
Yellow Jawbreakers (3) – Yellow 5 & 6	0.2	27

Notes: * AFC stands for artificial food colorant ** Assumes no alumina extender and 2 atoms of aluminum per molecule of colorant, except 3 for Yellow 5, and assumes a mixture of 4 colors to be approximately 10% aluminum.

Increase Dissolved Silica in Your Diet

In their 1997 book, "Prescription for Nutritional Healing", J. F. Balch, M.D., and P.A. Balch, C.N.C., pointed out:

> *"Silicon counteracts the effects of aluminum on the body and is important in the prevention of Alzheimer's disease and osteoporosis. Silicon levels decrease with ageing, and, therefore, are needed in larger amounts by the elderly"*

The dissolved mineral silica (OSA, $Si(OH)_4$, orthosilicic acid) is required by our body for both protection from aluminum absorption by our brains[455] and for maintaining bone mineral density (BMD) and collagen health by stimulating collagen type 1 synthesis[483-485]. Quartz (silicon dioxide, SiO_2) in contact with water very slowly dissolves to make a dilute solution of OSA. Silicon is an atom in OSA that comprises 29% of OSA by weight. Silicon should not be confused with silicones that are not natural and are used for lubricants and cosmetic implants.

Dilute solutions of OSA are available as mineral waters, with Starkey and Fiji having 20-36mg/L of silicon as OSA. When OSA is concentrated at higher levels it polymerizes. Only stabilized OSA can be sold as a concentrate in capsule or liquid form. The most common version is choline stabilized OSA sold under the trade name Biosil made by Natural Factors. Colloidal silica made by firms, such as Eidon, is 2.5% by weight polymerized silica that is minimally bioavailable (see table in this section). Colloidal solutions have a faint blueish haze because the colloidal particles of silica polymer scatter the blue portion of the visible light spectrum.

In 1988 Carlisle and Curran at UCLA School of Public Health were the first to find that 23 month old rats, having been feed an aluminum and low soluble silicon diet, accumulated aluminum in their brains while 28 month old rats, having been fed aluminum and high soluble silicon (OSA) diet, did not accumulate aluminum in their brains[455]. They concluded:

> *"Dietary silicon supplementation thus appeared to be protective against aluminum accumulation in an ageing brain."*

Carlisle and Curran also found that silicon in different brain regions of these 28 month old rats was independent of dietary silicon supplementation. They suggested that silicon is accumulated by the brain as an essential element in the brain[455]. Silicon's essentiality could stem from its' ability to protect the brain from aluminum neurotoxicity.

Kristien Van Dyke in 2000 measured the silicon (OSA) content of blood serum in different aged individuals[486]. She found very high levels of OSA in infants less than a year old and extremely low levels in pregnant mothers. Van Dyke came to a startling conclusion:

> "The explanation of the high silicon levels of the infant group, especially (<1yr), may be that pregnant mothers offer their silicon to the growing fetus ..."

The graph of the Van Dyke's data brings this into sharper focus in the following figure:

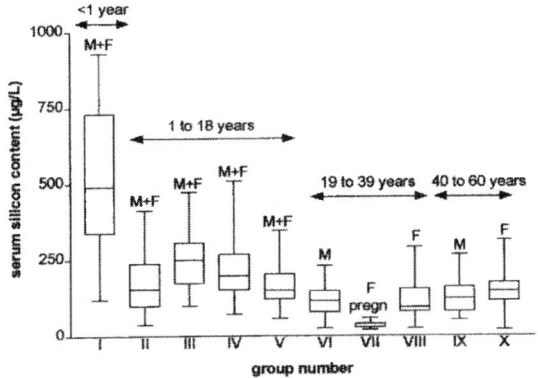

Figure 6 – Box plot of serum silicon content of various groups
(M: male; F: female; F pregn: pregnant women)[486]

Since soluble silicon in the blood serum is OSA, is it possible there are high levels of OSA in breastmilk? In 1990 Tanaka found levels of silica in breastmilk of 470 to 670ug/liter from 1 week to 1 month of birth[487]. These findings suggest that OSA is a required nutrient that mothers have evolved to supply to the fetus and infant. OSA not only lowers the levels of absorbed aluminum in the brain[455] but also improves bone mineral density (BMD) and strength[474,483]. Therefore regular OSA supplementation is recommended during and after pregnancy to protect the fetus and infant from aluminum absorption and improve their bone strength.

Silica from natural sources comes primarily from grains, vegetables, and products of grains, such as beer. The following table of unprocessed foods provides guidance on which foods have more silica content[488]. Note that high silica content does not necessarily mean that the silica is dissolvable, absorbed, and therefore bioavailable. The numbers in parenthesis are the percentage of absorbed and bioavailable silica in 100 grams of unprocessed food[469,489].

Unprocessed Food (100 grams)	**Silica Content (milligrams) & (% absorbed and bioavailable)**
Oats (oat bran includes husk/hulls)	595 (49%)
Millet	500 (49%)
Barley	233 (49%)
Potatoes	200 (21%)
Whole wheat grain	158 (49%)
Jerusalem artichoke	36 (21%)
Red Beets	21 (21%)
Corn	19 (21%)
Asparagus	18 (21%)
High bran cereal	10 (49%)
Rye	17 (49%)
Raisin (seedless)	8.2 (44%)
Banana (peeled)	5.4 (4%)
Corn Flakes	2.4 (49%)
Green Beans	2.4 (44%)
Whole Grain Bread	2.3 - 4.5 (49%)
Brown Rice (with husks)	2.1 (41%)
Beer (alcoholic or non-alcoholic)	1.9 (64%)

Fluids account for 20 to 30% of our dietary intake of silica and the ingestion of solid foods account for the rest. In order to be absorbed the solid foods must be hydrolyzed in our gastrointestinal (GI) tract. Since the kidney is the major route for silica excretion, urinary silicon levels are an indicator of silica absorption and bioavailability.

A semi-quantitative study was performed measuring the dietary intake of silica in foods eaten by members of the Framingham study[489]. A 126-item food frequency questionnaire was filled out to get a measure of what is consumed on average by members of the study. A second part of the study involved overnight fasting of healthy volunteers followed by ingestion of a test meal and then 6 more hours of fasting. Throughout this period of time the volunteers only drank ultra-high purity water containing negligible silicon content. Urine samples were taken and analyzed for silicon as a measure of silica absorption and bioavailability. The results indicated that between 13 and 62mg/day of silicon was ingested per day and 43% of this silicon was absorbed and bioavailable as dissolved silica (OSA). The major food sources for silica among women were bananas and string beans accounting for 17% of dietary silica intake. The major food source for silica among men was beer and bananas accounting for 25% of dietary silica intake. Women have less bioavailable silica than men because men consume more beer than women. For children the major dietary source of silica is from cereals (68% of total dietary intake).

Most of the silicon in the grains and vegetables we eat is in the husks, hulls, and skin. Processed foods have the silica rich husks, hulls, and skins removed thereby lowering their silica levels. Our paleo hunter gatherer ancestors had a diet much richer in silica than our modern diet. Note from the box plot in figure 6 that as we age our serum silicon levels decline. Intake of silica decreases significantly with age declining at a rate of 100μg/year of age[483,489]. This decline in serum silica at least partially accounts for why plasma levels of aluminum increase with age[53] resulting in an increased rate of aluminum accumulation in elderly brains[28].

Therefore OSA supplementation is recommended particularly as you age and when you are pregnant and breast feeding. OSA supplementation is also recommended for children.

The following table compares the bioavailability and daily cost of different silica supplements:

Silica Supplements[417,469]				
Supplement	Dose/Day	Silicon\Dose\Day	Bioavailable	Cost/Day
Mineral Water[A]	3 - 4 cups	25.5-34mg	11 – 14.7mg	$1.00 - $1.50
Silicade[B]	3 - 4 cups	25.5-34mg	11 – 14.7mg	$0.04 - $0.05[C]
Choline Stab OSA[D]	10 drops	10mg	1.7mg	$0.42
Choline Stab OSA[E]	2 veg caps	10mg	1.7mg	$0.83
Colloidal Silica[F]	30 drops	175mg	0.15mg	$0.60
Colloidal Silica[G]	10cc	163mg	0.40mg	$0.59
Bamboo[H]	1cap(300mg)	99mg	0.29mg	$0.10
Horsetail[I]	1cap(500mg)	16.5mg	0.11mg	$0.04
Diatomaceous Earth[H]	625mg	<2.9mg	0.07mg	$0.01

A. Fiji and Starkey – Mineral Waters; B. Silicade - preparation Chapter 5; C. Excluding cost of tap water; D. Biosil Choline Stab. OSA; E. Biosil Veg Caps; F. Eidon – Ionic Minerals Silica Concentrate; G. Saguna – Silicolgel Colloidal OSA; H. Swanson; I. Swanson; J. Swanson

Safety of Silica Supplementation

OSA is the monomeric bioavailable form of silica commonly found in rivers, lakes, aquifers, and drinking waters around the world[490]. The amount OSA in drinking water varies widely depending upon the source (see Chapter 5). In the U.S. 160mg per liter of dissolved silicates, such as OSA, are generally recognized as safe (e.g. GRAS) in drinking water[462]. 160 mg per liter of OSA corresponds to 47mg per liter of silicon and 100mg per liter of silica as SiO_2. The adequate intake of water per day is 3 liters for men and 2.3 liters for women. This level of water intake corresponds to a maximum safe level of silicon intake per day of 141mg for men and 108mg for women. Therefore, drinking 3 to 4 cups of supplemental silica water each day containing a total of 25.5 to 34mg of silicon is well below the GRAS level for dissolved silicates.

Biosil supplementation is a combination of 200mg of choline with 10mg of silicon. Note that only 17% of the silica in Biosil is bioavailable as compared with 43% bioavailability with mineral water and Silicade. Also there is a 70% greater risk of lethal prostate cancer with high (500mg/day) choline diets[471]. The European Food Safety Authority therefore recommends that liquid choline stabilized OSA be taken at a maximum dose of 10 mg. of silicon that is complexed with 200mg of choline per day[472,473].

Jarrow Formulas have developed a patent pending product called JarroSil that contains molecular clusters of stabilized silicic acid. Although JarroSil is less expensive per ounce than BioSil, JarroSil only contains 0.4 mg of silicon per drop as compared with 1 mg of silicon per drop in BioSil. Jarrow Formulas claims that JarroSil is "highly bioavailable". Note that colloidal silica is also clusters of stabilized silicic acid and only 0.25% or less of the silica in colloidal silica is bioavailable as compared with 43% bioavailability with mineral water and Silicade. Also silica colloids made synthetically and sold commercially as nanoparticles have been tested *in vitro* on four different types of human cells and shown to have cytotoxicity[474].

In Europe a company, Silicium Laboratories, is promoting a non-natural silica as a supplement called monomethyl silanetriol (MMST). MMST in water is absorbed by the gut and made 64% bioavailable when dissolved in alcohol free beer[469]. There is no data showing that MMST facilitates elimination of aluminum from the body. In addition, the lack of toxicity data on MMST makes it impossible to recommend MMST at the present time[491].

The safest strategy for silica supplementation at the present time is to use high silica mineral water or make and drink 3 to 4 cups a day of Silicade (see Chapter 5). Silicade is much less expensive than high silica mineral water, such as Starkey or Fiji Water.

Aerobically Exercise

We all know the difference between walking and running when we exercise. When walking both our heart and breathing rates are slightly increased and when running our heart and breathing rates are significantly increased. This increase in heart and breathing rates keeps the oxygen level of our blood, brain, and muscles constant. When performed regularly both of these aerobic exercises, walking and running, increase our aerobic fitness and endurance. When a several minute sprint is added to this aerobic exercise routine we push our heart and breathing rate to the limit where we can no longer get sufficient oxygen into our blood. This is called anaerobic exercise. It results in lower than normal oxygen levels in our brain and muscles and painful lactic acid build-up in our muscles.

Aerobic exercise when performed correctly is not painful and will prevent or postpone the onset of Alzheimer's. I recommend non-impact exercise performed by walking, rowing, stepping, and bicycling. In order to be effective aerobic exercise should be performed at least three times a week for 40 minutes with a heart rate of 60% to 75% of your peak heart rate reserve. Your peak heart rate reserve is the difference between your resting heart rate and your maximum heart rate. Your maximum heart rate is 220 beats per minute (bpm) minus your age in years. For example if you are 70 years of age with a resting heart rate of 50 bpm, your maximum heart rate is 220 – 70 = 150 bpm and your peak heart rate reserve is the 100 bpm difference between 50 and 150 bpm. In this example 60% to 75% of your peak heart rate reserve is therefore 110 to 125 bpm. Before beginning an aerobic exercise program I recommend a doctor supervised stress test.

The results of a multi-year study of 18,670 men and women were recently published in the Archives of Internal Medicine. The study, beginning in 1970, involved a mid-life fitness evaluation. Then 30 years later, when the participants were in their 70's and 80's, their medical records were checked. The results revealed that those who were most aerobically fit in their 40's and 50's suffered from AD only in the final five years of their lives. Those who were less fit in their 40's and 50's suffered from AD in the final 10 to 20 years of their lives. Even though both groups had the same frequency of getting AD, those who were most aerobically fit at mid-life lived longer and suffered with AD for a shorter period time than those who were less fit[492].

In our brains during aerobic exercise there is a choreographed production of biochemicals that are both neuron growth promoters and neuroprotective cleansing agents counteracting the effects of accumulated aluminum and associated Aβ plaques:

Neuropeptide YY (a.k.a. PYY) – Aerobic exercise stimulates the production of a small neuropeptide called PYY[493]. Injections of PYY in mice has been found to lower both aluminum absorption from the gut into the blood by 54% and aluminum accumulation in the brain by 86%[494]. This dramatic decrease in aluminum accumulation in the brain suggests that PYY not only decreases absorption but also cleanses the brain of aluminum.

In humans aerobic exercise increases PYY production by 23-24% both during and after acute and long-term exercise training[495,496]. In addition PYY levels remain high for an hour after exercise[495]. Rising PYY levels are observed during and after exercise in adolescents and adults with a normal body mass index (BMI) and in adolescents with a BMI in the 85th percentile or higher, but surprisingly not significantly in obese adults[493,496,497]. This is possibly due to obese adults having less PYY in their blood than those with normal BMI[498]. Lower PYY in the blood of obese adults may account for why each unit of BMI at midlife predicts earlier onset of AD by 6.7 months[209]. Lower PYY in the blood of obese adults results in more aluminum accumulation in their brains and a higher risk of AD.

In addition to lowering aluminum accumulation, PYY is a regulator of energy metabolism[496]. Protein consumption, but not carbohydrate consumption, also increases PYY production[498]. PYY is produced by cells in the stomach and released into the blood. When PYY reaches the hypothalamus in the brain, the feeling of hunger is decreased[493,496]. High PYY levels cause appetite suppression in those people with both normal and high BMIs[494-496,498]. Therefore for optimum appetite suppression eat some protein and eat slowly to allow the PYY to reach your hypothalamus.

Somatotropin and Somatostatin – In AD patients Aβ plaque accumulation is observed almost a decade before cognitive impairment. Removal of the Aβ plaque may postpone the onset of cognitive impairment. Somatotropin and somatostatin facilitate the removal of Aβ plaques from the brain. Physical exercise has been shown to stimulate the anterior pituitary gland of the brain to produce the peptide hormone somatotropin (a.k.a. human growth hormone)[500]. In response to high levels of somatotropin for periods longer than 15 minutes[501], the peptide hormone somatostatin is produced by the hypothalamus to inhibit somatotropin production. Therefore thirty minutes of aerobic exercise causes somatotropin levels to peak and decline and somatostatin levels to increase in the brain[500,502].

Neprilysin is a membrane bound zinc-dependent enzyme that degrades Aβ peptides and Aβ plaques. The activity of neprilysin is increased by aerobic exercise because somatostatin enhances neprilysin's activity[503]. Somatostatin levels decline with age and are reduced by 47% in the temporal cortex of the brains of AD patients as compared with normal brains[504]. These changes may contribute to the increase in Aβ plaques in the brains of AD patients. Aerobic exercise for 30 minutes increases the level of somatostatin that in turn increases neprilysin's rate of Aβ plaque degradation thereby postponing the onset of AD and possibly preventing AD.

Norepinephrine - Norepinephrine both counteracts the negative effect of aluminum on the working memory and improves the working memory in the frontal cortex of the brain[505-507]. Aerobic exercise increases norepinephrine plasma levels by as much as 14 fold in both men and women[508,509]. People who exercise regularly (i.e. trained people) produce more norepinephrine than people who do not exercise regularly (i.e. untrained people). More than twice the amount of norepinephrine is produced during equivalent aerobic exercise performed by trained versus untrained men and women of 22-45 years of age[509,510]. Trained 65 year old men produce 50% more norepinephrine than untrained men of the same age while aerobically exercising[510].

The locus coeruleus (a.k.a. LC, locus ceruleus), located in the brain stem, is the principle norepinephrine producing site of the brain[511]. In the brains of AD patients there is up to an 80% loss of the norepinephrine producing LC neurons[511]. For details on how norepinephrine counteracts aluminum's negative impact on working memory see "Neurochemistry of Memory Improvement by Exercise" at the end of this chapter.

Brain Derived Neurotrophic Factor (a.k.a. BDNF) - Aerobic exercise stimulates the production of BDNF in the brain that has been found to stimulate the process of neurogenesis. Neurogenesis is involved in creating a network of neuronal connections required for memory storage. Neurogenesis also adds volume to the hippocampus. Hippocampal volumes are larger in more-fit older adults and these larger hippocampal volumes are associated with improved spatial memory. BDNF levels are lower in the the brains of those 90+ year olds with dementia versus those without dementia[512].

The hippocampal region of the brain is where short-term memories are converted to long-term memories and where long-term episodic and spatial relationship memories are pre-sorted, processed, and stored. The dentate gyrus in the hippocampus is one of several regions in the brain where neural stem cells are converted to new neurons in a process called neurogenesis that continues to occur throughout one's lifetime. Neurogenesis in the adult human hippocampus was first observed in 1998 using a chemical label that permanently integrates into the DNA of dividing brain cells[513]. This finding was confirmed in 2013 by analyzing radioactive carbon in the DNA of brain cells. The amount of radioactive carbon in human DNA declined after 1963, due to the above ground nuclear test ban treaty, providing a marker to distinguish old from new DNA. From the amount of radioactive carbon in DNA of 55 deceased patients it was found that one third of the hippocampal neurons are renewed throughout one's life amounting to the addition of 1400 new neurons a day[159]. In spite of this increase in neurons, hippocampal volume declines 1-2% per year as a part of ageing. In individuals with mild cognitive impairment there is a larger decline than normal and with AD this decline in volume is much more pronounced.

In 2011 a study of 120 older adults was published[514]. In this study, the older adults were paid to excercise for one year. At 6 and 12 months their hippocampal volume, BDNF serum levels, and spatial memories were tested. Half of the study group (mean age of 67.6) walked aerobically for 40 minutes 3 days a week while maintaining 60-75% of their peak heart rate reserve. The other half of the study group (mean age of 65.5) did not aerobically excercise but instead non-aerobically exercised for 40 minutes 3 days a week with:

- four muscle toning exercises using dumbells or resistance bands
- two exercises designed to improve balance
- one yoga sequence
- one exercise of their choice

Hippocampal volume increased 2% over the year in the group that aerobically exercised by walking and declined by 1.4% in the other group. Also in the group that exercised aerobically by walking both spatial memory improvement and increased serum BDNF levels correlated with increased hippocampal volume. These results indicate that starting an aerobic exercise program in later life can lead to improvements in hippocampal volume, spatial memory, and cognitive function. **An aerobic exercise program will prevent or postpone the onset of AD.**

Aluminum Excretion by Sweating During Exercise – Perspiration is another way that aluminum is excreted by the body. Sweating while exercising lowers aluminum levels in the body[515]. It has been shown that a diet that includes a mineral water high in dissolved silicic acid facilitates this pathway for aluminum excretion[516].

Neurochemistry of Memory Improvement by Exercise

A neurochemical mechanism has been proposed to explain how norepinephrine, produced during aerobic exercise, improves one's working memory and counteracts the negative effect of accumulated aluminum on the working memory. Working memory is defined as the brain's capacity to retain, manipulate and utilize information. The prefrontal cortex is the location of working memory. In the prefrontal cortex co-located on the neuronal dendrites there are both:

- *Hyperpolarized cyclic nucleotide – gated ion channels (HCN)*
- *Alpha 2A adrenergic receptors (AAR)*

Cyclic adenosine monophosphate (cAMP) in the brain holds HCN channels open lowering synaptic efficiency and preventing information required for the working memory to be passed across synapses. Norepinephrine produced during aerobic exercise stimulates the AARs that inhibit cAMP biosynthesis from ATP. This lowers the cAMP concentration that in turn keeps HCN channels closed, thereby improving working memory in the prefrontal cortex[505].

Aging human brains have higher levels of cAMP and this holds HCN channels open in ageing brains. The accumulated aluminum in older brains inhibits the calcium/calmodulin complex from activating the enzyme PDE4A that normally degrades cAMP. Therefore aluminum increases the cAMP concentration in aging brains[506]. Agents like norepinephrine that inhibit cAMP production or close HCN channels can restore normal working memory in the prefrontal cortex and reverse the effects of accumulated aluminum[507]. Therefore aerobic exercise reverses the negative effect of accumulated aluminum on the working memory.

Another stimulant for AARs is guanfacine that also improves working memory and mental attention in the prefrontal cortex. Guanfacine is sold under the brand name Intuniv as a time-release pill. Resveratrol, sold for improved mitochondrial and cardiac function, increases cAMP and therefore can't be recommended[506].

Avoid Lack of Sleep

Enhance Aβ protein and aluminum clearance: Sleep does more than relieve the feeling of sleepiness. It has been found that both natural sleep and anesthesia induced sleep are associated with a 60% increase in the interstitial space in the brain. The interstitial space is the space between neurons. It is filled with interstitial fluid. This increased space results in a significant increase in convective exchange of cerebrospinal fluid with the interstitial fluid. This convective flux has been shown to increase the rate of beta-amyloid (Aβ) protein clearance during sleep as compared to the rate of Aβ clearance while awake[517].

Aβ protein as oligomers and plaque in the brain is complexed with metal ions including aluminum. Purging these metal laden Aβ protein complexes from the brain is an excellent way to lower levels of accumulated aluminum in the brain[137]. Factors that slow the rate of clearance of beta-amyloid (Aβ) from the brain account for its' build- up over time. Enhancing the rate of clearance will postpone the onset of AD and possibly prevent AD.

Consolidate Memories: Sleep has also been implicated in the off-line reprocessing of recently acquired memory. This process is called memory consolidation. The neurochemical mechanism for memory consolidation in mice has been found to involve a molecular cascade ending in the production of a molecule named P-CREB, that increases the transcription of genes responsible for brain derived neurotrophic factor (BDNF) production [179,180,518,519]. Rapid eye movement (REM) sleep has been found to speed up this molecular cascade in the mouse brain increasing P-CREB production[520] and improving long term memory, brain plasticity, and learning[181,182].

Lower Aβ Peptide and Plaque Levels: By increasing P-CREB production, REM sleep also increases the transcription of genes responsible for somatostatin production[179,180,518,519]. There is an inverse relationship between P-CREB levels and Aβ peptide in mouse brain. This is probably due to P-CREB increasing somatostatin levels that thereby increasing neprilysin activity that in turn lowers Aβ peptide and plaque levels. Therefore REM sleep can postpone the onset of AD by increasing both P-CREB and somatostatin levels in hippocampal neurons[103].

The beneficial effects of REM sleep can be negated by aluminum accumulating in the brain. It has been found that aluminum chloride in the diet of neonatal and postnatal rats inhibits P-CREB production by modifying the calcium/calmodulin complex[520]. This in turn lowers both hippocampal BDNF and somatostatin production resulting in long term memory impairment, spatial learning impairment, and Aβ peptide accumulation[101,102].

Sleep Better with Daytime Solar or Blue Lighting: Orexin (a.k.a. hypocretin) is a neurotransmitter produced in the hypothalamus by 10,000 to 20,000 orexin neurons that extend over the entire brain and spinal cord. Orexin promotes wakefulness and regulates arousal, wakefulness, and appetite. Circadian rhythms are controlled by high levels of orexin during the day and low levels at night. In AD, dysregulation of the orexinergic system results in too much orexin in the cerebrospinal fluid[521]. In mild and moderate AD this dysregulation causes more awakenings and less REM sleep during the night resulting in greater than normal daytime sleepiness. This condition is correlated with cognitive impairment in AD[146] possibly due to more Aβ protein accumulation and less Aβ clearance at night[521].

Melanopsin, like orexin, promotes wakefulness and is involved in neuronal communication with the brain's clock. The brain's clock controls circadian rhythms and is called the suprachiasmatic nucleus. Melanopsin, one of the three light-sensitive retinal opsin proteins in the human eye, is found in neurons in the retina called intrinsically photosensitive retinal ganglion cells (ipRGCs). Blue light photostimulates melanopsin in ipRGCs linked neuronally to the brain's clock[522]. The solar spectrum reaching the earth has a strong blue component. Therefore exposure to solar lighting during daytime hours is recommended to photostimulate melanopsin maintaining daytime wakefulness. This daytime wakefulness helps to maintain circadian rhythms and a good night's sleep resulting in less Aβ protein accumulation and more Aβ clearance.

Aβ oligomers complexed with aluminum compared with other metals are less prone to aggregate and are sufficiently small to scatter blue light[522]. The percentage of blue light being scattered to total blue light entering the eye increases as Aβ oligomer concentration rises in the retina[523]. Also ipRGC degeneration has been recently observed in AD patients[524]. Therefore some patients with AD need to see more blue light to compensate for both scattering and degeneration in order to maintain circadian rhythm. Thus it is not surprising that using lights with enhanced output in the blue spectral region during the day allows some elderly patients with AD to sleep better at night[525]. Moderation is called for as long-term blue light exposure can cause retinal damage. Mixing exposure to both solar and blue lighting during the day is a good compromise.

Sleep and Stroke Risk: Moderation may also be called for in the case of sleep. Recently 9,692 people's average nightly duration of sleep over a 9.5 year period was evaluated for correlation with risk of stroke. The participants were 41 to 82 years of age. During this time period there were 346 participants who had a stroke. It was found that people who routinely slept longer than 8 hours per night were 46% more likely to get a stroke as compared with those who routinely slept less than 8 hours per night[526]. The correlation was strongest for people 63 and over having an increased risk of hemorrhagic stroke by persistently sleeping for more than 8 hours.

A meta-analysis was performed on six studies including 559,252 people in 7 countries. Over the 7 to 34 year periods of these studies the participants had 11,695 stroke events. This meta-analysis came to the same conclusion that people who sleep longer than 8 hours are 45% more likely to have a stroke[526].

Sleep may be an indicator of increased stroke risk and not be a cause of stroke. For instance the duration of sleep has also been correlated with both carotid artery atherosclerosis, as measured by artery wall thickness, and atrial fibrillation[527,528]. This makes sense as the heart must pump harder with atherosclerosis and a-Fib, which requires more sleep for the heart's daily recovery. As discussed in Chapter 2, atherosclerosis and a-Fib are increased risk factors for stroke.

Avoid Head Trauma

Head trauma usually results from accidents and lifestyle choices that impact the frequency and severity of head trauma. For instance, the severity of accidental head trauma can be lowered by wearing a seat belt while driving or a helmet while biking or motorcycling. The frequency of accidental head trauma can be decreased by avoiding contact sports such as football and soccer. Since falls result in 2/3 of traumatic brain injuries, avoid falling by keeping walkways free of objects, loose rugs, and pets and by using a walking or balancing aid, such as a pole, walking stick, cane, or walker. The use of metal studded over-boots when walking on snowy or icy surfaces is recommended.

Acute Traumatic Encephalopathy

A study was done in California with 164,661 patients. Participants were limited to patients:

- with a single traumatic brain injury (TBI) or
- with non-TBI trauma (NIT)
- who were 55 years or older between 2004-2005
- who did not have baseline dementia
- who were not diagnosed with dementia less than a year after the initial trauma
- who did not die during hospitalization

The patients were identified in a California statewide administrative health database of emergency department and inpatient visits and were followed until December 31st of 2011. The NIT group was used as the control population. Of the 51,799 patients who had TBI 4,361 (8.4%) developed dementia, while of the 112,862 patients who had NIT only 5.9% developed dementia. Those with moderate to severe TBI at 55 years or older or mild TBI at 65 years or older had an increased risk of developing dementia. Since 66.4% of the cases of TBI were due to falls, preventive measures are strongly recommended[529].

Chronic Traumatic Encephalopathy (CTE)

A post mortem analysis of brains from 84 individuals (mean age 59.5 years) with repetitive mild brain injury was compared with the brains from 18 age-matched and gender-matched individuals who had no history of repetitive mild brain injury. CTE was found to be characterized by an ordered and predictable progression of HPτ and NFT accumulation through the nervous system that occurs with widespread axonal lesions and loss. CTE was the sole diagnosis in 43 of the 84 individuals. CTE with motor neuron disease was diagnosed in 18 cases, CTE and AD in 7 cases, CTE and Lewy body disease in 11 cases, and CTE and frontotemporal lobar degeneration in 4 cases. Most of these cases of CTE were formerly athletes who engaged in a contact sport[530].

The scientific evidence that CTE does increase the risk of dementia is just beginning to reshape our sports culture. Parents are beginning to consider if their children should participate in a contact sport. Sports teams who hire professional athletes are coping with the potential of a class action suit from former athletes who have dementia or their families, if the former athletes committed suicide.

Conclusion of Lifestyle Choices and Dementia

Stop Smoking: Smoking 2 pack of cigarettes a day is correlated with an increased risk of vascular dementia and AD. Even though the nicotine derived from smoking may improve your concentration and long-term memory, the risk is not worth the reward. Smoking volatilizes aluminum in tobacco and cannabis adding to the body burden of aluminum. Cigarette smoking is the single largest cause of premature death in the U.S., killing approximately 490,000 people a year.

Enjoy Periodic Moderate Alcohol Consumption: Chronic moderate alcohol drinking has been shown to lead to higher levels of homocysteine and high blood pressure. Make drinking alcohol a special occasion not a daily routine.

Avoid aluminum ingestion: Aluminum is a known neurotoxin that should not be ingested.

- **Avoid aluminum containing pharmaceuticals** – Read labels and lists of ingredients. Do not use antacid tablets containing aluminum

- **Filter your drinking water** - Use a Brita pour-through pitcher system with filter number OB03 to remove aluminum from your tap water.

- **Avoid using aluminum cookware** – Use stainless steel and cast iron for cooking. Use non-stick aluminum foil with the non-stick surface against food or use a layer of plastic wrap between aluminum foil and food.

- **Use aluminum free antiperspirants and astringents** - Use either Arm & Hammer's "Essentials" or Tom's of Maine "Original" deodorants that are both aluminum free. Use Epsom salts and avoid aluminum containing astringents for mild skin irritation.

- **Don't purchase and store beverages or food in aluminum containers** - as they will slowly add aluminum to the water and beverages. Purchase and store beverages and food in glass or plastic.

- **Avoid using soy-based infant formula** – Purchase non-soy based formula.

Increase Dissolved Silica in Your Diet: Add some dissolvable silica to your diet as a daily supplement in order to increase your aluminum excretion and lower aluminum absorption by your brain.

Aerobically Exercise: Aerobic exercise has the following benefits:

- Results in the destruction and clean-up of amyloid plaque in the brain
- Increases neurogenesis in the dentate gyrus of the hippocampus resulting in larger hippocampal volume and increased memory
- Stimulates production of PYY that lowers aluminum absorption and accumulation.
- Reverses the effect of aluminum in the prefrontal cortex thereby improving working memory

Aerobic exercise has been shown to perform these benefits in older adults even when the exercise program is begun in later life. This method of postponing the onset of AD and possibly preventing AD involves an investment of time but not money. These benefits of aerobic exercise are available to anyone mobile enough to achieve 60-75% of their peak heart rate reserve through aerobically exercising for 40 minutes at least three times a week.

Avoid Lack of Sleep: Research suggests that the restorative function of sleep may be due to increased neurogenesis and the enhanced removal of neurotoxic waste products, such as metal laden $A\beta$ protein from the brain. This occurs by three mechanisms:

- Increased convective exchange of cerebrospinal fluid with the interstitial fluid
- Increased BDNF production that stimulates neurogenesis
- Increased neprilysin activity that degrades $A\beta$ protein in the brain

REM sleep increases P-CREB production that in turn increases somatostatin production. Somatostatin increases neprilysin activity and BNDF production, both of which may be responsible for the observed memory consolidation during REM sleep.

AD is associated with dysregulation of the orexinergic system causing a lack of sleep resulting in higher levels of $A\beta$ peptides in the brain and less memory consolidation. Exposure to normal solar lighting is recommended to stimulate melanopsin production during the day. This helps to maintain circadian rhythms and a good night's sleep. Daytime lighting with a strong blue spectral component results in AD patients having better quality sleep, but can't be recommended routinely due to blue light induced retinal damage.

Avoid Head Trauma: Acute and chronic head trauma increases the risk of dementia. Therefore avoiding both falls and contact sports is strongly suggested. Since falls result in 2/3 of traumatic brain injuries, avoid falling by keeping walkways free of objects, loose rugs, and pets and by using a walking or balancing aid, such as a pole, walking stick, cane, or walker. The use of metal studded over-boots when walking on snowy or icy surfaces is recommended.

Chapter 7– Drugs for Alzheimer's Disease

"Medicine is only palliative, for back of disease lays the cause, and this cause no drug can reach." Wier Mitchel, M.D.

Knowing the cause of Alzheimer's disease (AD) is aluminum gives us ways to prevent, slow the progression, and combination therapies to reverse the progression of AD. But there are no known cures for AD making it a terminal disease. However there are palliative measures to relieve the symptoms of AD. This chapter reviews drugs available for slowing the progression of AD, combination therapies to reverse the progression of AD, palliative measures for AD, and future cures for AD now under development.

The current state of AD drug-development focuses on drugs for palliative relief and slowing the cognitive decline. In general there is a lack of understanding about identifying symptoms versus causes of AD. For instance the build-up of amyloid plaque in the brain is a hallmark of AD. However many people who have amyloid plaque in their brains have no cognitive decline. As described in Chapter 1 amyloid plaque is a symptom not a cause of AD.

Aβ oligomers, the precursors of amyloid plaque, are neurotoxic because they promote excessive calcium ion diffusion into neurons as discussed in Chapter 1. This neurotoxicity is enhanced by both aluminum forming complexes with Aβ oligomers and increased levels of Aβ oligomers for complexing with aluminum. Does a cure for AD involve lowering either or both Aβ oligomers and the amount of aluminum in the brain? Only longitudinal studies with drugs that lower either or both Aβ oligomers and aluminum will answer this question.

Aluminum is the primary cause of Alzheimer's, autism, and stroke because of the number of neurotoxic effects it has on the brain (see Chapters 1, 2, and 9). Therefore lowering aluminum ingestion, absorption, and accumulation in the brain is a recommended precaution that should be taken to prevent Alzheimer, autism and stroke.

Drugs for Slowing or Reversing the Progression of AD

Aluminum Chelators for Preventing and Reversing the Progression of AD

Desferoxamine: An AD treatment that has been shown to slow the rate of deterioration in activities of daily life is desferoxamine (a.k.a. DFO, desferrioxamine) injections. Cognitive decline in AD was slowed by 50% when 125 mg of DFO was administered intramuscularly for five days a week for two years[71]. In 1998 it was demonstrated that DFO could reverse the formation of NFTs in white rabbits from New Zealand that had been previously injected with aluminum[24]. DFO removes aluminum from the aluminum/HPτ complex and allows HPτ degradation by calpain. The degradation of HPτ reverses aluminum-induced neurofibrillary tangles (NFTs)[24]. DFO chelates both aluminum and iron trivalent ions and is FDA-approved for treatment of acute iron poisoning. But in the U.S. DFO is not FDA-approved for treatment of aluminum toxicity or AD. The problems with DFO are the number of required injections and its' ability to remove not only aluminum but also iron from the body. A more ideal candidate for slowing or reversing AD would be a complexing agent for aluminum that can be taken orally and does not complex iron.

Dissolved Silica: Dissolved silica (a.k.a. OSA, orthosilicic acid) taken orally binds tightly to aluminum in the blood and facilitates its excretion but does not facilitate the excretion of iron. Thereby OSA lowers aluminum level in the blood and decreases aluminum retention by the brain[51,452,454,455] without effecting iron levels[37,38]. It is theorized that dissolved silica in the brains of AD patients will also bind to aluminum in the brain. This will lower aluminum levels in the brain and improve cognition as does DFO.

This theory was tested in 2013 when fifteen AD patients were given 1 liter/day of silicon rich mineral water for 12 weeks. This treatment was shown to facilitate the removal of aluminum via urination without any concomitant affect upon the urinary excretion of the essential metals iron and copper. Over the 12 weeks of silicon-rich mineral water therapy the body burden of aluminum fell in individuals with Alzheimer's disease. At the same time cognitive performance showed clinically relevant improvements in at least 3 out of 15 individuals[37,38]. This reversal in cognitive decline is encouraging but what about larger and longer term studies?

A 15 year study (e.g. Paquid) was conducted in the Gironde and Dordogne parishes of France by measuring the dissolved silica and aluminum levels in tap and bottled water drank by 1,925 people and their incidence of dementia or AD[76,414]. The dissolved silica levels in tap water ranged from 4.2 to 22.4mg/L and in bottled water they ranged from 2 to 77.6mg/L. The aluminum levels in tap water varied from 1 to 514mcg/L. Mean consumption of water was 0.94L/day with a standard deviation of 0.49L/day. The study came to two conclusions:

- The risk of AD and dementia are both twice as high after drinking water with $\geq$100mcg/L of aluminum.
- The risk of AD is lower after drinking water with $\geq$11.25mg/L of dissolved silica.

The data from the first 8 years of the Paquid study in France[414] were analyzed looking at the following five variables in the drinking water[451,461]:

- Aluminum
- Silica
- Calcium
- pH
- Aluminum – pH Interaction

The conclusions of this study are that drinking water with aluminum at low pH and with low silica levels lowers cognition more than at high pH and high silica levels[451]. Also calcium at concentrations $\geq$75mg/L ($\geq$75ppm) has a significant protective effect on cognition[451,461]. Aluminum has deleterious effects on cognition at concentrations as low as 3.5mcg per liter at low pH and with low silica and calcium levels[451]. Aluminum is most complexed with dissolved silica at high pH not at low pH (see Chapter 5 "Chemistry of Orthosilicic Acid Complexation with Aluminum"). Therefore aluminum is more bioavailable (i.e. absorbed by the gut) at low pH in spite of dissolved silica being present. Also since calcium and aluminum compete for absorption in the gut[310], it is not surprising that high levels of calcium in drinking water lower aluminum absorption and thereby protect cognition.

A second long term study (e.g. EPIDOS) was performed over the period 1992 to 2000 on a cohort of 1,462 women aged 75 and older living in Toulouse, France[531]. Dissolved silica acid was mainly supplied by bottled water with concentrations ranging from 8.6 to 36.4mg/L. Aluminum varied from 63mcg/L in their tap water to 3 to 32mcg/L in their bottled water. The silica levels in the women's water and their cognitive performance or diagnosis of AD were statistically evaluated for a correlation. Women drinking water higher in silica were less likely to be diagnosed with AD and had higher cognitive performance than women drinking water with low silica levels. In this study the aluminum levels in the women's drinking water averaged at 23mcg/day and ranged from 3 to 63mcg/L[531]. It is surprising that even at these low aluminum levels a correlation between lower AD incidence and high levels of silica was observed.

Dicarboxylic and Tricarboxylic Acids: Researchers at the University of Barcelona found that citric, malic, and succinic acids were all effective as *in vivo* chelating agents for aluminum[532]. After mice were given daily doses for five weeks of aluminum nitrate (0.27mmol/kg) by injection into the body cavity (a.k.a. intraperitoneal), chelating agents were administered intraperitoneally for two weeks at doses equivalent to one quarter of their LD50. Each of the three acids significantly increased the excretion of aluminum and reduced its concentration in various organs and tissues. When compared with DFO it was found that both malic acid and DFO were most effective at increasing urinary excretion of aluminum. Also citric acid was found to be the most effective at increasing fecal excretion of aluminum[533]. Malic and succinic acids were found to be most effective at increasing survival rates in mice exposed to aluminum, and in removing four different types of aluminum from the spleen and liver of rats and mice[534].

Currently there is no human data available on the effectiveness of this class of aluminum chelators. Also there is no data on how these chelators effect aluminum levels in the brain. However there is experimental evidence in humans that OSA at 10mg/liter is more effective than citric acid at approximately 17gr/liter[535] in orange juice at lowering the concentration of aluminum in the blood after ingestion (see Figure 4)[51].

Combination Therapy to Reverse the Progression of AD

This book proposes a system for preventing AD with 7 supplements, 7 lifestyle choices, and a dissolved mineral for aluminum chelation. This raises the question that since this system prevents AD can it also act as a combination therapy for reversing mild cognitive impairment (MCI) caused by AD. Combination therapy has been shown to be effective against other chronic diseases such as cancer and HIV so why not AD?

By combining supplements, such as D3, taurine, and metal chelators like OSA, that combat the cause of AD (e.g. aluminum) with supplements that improve AD's neuro-metabolic dysfunction by increasing brain energy and memory, such as PQQ and CoQ10, and with supplements that keep your blood flowing smoothly through your brain, such as vitamin B12, 5-MTHF, vitamin K2-MK-4 and, if necessary TMG, we may have a better chance of reversing MCI caused by AD than with monotherapies involving a single drug.

In 2014 Dale E. Bredesen published the results of a study that tested if the progression of AD could be reversed by combination therapies[536]. Bredesen's study involved most of the same supplements and 2 of the 7 lifestyle choices described in this book in addition to several other supplements and lifestyle choices to achieve "metabolic enhancement for neurodegeneration (MEND)". The MEND study had 10 AD patients with MCI or subjective cognitive impairment (SCI). This anecdotal study showed that an individually tailored combination therapy involving supplements and lifestyle choices can reverse the progression of AD in 9 out of the 10 patients. Subjective or objective improvement in cognition was seen within the first 3 to 6 months of treatment. The tenth patient with late (4th) stage AD did not show improvement during the treatment. All six of the patients whose cognitive decline had a major impact on job performance returned to work during the MEND study. An important part of the individual tailoring involved checking for serum homocysteine levels as recommended in this book.

Mono Drug Therapies for Treating and Reversing AD

Allopregnanolone (Allo)) lowers the levels of intercellular Aβ peptides and reverses cognitive deficits and both the learning and long-term memory loss associated with AD in mice genetically modified to simulate AD[537]. Allo has also been shown to increase neurogenesis in the hippocampus of mice genetically modified to simulate AD[538]. Levels of Allo are reduced in the prefrontal cortex of AD patients[539]. Allo is only effective in the early stages of AD before extracellular Aβ peptides start to form plaque[537]. Allo is deemed safe in humans as it is biosynthesized in human brains. In women Allo production rates reach 100mg per day during the third trimester of pregnancy. Other than inducing drowsiness, Allo has no adverse effects. Allo can be administered intravenously and readily penetrates the blood-brain barrier.

In July 2013, at the Alzheimer's Association International Conference in Boston, Professor Roberta Diaz Brinton of the USC School of Pharmacy described her proposed work on a phase 1 human trial of Allo in participants with mild cognitive impairment due to AD and mild AD.

Memantine – Memantine blocks excess calcium diffusion through NMDA receptor channels as discussed in Chapter 1. There is increasing evidence that for some people memantine (trade name Namenda) may be an effective treatment for behavioral (i.e. aggression and agitation) and psychological symptoms in AD. Memantine has the advantage of being a safe treatment, with benefits for daily living and memory. Further research is still needed to confirm how effective memantine is in treating behavioral and psychological symptoms, but the evidence shows it is more effective than using antidepressants or anticonvulsants.

Cholinergic drugs affect acetylcholine and portions of the nervous system that use acetylcholine which is an important neurotransmitter required for memory[540]. Many common drugs and pharmaceuticals are anticholinergic and lower the concentration of acetylcholine in the body leading to mild cognitive impairment. Cholinergic drugs, such as a precursor of acetylcholine, increase the concentration of acetylcholine. Examples include:

- **Choline** has been shown to improve long-term memory and decrease the amount of leukoaraiosis (i.e. small brain regions with diminished blood flow) in human studies[541]. Note that low choline supplementation (200mg/day) may have benefits but there is a 70% greater risk of lethal prostate cancer with high (500mg/day) choline diets[471].

- **Dimethylaminoethanol** (DMAE), a natural product found in fish, has shown promise in improving concentration[542].

- **Meclofenoxate** (a.k.a. Lucidril) is a synthetic ester of DMAE and is approved by the FDA to treat the symptoms of senile dementia and AD by improving memory[543].

Administration of a cholinesterase inhibitor increases the concentration of acetylcholine by inhibiting its breakdown. Examples of cholinesterase inhibitors are:

- **Galantamine** (trade name Razadyne) is approved by the FDA for treatment of vascular dementia and mild to moderate AD. It enhances memory in brain-damaged adults[544].

- **Rivastigmine** (trade name Excelon) is approved to for mild and moderate AD.

- **Donepezil** (trade name Aricept) is approved to treat all stages of AD.

Rivastigmine and donepezil may also reduce the severity of some behavioral and psychological symptoms in dementia and help delay their onset. Cholinesterase inhibitors are especially effective in Lewy body dementia and dementia related to Parkinson's disease. These drugs treat agitation, apathy and psychotic symptoms including delusions, hallucinations, and disordered thought. People with AD and Lewy body dementia should be offered cholinesterase inhibitor treatment only if their behavioral and psychological symptoms are causing them significant distress. However, this should only be used if non-drug approaches have already been tried and were ineffective, or they are thought to be inappropriate. People with dementia that is entirely due to vascular disease and is not a mixed form (i.e. dementia that is caused by both vascular disease and AD or Lewy body dementia) should not be prescribed cholinesterase inhibitors for behavioral or psychological symptoms.

Future Drugs for Curing AD

The number of Alzheimer's cases in the U.S. in 2002 was 2.7 million. That number is expected to more than double by 2050 as the nation's demographic profile continues to gray. With these statistics it is clear why considerable time and money has been and is being spent looking for ways to cure or reverse the effects of AD. The focus has been on neural clean-up strategies involving drugs that dissolve amyloid plaques and/or lower the levels of Aβ peptides[545].

In the 1990s the apolipoprotein E (apoE) gene was identified. It comes in several versions. The apoE4 variant, is linked to increased risk of AD. People with the apoE4 allele have a 60% chance of having AD by age 80 versus a less than 10% overall risk of AD at this age in the general population. The apoE4 carriers, about 20% of the population, may be more vulnerable to AD because they have an increased ability to produce an Aβ chaperone molecule called apolipoprotein E4 (apoE4). ApoE4 disrupts Aβ peptide clearance at the blood-brain-barrier by redirecting the clearance from a faster to a slower Aβ chaperone receptor[12].

Bexarotene: One strategy for dissolving amyloid plaques in AD patients is to enhance the production of the faster Aβ chaperone. Recently a drug named Bexarotene has been found to have the following effects in demented mice:

- Increases Aβ chaperone production
- Lowers the Aβ peptides in the brain by 25% within 6 hours
- Reverses cognitive impairment within 72 hours of oral administration

The mice were bred to have increased amyloid plaque in their brains but did not have the other neuronal changes seen in AD. This work with Bexarotene was performed at Case Western Reserve University. The effectiveness of Bexarotene seems to wear off after 90 days and it raises levels of triglycerides implicated in strokes, cardiovascular disease, and diabetes. Human studies with Bexarotene are underway by a company named ReXceptor Therapeutics.

Monoclonal Antibodies (MABs): The concept behind these drugs is to engineer a MAB that will bind to a soluble Aβ preventing it from forming into an insoluble plaque. There are several MABs under development but the results so far are not encouraging:

- Aducanumab (a.k.a. BIIB037) – Biogen Idec – In Phase III trials despite side effects.
- Solanezumab – Eli Lilly – Targets Aβ oligomers – Failed trials & abandoned in 2016.
- Crenezumab – Hoffman-La Roche – Targets soluble Aβ oligomers – Failed Phase 2 trials but still launching a Phase III trial.

BACE Inhibitors: A third strategy involves inhibiting Aβ production in the brain of AD patients. Aβ is produced as a result of two sequential cleavages of the amyloid precursor protein (APP). The enzyme β-secretase (BACE1) cleaves APP creating a soluble fragment and membrane bound fragment referred to as C99. Cleavage of C99 by γ-secretase produces amyloid-β.

- **MK-8931** is an experimental drug that inhibits BACE1. MK-8931 was tested in phase 1 trials by Merck and was shown to reduce amyloid-β in cerebral spinal fluid by as much as 90 percent with no sign of dose limiting side-effects. Merck's new trials beginning in 2014 seek to enroll more than 3,000 people and will run from 18 months to two years.

- **AZD3293** (a.k.a. LY3314814) is an experimental drug that inhibits BACE1. AZD3293 is being co-developed by Eli Lilly and AstraZeneca. AZD3293 is tested in a pivotal phase II/III clinical trial called AMARANTH that started in late 2014 and plans to recruit 1,500 people by 2019.

- **E2609** is an experimental drug that inhibits BACE1. E2609 is being tested jointly by Biogen Idec and Eisai Co. Ltd. (Tokyo). E2609 was discovered in-house by Eisai Co. and in 2015 it entered Phase II clinical trials.

Chapter 8 – Alzheimer's and Stroke as Mismatch Diseases

"... indeed the brain held out as well or better than other organs" G. M. Humphry 1889

Aluminum is the third most common element in the earth's crust. Did we evolve a protective mechanism for our brains from the neurotoxicity of aluminum and, if we did, why has it failed? In order to answer this we must step back in time and look at a series of two evolutions:

- First the geochemical evolution of the earth
- Second the evolution of life resulting in our species *Homo sapiens*

In addition to these two evolutions, that took place over a period of 4 billion years, there have been culture driven dysevolutions that have occurred in the last 130 years. Cultural life-style changes made by our species that become harmful (i.e. dys) and impair the earth's geochemical evolution or our evolutionary advantage are called dysevolutionary. These dysevolutionary changes increase our risk of diseases such as Alzheimer's and stroke.

Geochemical Evolution

Over the billions of years in which the geochemical evolution of the earth occurred and before life began the second most common element in the earth's crust, silicon, reacted as silicic acid (a.k.a. silica) with aluminum oxides (a.k.a. alumina) and hydroxides to form stable crystalline complexes called hydroxyaluminosilicates (HAS). HAS has extremely low water solubility at neutral pH and is very slowly dissolved in acid. HAS is nontoxic because any HAS ingested by animals is not bioavailable and is therefore not absorbed but excreted.

Homo Sapiens Evolution

Our ancestors evolved on the earth as hunter-gatherers and there is archaeological evidence that by 1.9 million years ago they were hunting wildebeest sized animals. There is also evidence that the simplest stone spear point was not invented until 500,000 years ago and the bow and arrow was not invented until 100,000 years ago. So how did our ancestors evolve to kill, at close range, large animals that could gallop faster than our ancestors could run?

It is theorized that for over a million years our ancestors ran down the animals they killed using what has been called persistence hunting. There is evidence that by the time of *Homo erectus* our ancestors had evolved the ability to run long distances at moderate speed. In addition they had evolved very short and thin body hair, sweat glands, and an arched nasal passage to conserve water. All of these changes allowed them the evolutionary advantage of being able to keep cool while running long distances in the heat of the day. Their prey on the other hand could gallop faster but had long thick hair, had to pant in order to keep cool, and could not pant and gallop at the same time[546]. The niche filled by our ancestor's evolution was persistence hunting that involved running after and killing swifter animals by forcing them to gallop during the heat of the day until they collapsed of heat exhaustion[547,548].

Persistence hunting required considerable aerobic and anaerobic exercise coupled with deductive reasoning and tracking skills that had to be performed while the brain was not fully oxygenated. It is not surprising that our ancestor's brains evolved to not only become larger but also to switch on biochemical pathways to increase the production of taurine, glutathione during anaerobic exercise, and production of PYY, somatostatin, norepinephrine, and BDNF under aerobic conditions as described earlier in this book. This self-medicating neuroprotection is vital to protect the brain and keep it working under both aerobic and anaerobic conditions. In addition persistence hunting would have evolved cultural life-styles that included daily aerobic and anaerobic exercise with sleep cycles that allowed for self-cleaning of the neurotoxic chemicals that built-up in the brain.

Human mother's evolved a protective mechanism for their children during pregnancy and during the period of breast feeding. This mechanism lowered the mother's serum silica levels while making silica available at high levels to the developing child in the womb and to the new born infant being fed on silica rich breastmilk. Silica not only strengthens bones but even more importantly lowers aluminum levels in the child. This evolutionary protective mechanism was in response to aluminum's neurotoxicity on developing brains.

Geochemical Dysevolution

Bauxite is an aluminum rich mineral containing only a small amount (1-2%) of silica. The first commercial extraction of alumina from bauxite has been attributed to Henri Sainte-Claire Deville in 1854. In 1888, Karl Joseph Bayer described what is now known as the Bayer Process. This process resulted in a dramatic reduction in the cost of producing aluminum metal. Because of this development humans began producing aluminum from bauxite and manufacturing it into metal products like aluminum cookware and converting it into chemicals, such as aluminum sulfate used for fertilizer and water purification, aluminum chloride, used for antiperspirants, and other aluminum compounds used in pharmaceutical formulations. All of these products facilitate aluminum absorption by our brains.

In 1824 Joseph Aspdin took out a patent on the manufacture of Portland cement that involved heating a mixture of clay and crushed limestone in a kiln and then grinding the resulting clinkers into a powder. When the powder is mixed with water it hardens into hydraulic cement. Chemical investigation of the Portland clinkers started in 1882 with Le Chatelier and revealed the composition to be celite (a.k.a. tricalcium aluminate) and three other aluminates and silicates. Portland cement allowed a water pipe to be internally coated with cement, sand, and water mixture, called mortar, while spinning on its axis. Because of these developments mortar lined water pipes have been used for the last 150 years and have become the most commonly used lining for water pipes around the world. A mortar lining only lasts for 50-100 years because of leaching of the celite into the water as aluminum and calcium ions. This, coupled with fluoridation, facilitates aluminum absorption by our brains from drinking water.

The earliest known oil wells were drilled in China in 347AD. In North America the first commercial oil well was drilled in 1858 in Oil Springs, Ontario. The development of oil fired engines created a large market for oil starting in the early 1900's. By the end of World War II the burning of a large amount of sulfur containing fossil fuel in cars and power plants began to acidify the planet's rain. Acid rain breaks down non-bioavailable HASs into bioavailable aluminum that finds its way into our water supplies.

Our refining of aluminum, use of Portland cement to line water pipes, and burning of fossil fuels, have all resulted in a culturally driven geochemical dysevolution. We have opened a Pandora's Box of bioavailable aluminum in our drinking water, food, and pharmaceuticals. It is not surprising that since the first case of Alzheimer's was reported in 1907 there are more than 2.7 million cases in the U.S. and more than 24 million cases worldwide. These numbers will overwhelm our medical systems and economies if we do not take the steps required for prevention.

Homo Sapiens Dysevolution

Homo sapiens evolved on the earth during the last million and half years as hunter-gatherers. For over a million years *Homo sapiens* used persistence hunting without tools to kill animals for food. This type of hunting required considerable aerobic and anaerobic exercise coupled with deductive reasoning and tracking skills. Our biochemistry and large brain evolved during this time to perform best on an omnivore diet with hours of sleep and both daily aerobic and anaerobic exercise.

When some of our ancestors became farmers they still performed aerobic exercise by spending long hours working their fields. Their diet changed to become dependent upon a primary staple grain. This was culturally dysevolutionary with respect to their evolved biochemistry that relied upon an omnivore diet consisting of meat and fish (66 to 75% of the diet) a variety of fruits, nuts, and grains (26-35% of the diet)[549]. A practice that is culturally dysevolutionary can lead to a mismatch disease where human's evolved biochemistry is no longer matched to their diet.

Harvard Professor Daniel E. Lieberman defines mismatch diseases as:

"Diseases that result from our Paleolithic bodies being poorly or inadequately adapted to certain modern behaviors and conditions"[210]

Pellagra as an Ancient Mismatch Disease

An example of a mismatch disease was experienced by the Mesoamericans who grew corn (i.e. maize) as their primary staple grain. Corn is the only grain low in digestible niacin (a.k.a. vitamin B3). Therefore Mesoamericans suffered from a mismatch disease caused by chronic niacin deficiency with dementia as a symptom. We now call this condition pellagra and it is a type of metabolic dementia (see Appendix II). Niacin (a.k.a. vitamin B3, nicotinic acid) is required for human metabolism to produce energy from food. The Mesoamericans developed technology to prevent the mismatch disease pellagra by modifying their cultural practice of cooking corn. They developed a special cooking technique called nixtamalization between 1500 and 1200 BC. Nixtamalization uses an alkaline (i.e. basic pH) water solution to hydrolyze or release the niacin from corn meal. The Mesoamericans used calcium hydroxide (a.k.a. slaked lime) and potassium hydroxide (a.k.a. potash) from the ashes of wood fires in order to make the alkaline solutions. Nixtamalization made niacin bioavailable and allowed the ancient Aztec and Mayan cultures to develop by preventing pellagra[550].

Lead Poisoning as an Ancient Mismatch Disease

Another example of a mismatch disease occurred during the Roman Empire. The people of this period used lead to make water pipes, cookware, and cosmetics. Corrosion of lead in contact with their drinking water and application of leaded cosmetics to their skin resulted in lead accumulation in their bones as shown by examination of the skeletal remains of these people as shown in Figure 7[141]. Judging from the amount of lead found in their bones, these people suffered from mild to severe lead poisoning resulting in brain swelling that caused severe headaches, confusion, irritability, seizures, and possibly death.

The data in Figure 7 was acquired by analyzing human bones exhumed from cemeteries in two suburbs of ancient Rome that were used from 0 to 300 AD, and from 200 skeletons found in Britain from 300 BC through the Late Medieval period ending in 1500 AD[141]. A portion of ingested lead is stored in bone during a person's lifetime. These data gives us a good idea of how both the cultural use of lead and the body burden of lead steadily increased in these two regions over an 1800 year period. A body burden of one milligram per kilogram of lead is the World Health Organization's (WHO's) level of concern and ten milligrams per kilogram of lead is WHO's level of severe lead poisoning. Therefore mental impairment resulting from lead is another example of a mismatch disease due the cultural use of a neurotoxic metal.

We are still living with the dysevolution of lead mining, refining, and usage. Our culture has banned or strongly discouraged the use of lead in certain products including:

- Lead buckshot
- Lead sinkers for fishing
- Lead in paint
- Lead in gasoline
- Lead solder in electronic circuit boards

The parallels between lead and aluminum are striking. Both lead and aluminum have some unique and advantageous properties that make them highly desirable by our cultures. Because of this it takes longer to make cultural changes that will lower these metals impact on our mental health. If this information is discouraging you from working toward making the cultural changes required to lower our aluminum ingestion, I recommend taking a little dissolved silica in water and you will feel better in the morning.

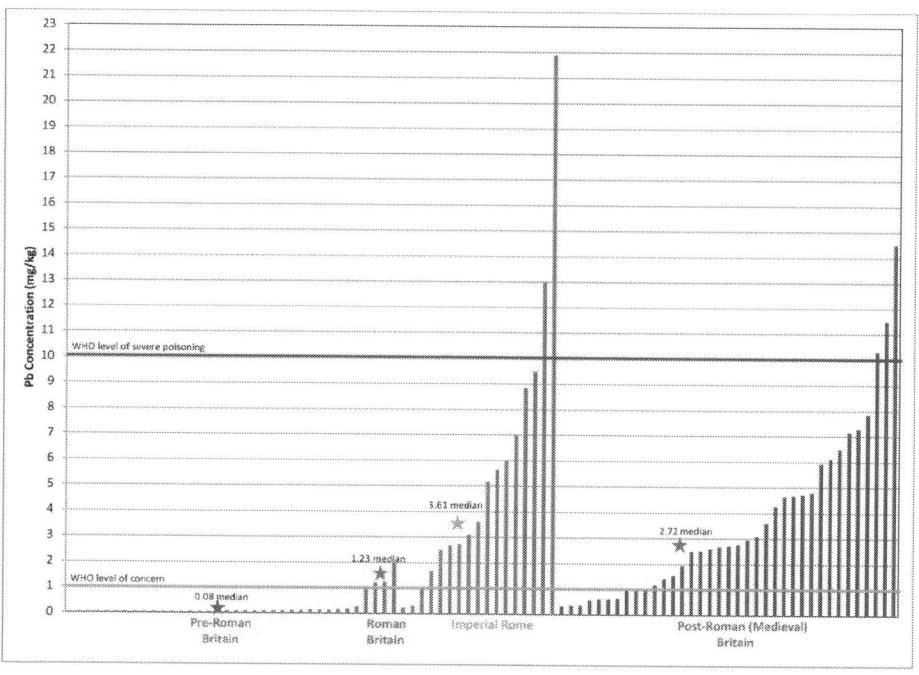

Figure 7 - Lead in old bones

Lead concentration in skeletons from Britain and Rome. Raw data from Montgomery et al. 2010[141] tables 11.2, 11.3, 11.4, as graphed by K. Killgrove[551].

Alzheimer's and Stroke as Modern Mismatch Diseases

In the last hundred years the industrial and technological revolutions have given us the automobile. The auto has propelled us into a more sedentary life-style involving much less aerobic and anaerobic exercise. And with the advent of the electric light, we can ignore natural circadian rhythms depriving ourselves of sleep. In addition, cultural behavior has resulted in more aluminum absorption by our brains due to:

- aluminum cookware
- fluoride added to drinking water
- aluminum in:
    - food
    - drinking water
    - pharmaceuticals
    - vaccines
    - toothpastes
    - antiperspirants
- use of mortar containing Portland cement to line water pipes
- use of alum to:
    - fertilize tea plants
    - purify water
    - make pickles crunchy

All of these cultural life-style changes are harmful and counter to our hunter-gatherer evolution and can be called "dysevolutionary" as they impair our ability to prevent AD and stroke.

As a Boy Scout I learned how to track animals and hike long distances by taking many 5 mile hikes and three 20 mile hikes (e.g. the Blackhawk, Hoover, and Lincoln trails) under the hot

Midwestern summer sun. Like my Paleolithic ancestors I was evolved to perform well under these conditions and even enjoy them. While camping out after a long day spent hiking, I was introduced to the Boy Scout culture of cooking in aluminum foil. For dinner we wrapped a hamburger, slice of onion, potatoes, and some sweet pepper into to a tightly closed aluminum foil package and laid it on hot coals for 20 minutes. We consumed this delicious meal including its dissolved aluminum and were totally unaware of its dysevolutionary cultural aspects including the harm being done to our young brains.

Looking back in time it can now be demonstrated that geochemical and cultural dysevolution occurring over the last 130 years have resulted in an increased percentage of elderly humans with dementia. The mental health of older people living between 1896 and 1899 is described in the monograph "Old Age" published in Cambridge England in 1889[7]. The monograph summarizes the results of British general practitioners studying the mental health of their oldest patients during the mid-1880s. The study group was 900 subjects who were 80 or older including 74 centenarians. The monograph's author concludes that dementia:

> *"... was witnessed only in two of our centenarians ... indeed the brain held out as well or better than other organs"*

This 3% rate of dementia among centenarians in the mid-1880s can be compared with a study 125 years later. In 2000 a study was done of people in three Dutch towns with populations greater than 250,000. Of the 17 centenarians found in this more recent study 15 had dementia for an 88% rate of dementia. The other 2 centenarians could not be examined[8].

AD and stroke may therefore be thought of as both modern diseases and mismatch diseases in that our behaviors and cultures have changed both our environment and life-style making them more harmful than what our ancestors experienced during their evolution.

Conclusion of Alzheimer's and Stroke as Mismatch Diseases

In our culture the profusion of new technology and products occurs at such a fast pace that there is a high probability of dysevolutionary cultural practices resulting in mismatch diseases. The information in this book provides a new lens through which our cultural practices should be examined so that mismatch diseases can be identified and possibly prevented in the future. Discovering how to prevent and cure these mismatch diseases requires money for research, time, and persistence.

Cultural evolution involves no genetic change but instead changes in values that cause groups of us to think and behave differently. Culture is the most unique characteristic differentiating *Homo sapiens* from other species. We have developed complex and diverse cultures with different customs, food, clothing, art, and tools. We have also developed the capacity to modify our culture on a time scale much faster than genetic evolution. The Mesoamerican's demonstrated this capacity between 1500 - 1200 BC when they developed nixtamalization and incorporated it into their culture in order to avoid dementia caused by pellagra. Modern Americans, and for that matter all modern cultures, are now at a similar crossroads. We must develop a cultural modification to remove aluminum from our food, drinking water, air, vaccines, and pharmaceuticals in order to prevent dementia and autism. Otherwise we will accept the consequences of inaction. Information is frequently the catalyst for cultural modification and hopefully the information in this book will facilitate a cultural change in behaviors that will ultimately prevent mismatch diseases such as Alzheimer's and stroke.

Chapter 9 – Autism as a Mismatch Disease

"... the genetic and environmental causes of autism are obscure making it challenging to figure out whether the disease is caused by a mismatch between ancient genes and modern environment." Professor Daniel E. Lieberman 2013[210]

In this chapter we will accept Lieberman's challenge[210] and discuss why autism spectrum disorders (ASD) are another example of mismatch diseases[383]. Children's brains during their first years of life create neural networks that can last for their lifetime. We as a culture have the responsibility to not derail this natural development of their brains.

Autism was first described in 1943 by a physician, Leo Kanner, who suspected it was a new syndrome that he first observed in 1938. In 1938 Kanner was 44 years old and had been working for 8 years developing the first child psychiatry service in a pediatric hospital at John Hopkins Hospital in Baltimore. By 1943 Kanner had identified 10 more cases of autism. Kanner believed that autism is a modern disease and his belief is supported by the fact that it took him 8 years working as a child psychiatrist to find his first case. A child psychiatrist working in a similar position today would probably find his first case of autism within a week, if not sooner.

Autism is defined as a pervasive developmental disorder occurring in the first three years of life. Autism is characterized by the presence of markedly abnormal or impaired development in social interaction and communication. The symptoms of autism include:

- Sensory processing difficulties
- Limited social interaction
- Deficits and delays in language development
- Unusual or problematic behaviors

It has been found that 85% of children with ASD have either low (i.e. hypo) or high (i.e. hyper) sensory arousal[6,142,552]. Abnormally early frontal lobe enlargement (i.e. hyperplasia) in children

2 to 3 years of age has also been found to be a hallmark of ASD[553]. Research has shown that there is an over-connectivity in the frontal cortex in children with ASD and there is also a long-distance under-connectivity of the frontal cortex with other areas of the brain[554]. It is theorized that this under-connectivity impairs both the frontal cortex's function of integrating information from sensory input and providing feedback for guidance, and control to lower-level systems in the body[554].

Although there may be genes that facilitate changes in the brains of children with ASD, no genetic syndrome associated with ASD has been shown to cause the disease. An example is fragile X syndrome that is associated with ASD, but only 30% of the children who are carriers of the fragile X gene actually develop autism accounting for only 5% of children with ASD[326,555]. Also the rapid rise in autism rates since 1938 indicates that autism is a modern disease and genetics cannot be the cause of a rapidly increasing modern disease, as described in Chapter 1[326]. It has become clear that ASD is caused by an environmental factor not by a genetic syndrome[556].

Homo Sapiens Evolution

Hunting and gathering food was the subsistence strategy used by *Homo erectus* beginning 1.8 million years ago and continued in use by *Homo sapiens* beginning about 200,000 years ago. Hunter-gatherer mothers typically weaned their children after 3 years and had children every 3 to 4 years. This resulted in not only three years of breast feeding but also a slow rate of population increase with the population estimated to double every 5000 years. From available archeological data it has been found that vegetable foods were 26 to 35% of the hunter-gatherer diet[549]. The hunter-gatherer diet included roots, leaves, stems and hulls of plants[557]. These parts of unprocessed plants have high levels of orthosilicic acid (OSA) to afford the plant protection from a number of stressors including metal toxicity[558]. Because OSA is commonly found in xylem sap of the roots, leaves, stems and hulls of plants[558], hunter-gatherer mothers had ample dissolved silica in their blood and breastmilk. This dietary silica decreased dietary aluminum absorption and aluminum levels in both mother and child (see Chapters 5 and 6).

Did we evolve the silica transfer from mother to child for both improved bone strength and neuroprotection from aluminum in the child? If we did, it implies there was sufficient aluminum in the hunter-gatherer diet to require neuroprotection in children. Dietary sources of aluminum in the hunter-gatherer diet would have included the same types of plant material in which OSA is found, and soil on unwashed fruits and vegetables. The sources of aluminum in our diet today are much more varied than during the hunter-gatherer period and usually don't contain OSA for protection against aluminum neurotoxicity (see Chapters 4 and 5).

The outdoor lifestyle of the hunter-gatherer meant the both mothers and children were exposed to ample sunlight and therefore had high vitamin D levels. Modern hunter-gatherers in equatorial Africa have average vitamin D serum levels of 115nM, including one pregnant woman with a level of 273nM[559,560]. It is estimated that for an indoor worker to have these serum levels of vitamin D would require supplementation with 5,000 IU of vitamin D per day[326]. Vitamin D lowers the absorption of aluminum in children even those children with high levels of aluminum due to aluminum ingestion or kidney disease[289] (see Chapter 3). Therefore, with a diet high in dissolved silica and with exposure to ample sunlight, the brains of children of hunter-gatherers were protected against the neurotoxicity of aluminum during gestation and their first three years.

Homo Sapiens Cultural Evolution

Twelve to ten thousand years ago some hunter-gatherers began early attempts at agriculture and living in permanent settlements. As the availability of food increased due to this agriculture, harvested food was increasingly processed by removing some previously eaten roots, stalks, and hulls that are rich in OSA[561]. This trend has continued to the present day by food processing technology that alters food from plants so that more energy can be ingested per day at the expense of ignoring key minerals such as OSA[562].

Farmer mothers had sufficient food to wean their children after only 1.5 years and not the 3 years required by the hunter-gatherer mothers. This meant farmer mothers could have children every 1.5 to 2 years. This resulted in farmer mothers giving birth every 1.5 years leading to both shorter period of breast feeding and a faster rate of population increase with the population estimated to double every 2,500 years. This cultural trend of early weaning has continued until 1970 when only 5% of babies at 6 months were being fed some breastmilk. During the period from 1970 to 2015 there has been an increase in breast feeding. By 1982 breastfeeding at 6 months had increased to 25% and, after a slow decline to 20% by 1990, the percentage of babies being breastfed at 6 months slowly rose to 31.4% by 2000[563,564].

The rapid population growth during the last ten thousand years was made possible by farmer mothers weaning their children at an earlier age. This population growth coupled with higher density living conditions in permanent settlements fostered new infectious diseases. Living in less densely populated encampments our hunter-gatherer ancestors had not evolved protection from these infectious diseases. Therefore as farmers we were evolutionarily mismatched to protect ourselves from these new infectious diseases. Cultural evolution was required to find protection from these infectious diseases. This protection has taken the form of improved sanitary conditions and vaccines. Once fully immunized to a specific disease, a large population living in close proximity is no longer susceptible to the disease. Therefore our farming lifestyle requiring community living has forced humans to improve their sanitary living conditions and immunize themselves to avoid infectious diseases.

Aluminum a Causal Factor of Autism

Aluminum absorption by the brain begins early in life. Aluminum is transferred from the maternal blood circulation to the fetal blood circulation via the placenta[565]. The brains of three fetuses, one full-term infant and three infants from two to six months were analyzed for aluminum. The results were that these brains have a mean aluminum concentration of 1.2mcg per gram dry-weight of brain tissue with a standard deviation of 0.2mcg per gram[74]. Aluminum levels have been found to rise in the brains of fetuses during gestation and they rise the highest immediately after birth[566]. The blood-brain barrier which protects the brain is incompletely developed at birth and is even less mature in the fetus. The rate of aluminum uptake into the brain dramatically slows approximately 10,000 times with maturation of the blood-brain barrier[567].

Approximately 50% of children with autism have increased intestinal permeability that is not seen in children without autism[568]. After a metal ion such as aluminum is ingested and absorbed by the intestine it becomes dissolved in the blood. Some of the metal is absorbed from the blood by both the brain and hair.

In 2012 an analysis was performed on hair from 44 children, age 3 to 9 years, diagnosed according to DSM-IV with ASD. It was discovered that the mean value for aluminum in the hair of autistic children (15.2mg/kg) was 90% higher than aluminum in the hair of non-autistic children (8.0mg/kg)[569]. This was the first analytical data linking high levels of accumulated aluminum to autism. In 2015 a second study demonstrated that aluminum levels in the hair of autistic children are higher than aluminum levels in non-autistic children. In this study the source of aluminum was traced to the use of aluminum cookware[570].

In 2017 an analysis was performed on the brains of 5 individuals with confirmed ASD, 4 males and 1 female. The mean and standard deviation (in parenthesis) of aluminum content across all five individuals for each lobe were 3.82(5.42), 2.30(2.00), 2.79(4.05) and 3.82(5.17) mcg per gram dry weight for the occipital, frontal, temporal and parietal lobes respectively. These are some of the highest aluminum levels in the brain yet recorded[571].

In the brains of those with autism it has been found that the brain regions most impacted include the hippocampal complex and entorhinal cortex[95]. These areas of the autistic brain have smaller and less complex neuronal networks than normal[95]. This suggests a curtailment of normal neuron development and neuronal connectivity. These areas of the brain are also responsible for memory, learning, and emotion and behavior, disturbances of which comprise the core clinical features of autism[96]. Most importantly these are the same brain regions found to be hot spots for aluminum accumulation[86].

Aluminum in the body creates a characteristic biochemical fingerprint that can be measured by taking a blood sample. This fingerprint is made by aluminum inhibiting the activation of the enzyme MS that converts homocysteine to methionine. Based upon this biochemical fingerprint aluminum is suspected as a causal agent for autism as summarized in the following table.

Similar Biochemical Markers in AD and Autism			
Biochemical	**Aluminum Inhibition of MS**	**AD**	**Autism**
Homocysteine Level	Above Normal	Above Normal [A]	Above Normal [B]
SAM Level	Below Normal	Below Normal [C]	Below Normal [D]
Glutathione (GSH) Level	Below Normal	Below Normal [E]	Below Normal [F]

A) Homocysteine in AD patients[572-574] B) Homocysteine in autistic children[575] C) SAM in AD patients[576] D) SAM in autistic children[577] E) Glutathione (GSH) in AD patients[578] F) Glutathione (GSH) in autistic children[579-582]

In addition to the data in this table, the prevalence of mitochondrial disease is significantly higher than normal in both autistic children[583] and patients with Alzheimer's disease[55]. The mitochondria are responsible for producing NADH and ATP required for providing the brain with energy. Aluminum may be the culprit since it lowers brain energy by lowering the expression and activity of six Krebs cycle (a.k.a. TCA cycle) enzymes in the mitochondria. These enzymes include α-ketoglutarate dehydrogenase and isocitrate dehydrogenase that are two Krebs cycle enzymes involved in NADH production[56,57,584].

Aluminum also has the means to cause the long-distance under-connectivity observed between the frontal cortex and other areas of the developing brain of children that are hallmarks of autism. Long term potentiation is the process whereby neurons make permanent connections between themselves to store memories and make those memories available to the frontal cortex. Aluminum inhibits long term potentiation as described in Chapter 1.

Aluminum also inhibits the production of brain derived neurotrophic factor (BDNF) in the hippocampus that in turn inhibits the growth of neuronal connections. These connections are required to make the neuronal networks in the infant's rapidly developing brain. Aluminum in the diet of neonatal and postnatal rats lowers hippocampal expression of BDNF resulting in impairment of both long term memory and spatial learning[101,102].

When our right eye is simultaneously exposed to a different image than our left eye, there is a rivalry between each eye for dominance. What we see alternates approximately every 3 seconds between the right and left image. This is called the rate of binocular rivalry and this rate is slower as the severity of autistic symptoms increase[585]. Neurochemical hallmarks of autism include imbalance between excitatory and inhibitory neurotransmissions leading to a slower rate of binocular rivalry and either hypersensitivity or hyposensitivity[552,585,586]. The modulation of $GABA_A$ receptor-mediated currents in neurons by amplifying or attenuating sensory signals can create these symptoms. This mechanism of neurochemical signaling is called GABAergic signaling. Aluminum accumulation and modulation of GABA receptors in the brain is a cause of GABAergic signaling being out of balance in both autism and AD (see page 58 of this book).

There are two aluminum binding sites on $GABA_A$ receptors[587]. One binding site has a high affinity for aluminum. Low levels of aluminum (e.g. less than 100mcM) at this site can bind to and increase the $GABA_A$ receptor-mediated current in neurons[587]. This can result in hyposensitivity. There is a second site with a low affinity for aluminum. High levels of aluminum (e.g. greater than 300mcM) at both sites bind to and block $GABA_A$ receptor-mediated current in neurons[587]. This can result in hypersensitivity. Both hyposensitivity and hypersensitivity are counterproductive to creating long term neural connections in the brain.

There are gender differences in embryonic development of rats that may be occurring in human embryonic development that can help us understand why autism is more common in boys than girls[298]. In the developing embryo and early postnatal brain of rats and humans there are two chloride ion transporters associated with the $GABA_A$ receptors, one with decreased and one with increased ion transport. Since chloride ions are required for filtering out unwanted neuronal signals, the increased ion transporter makes $GABA_A$ receptors better filters. The early rat embryo shifts from using the decreased ion transporter to the increased ion transporter during development. In rat embryos, females make this shift to better $GABA_A$ filters 10 days earlier than males. This gives females a 10 day head start in making improved neuronal connections[588]. If the timing of this shift is similar in humans, this could be one of the reasons why autism is more common in boys than girls.

Homo Sapiens Cultural Dysevolution and Autism

Autism is a spectrum of disorders (ASD) that delays the development of immature brains. Although all the disorders on the spectrum share some symptoms there is variation in developmental timeline and severity of the disorders. Currently it is estimated that 1 in 68 children born in the U.S. has autism. Autism is measured in the U.S. by the CDC that analyzes how many children have autism at age 8 as measured by the criteria described by the then current Diagnostic and Statistical Manual of Mental Disorders (DSM). In order to measure how autism increased between children born in 1980 versus those born in 2000 we need to compare the CDC's number of autistic 8 year olds diagnosed with autism in 1988 and 2008. In 1988, 1 in 1,000 children had been diagnosed with autism at age 8. By 2008, 11 in 1000 had been diagnosed with autism at age 8 in the U.S.[589]. This corresponds to an 11 fold increase in autism in U.S. children born in the twenty year period between 1980 and 2000.

The 11 fold increase in autism nationwide, as measured by the CDC in children born from 1980 to 2000, occurred against a backdrop of changes in diagnostic criteria for autism. In 1987 the criteria for autism was changed in the DSM-III-R. This increased the number of children being diagnosed with autism. In 1994 DSM-IV added pervasive developmental disorder (PDD) to the autism spectrum. Thus some portion of the 11 fold increase in autism is due to these changes.

Irva Hertz-Picciotto, an epidemiology professor at the University of California, led a study looking at autism rates in California[590]. In 1990, 6.2 of every 10,000 children born in California were diagnosed with autism by the age of five. In 2001, 42.5 in 10,000 children born in California were diagnosed with autism. Therefore the rate of autism in children born between 1985 and 1996 in California increased 7 fold. The following changes occurred in this 11 year period that impacted the measured rate of autism in California:

- Changes in the diagnostic criteria accounted for a 2.2 fold increase
- The inclusion of milder cases of autism accounted for a 1.56 fold increase
- Earlier age diagnosis for autism accounted for a 1.24 fold increase

The total effect of these changes account for a 4.3 fold increase in autism in California in the children born from 1985 to 1996. Since there was actually a 7 fold increase, the rate of autism actually increased by 1.6 fold (60%) in California during this 11 year period. A genetic defect called the fragile X syndrome accounts for approximately 5% of all autism cases[555]. But the autism rate is rising too fast to be attributed to any genetic defect moving through the population. Therefore the primary cause of the rise in autism must be environmental.

Since autism is becoming more common in many developed countries including the U.S., the environmental factors responsible for the rise in autism must be increasing in all developed countries. Because of autism's early onset of symptoms, the environmental factors must affect either or both the fetus and the infant. Several environmentally related factors that could be involved in making autism a mismatch disease and meet the criteria of significantly increasing through the period of 1980 to 2000 in the U.S. and a number of other developed countries are:

- Increased baby formula usage
- Increased vitamin D deficiency due to:
    - Increased air pollution
    - Increased sunblock and sunscreen usage
- Increased premature birth
- Increased number of infant vaccinations

There is a common thread in all of these environmentally related factors. As we will see they all result in an increase in aluminum accumulation in brains of infants. This is in spite of the fact that the aluminum is not necessarily a component of the air pollution, sunscreen, or sunblock.

Increased Baby Formula Usage

The trend in the U.S. of increased breast feeding beginning in 1971 was associated with a decrease in formula feeding in the first 2 to 3 months of life[591]. However, between 1980 and 1998 the increase in breast feeding was accompanied by a deferment in the average age of introduction of foods other than formula. This resulted in increased formula usage between the ages of 3-12 months as diagrammed in the following figure[591]:

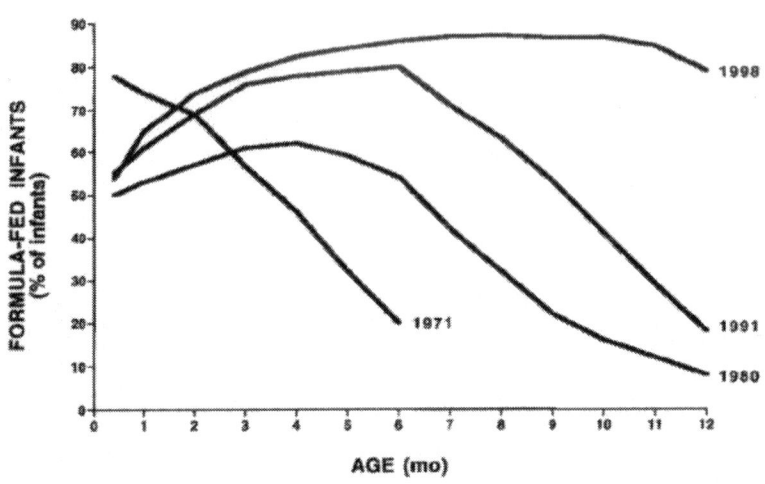

Figure 8 – Formula-fed as a percentage of infants versus age in the U.S.

Figure 8 shows that between 1980 and 1998 there was a 22% increase in baby formula feeding at 3 months of age, 33% at 6 months, and 64% at 1 year[591]. Note that this increase in baby formula usage between 1980 and 1998 is sufficiently large to entirely account for the 60% increase in autism observed during this same time period in California[590].

Soy based infant formula was originally introduced in the U.S. from Asia and Japan in the 1970's for the 1 to 2% of the infant population allergic to cow's milk. In 1988 the three main manufactures of infant formula split their alliance with the medical profession and began an independent commercial advertising campaign not guided by the medical profession. This led to a dramatic increase in formula usage with soy based infant formula sales reaching 25% of U.S. infant formula sales by 2000[592].

Link Found Between Formula Feeding and Autism

Four independent studies have shown a correlation between formula feeding and autism:

- The largest study of the effect of exclusively breast fed versus bottle fed babies and autism was carried out by S. T. Schultz and the University of California, San Diego, School of Medicine. In this 2005 study a survey was conducted by contacting parents of 861 children with ASD and 123 control children. Parents were asked to describe how they fed their babies and for how long they were fed. The study found that formula feeding in the absence of breastfeeding for the first 6 months significantly increased the odds of autistic disorder[593].
- This study was repeated in Oman in 2012 with 102 ASD cases and 102 healthy matched controls with the same results and an observation that the risk of ASD decreased in a dose dependent manner with increasing breastmilk feeding[594].
- Another parent survey done in River Side California in 2014 with 145 parents responding with 60 children with ASD and 85 children without ASD showed that increasing the duration time of breastfeeding versus formula feeding is associated with a decline in ASD[595].
- In 1989 a study done in Japanese of the weaning times of 145 children diagnosed with ASD (per DSM-III) and 224 normal children in the same catchment area were compared. It was found that 24.8% of the ASD children were weaned from breastmilk by the end of the first week after birth versus 7.5% of the controls[596].

Aluminum in Breastmilk and Baby Formula

The amount of aluminum in breastmilk has been found to vary in the U.K. from 3 to 79μg/liter[597] and in Spain from 14 to 33μg/liter[393]. These levels can be compared with 200μg/liter that is the World Health Organization's maximum level of aluminum in drinking water[68]. Although not insignificant, 3 to 79μg/liter of aluminum in breastmilk is significantly lower than the amount of aluminum in both soy and non-soy based infant formula[384,385,393]. This is most likely the reason why formula feeding has been found to correlate with the incidence of autism.

Soybeans prefer acidic soil for growth. Acid soil contains more bioavailable aluminum than basic soil. The bioavailable aluminum in the soil is absorbed by the soybean plant during growth leading to high levels of aluminum in the soybean. In Japan, the soybeans were found to contain 12mg/kg of aluminum and soy based freshly mixed instant baby formula was found to contain 1mg/liter of aluminum[592]. Therefore it is likely that the aluminum in baby formula originates from the soybean with the possibility of added aluminum during processing. In the U.K. and Canada soy based instant baby formula freshly mixed was found to contain 0.6 to 0.7mg/liter of aluminum[384,385,403]. This amount of aluminum is more than 3 times higher than the World Health's recommended maximum level of aluminum in drinking water[68].

The problem with aluminum in baby formula extends to cow's milk based formula as well as soy based formula. The amount of aluminum in ready-made infant formula milks in the U.K., Spain, and Canada ranges from 155 to 422μg/liter that translates to ingesting 78 to 350μg/day for a 6 month old baby[385,393,403]. The amount of aluminum absorbed by the body from baby formula is 0.1 to 0.3% of the aluminum in the formula[131,391]. This is called the bioavailable aluminum and its level in the blood peaks 8 to 9 hours after ingestion[131,391].

Dissolvable Silica as a Supplement and in Baby Formula

Does dissolved silica in drinking water have the same effect on both the incident rate of autism and AD? There are high levels of dissolved silica in drinking water from Malaysia and Singapore and high levels of aluminum in drinking water from Iceland. Therefore there is a correlation between aluminum and autism and AD in Iceland and between silica and autism and AD in Malaysia and Singapore (see Orthosilicic acid in Drinking Water in Chapter 5).

Autism Rate and AD Death Rate by Country		
Country	Autism Rate (per 100,000)*	AD Death Rate (per 100,000)**
United States	1470 (2014)	45.6
Iceland	1200 (2013)	34.1
Malaysia	160 (2008)	0.7
Singapore	100 (2001)	0.2

*Autism rate data from references 598-601, **AD death rate data 2016 worldlifeexpectancy.com

Dissolved silica facilitates the excretion of aluminum as described in Chapter 5. For this reason humans evolved to make dissolved silica available to the fetus and infants in breastmilk as explained in Chapter 6. Pregnant mothers are depleted of silica during pregnancy as diagrammed in figure 6. This accounts for why having two babies within 12 months or less, results in the second baby having a 50% higher risk of autism[602]. Mothers likely require more than a few months to restore silica levels to normal. The result of short interpregnancy periods is less silica being available for protection against aluminum in the second baby. Since silica declines with age in humans it is not surprising that having two babies greater than 10 years apart also results in the second baby having 44% higher risk of autism[602].

Dissolved silica facilitates the removal of aluminum from the infant's body and makes bones stronger. A silica supplement is recommended for pregnant mothers, infants and children (see Chapter 5). Since adding silica to formula is inexpensive, there is no reason to continue the dysevolutionary practice of not fortifying baby formula with dissolved or dissolvable silica.

PQQ in Baby Formula

Biochemical characteristics of both aluminum in the brain and autism include activation of inducible nitric oxide synthase (iNOS) in glial brain cells with increased production of oxidative chemicals (ROS)[49,58,280]. This is a neuro-inflammatory process leading to local cell damage, synapse destruction, and brain under-connectivity[280]. PQQ prevents this situation by decreasing the expression of iNOS and reducing ROS[121,261-265]. PQQ also prevents brain under-connectivity by enhancing nerve growth factor (NGF) production that in turn stimulates the growth of neuronal connections[268-270]. It is therefore not surprising that PQQ is found in mother's milk at a concentration 5 times higher than found in any other food[279]. However PQQ is not found as an ingredient in any currently available baby formula. Since an amount of PQQ equivalent to 160 nanograms per gram of mother's milk is inexpensive, there is no reason to continue the dysevolutionary practice of not fortifying baby formula with PQQ.

Increased Vitamin D Deficiency

In 2008 Doctor J. J. Cannell theorized that the rise in the rate of autism from 1988 to 2008 was caused by an increasing vitamin D deficiency[298]. The hypothesized links between autism and vitamin D are as follows[298,326].

- Children with rickets have several autistic makers that disappear with vitamin D supplementation.
- Consumption of fish containing vitamin D during pregnancy reduces autistic symptoms in offspring.
- Autism is more common in areas of impaired UVB radiation from the sun, such as nearer the poles, urban areas, and areas with high air pollution.
- Both autism and severe maternal vitamin D deficiency is common in dark-skinned people.

In 2012 Cannell's theory was tested by researchers who studied vitamin D2 levels in 50 autistic children comparing them with 30 healthy children age 5-12. Both groups had equal sun exposure and no vitamin D3 supplementation. The results conclusively showed that autistic children have lower vitamin D2 levels than non-autistic children and the lower their vitamin D2 level the more severe the autism[603]. Vitamin D2, the precursor of vitamin D, circulates in the blood throughout the body and is therefore easy to analyze.

In 2015 Doctor Elisabeth Fernell at the University of Gothenburg in Sweden published a study that looked at vitamin D2 levels of 58 sibling pairs, in which one child had ASD and the other did not have ASD. The children's vitamin D2 levels were measured within 4 weeks of birth. The children with ASD had significantly lower vitamin D2 (24nM) as compared with their non-ASD siblings (32nM)[290]. Doctor Frenell concluded that low prenatal vitamin D2 may act as a risk factor for ASD.

The prevalence of vitamin D deficiency is dramatically rising in the U.S. and Denmark. A study conducted in the U.S. was published in 2009 comparing the mean serum vitamin D2 levels of 18,883 participants measured in 1988 to 1994, with the mean serum vitamin D2 level of 13,369 participants, measured in 2001 to 2004. The mean level of vitamin D2 in the U.S. fell from 29.5ng/cc to 24ng/cc. This represents an 18.6% decline in vitamin D2 levels in the period from 1988 to 2004[302,604]. A similar study of medical records in Denmark found that vitamin D2 levels have declined even more than in the U.S. The Denmark study found average vitamin D2 levels declined from 25ng/cc in 1994 to 20mg/cc in 2001 and 17ng/cc in 2008. This represents a 32% decline in vitamin D2 levels in the period from 1994 to 2008[605,606].

Vitamin D3, the precursor of vitamin D2, is either made in the skin by UVB radiation (i.e. high energy UV in sunlight) induced dermal synthesis from 7-dehyrocholesterol or ingested in food or supplements. Vitamin D was first discovered in an effort to find the dietary substance lacking in rickets, the childhood form of osteomalacia. Rickets causes soft or easily broken bones in children. Rickets can be prevented with vitamin D3 supplementation.

In order to achieve an optimal level of vitamin D3 supplementation it is recommend that mothers take 4,000 IU/day while pregnant and 6,000 IU/day while breastfeeding. If baby formula is used, its level of vitamin D3 should be supplemented with vitamin D3 corresponding to the ingestion of 400 IU/day for infants and 800 IU/day for children. This vitamin D3 should come from their diet, exposure to sunlight when possible, and an added 600 IU per day of supplementation. The U.S. Code of Federal Regulations currently requires at least 40 IU and sets a maximum of 100 IU of vitamin D3 per 100 kilocalories (a.k.a. Calories) of infant and baby formula[607]. This amount of formula is equivalent to 5 fluid ounces. Usually to reach 800 IU/day of vitamin D3 requires additional D3 supplementation that can be added to the formula as drops, such as Baby D3 sold by California Gold Nutrition with 400 IU per drop.

Beyond its prevention of rickets, vitamin D has been shown to facilitate the lowering of aluminum levels in the serum of children and the bones, liver, and brain of rats with high levels of aluminum due to kidney disease[289,608]. Kidney disease results in both lower levels of vitamin D and higher levels of aluminum in serum. During 2009, 10 pediatric patients with kidney disease and 20 healthy controls were studied. It was found that 4 weeks of active vitamin D supplementation (not D3 supplementation) at a level of 15-45ng/kg/day (dosed according to their parathyroid hormone levels) resulted in serum aluminum concentrations declining from a median level of 27.2ng/ml to 3.8ng/ml as compared with a median level of 2.5ng/ml for healthy controls[289]. There was also a reversal of high aluminum levels in the tissues, including the brains, of the children with kidney disease[304,609]. Figure 9 emphasizes this dramatic reversal:

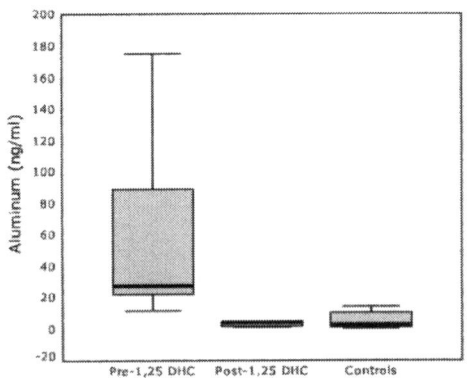

Figure 9 – Vitamin D lowers elevated aluminum levels in children[289]

Kidney disease frequently goes undiagnosed. This can be because a marker for kidney disease, parathyroid hormone – PTH, at first enhances aluminum absorption and aluminum accumulation in the brain and bones[304,305]. Once the aluminum levels get sufficiently high in the parathyroid gland, the aluminum disguises the kidney disease by then inhibiting PTH production by the parathyroid gland[610]. Aluminum also inhibits the production of active vitamin D from D2 in the kidneys of rats, dogs, and humans[300,301,611]. Therefore aluminum absorption may be one of the reasons for the prevalence of active vitamin D deficiency in the U.S. population[302].

Several reasons for why vitamin D prevents autism have been proposed but the most likely reason is that vitamin D helps to keep aluminum levels low in children.

UVB radiation in sunlight is required for converting 7-dehydrocholesterol to vitamin D. Therefore, in addition to aluminum inhibition of vitamin D biosynthesis, the following environmental factors have resulted in an 18% increase in vitamin D deficiency due to a loss of solar radiation penetrating the skin of mothers and their children from 1988 to 2004[302]:

- Increased Air Pollution
- Increased use of sunscreen and sunblock

Increased Air Pollution

Global dimming is the gradual reduction in the amount of solar radiation reaching the earth's surface due to pollution in the atmosphere. Pollution that has reduced the amount of UVB radiation reaching the earth's surface includes carbon dioxide, resulting from burning fossil fuels. Also increased atmospheric water vapor due to carbon dioxide induced global warming has reduced the amount of UVB radiation reaching the earth's surface.

The amount of global dimming from 1980 to 2000, as estimated from accurate measurements made by thermopile pyranometers, is 5.4%[612]. Global dimming increased from 1980 to 2000 due to man-made changes in atmospheric pollution and water vapor. This increase in global dimming reduces the amount of vitamin D being produced by people and has been partially responsible for creating a vitamin D deficiency in the population.

Increased Use of Sunblock and Sunscreen

Between 1980 and 2000 U.S. sales of sunblock and sunscreen adjusted for inflation during this period increased by 26%[613-615]. The fear of skin cancer, due to the enlarging ozone-hole, stimulated sales of UVB sunblock and sunscreen. The first UV sunblock was "Coppertone - For Faces Only" introduced in 1980. By 1993 more than 125 sunblocks and sunscreens had the Skin Cancer Foundation's seal of approval[616]. A sunscreen with a SPF of 15 blocks 93% of UVB radiation from skin and a SPF of 50 blocks 98%. Usage of sunscreen and sunblock increased significantly from 1980 to 2000. This was due to the fear of overexposure to UV radiation from the sun caused by the man-made lowering of atmospheric ozone. This increased usage of sunscreen and sunblock has created a dysevolutionary vitamin D deficiency in the population. This vitamin D deficiency has left children less protected from aluminum absorption and aluminum accumulation in their brains.

Increased Premature Birth

Premature birth complications are estimated to be responsible for 35% of the world's 3.1 million annual neonatal deaths[617]. ASD has been found to be three time more prevalent in children born extremely premature at less than 27 weeks. Each week of shorter gestation was associated with an increased risk of ASD[618]. The U.S. is one of ten countries in the world with the highest rate (e.g. 12%) of premature babies[614]. Broken down by race that rate of premature babies is 10.9% for white Americans and 17.5% for black Americans. Rates of premature birth are rising worldwide and from 1990 to 2010 they increased by 0.7% in the U.S.[617]. Even though the increasing rate of premature births in the U.S. is too small to account for the rise in autism rates, it may account for some percentage of autism.

The amount of aluminum in the blood of premature infants is more than that of full-term infants[566,619]. Aluminum levels in the blood of the fetus increases between 4 and half and 6 months, and again at 8 months gestation[566,619]. Also, the breastmilk of mothers with premature infants contains more aluminum than that of mothers who carried their babies to full term[566,619-621]. At delivery the blood of full term infants usually contains higher aluminum levels than the mother's blood[566,622]. These high levels of aluminum decrease shortly after delivery, if the full-term infant's kidneys are functioning normally[566,619]. However, because the kidneys of premature babies have not fully developed, the aluminum consumed is not fully excreted. If infants and premature babies with decreased kidney function are fed an intravenous feeding solution directly into their bloodstream with aluminum in excess of 25μg/liter[623], they can suffer from impaired neurologic and mental development including dementia. The level of aluminum in intravenous feeding solution is government-regulated such that solutions used for intravenous feeding can only have up to 25μg/liter of aluminum[623].

This aluminum limit is too high and should be adjusted down to a level commensurate with the amount of aluminum in the blood of an infant resulting from being fed 100% breastmilk. Aluminum in breastmilk has been found to vary in the U.K. from 3 to 79μg/liter[599] and in Spain from 14 to 33μg/liter[393]. A baby's daily consumption of milk and their blood volume are both correlated with their weight. Five pound babies consume 400cc of milk per day and have 180cc of blood and 13 pound babies consume 1300cc of milk per day and have 470cc of blood. Approximately 0.04μg of aluminum in 400cc of milk and 0.13μg of aluminum in 1300cc of milk (e.g. 0.2% of 50μg/liter aluminum in this milk) is absorbed into the baby's blood stream within a few hours after ingestion of breastmilk. This corresponds to an aluminum level in the blood of a breast fed baby of 0.1μg/liter that is 250 times lower than the U.S. government level for intravenous feeding solutions of 25μg/liter. A new government standard for intravenous feeding solution should limit the aluminum to less than 0.1μg/liter.

Increased Number of Infant Vaccinations

The number of vaccinations required for school entry increased from 10 in the late 1970's to 32 in 2010. As these vaccines have become available they have been adopted by developed countries around the world. Of the 32 vaccinations currently required for school entry, 18 vaccinations that are given in the first 72 months contain an aluminum salt as a helper or adjuvant for the vaccine (see table below on aluminum containing vaccines).

Vaccines without aluminum do not cause autism. A 2014 meta-analysis of a number of studies of MMR (mumps, measles, and rubella) vaccinations in 1.2 million children found no correlation between MMR vaccination and autism[624]. The study concluded that all vaccines were therefore safe. The study's reassuring conclusion was widely publicized without mentioning the results were only for the MMR vaccine that does not contain aluminum. The results of this study prove that in the case of the MMR vaccine, vaccination is safe with regard to autism since MMR contains no aluminum adjuvant. Vaccines have significantly lowered the prevalence of a variety of serious diseases, improved the quality of life, and increased the longevity of humans. Therefore we should continue to use vaccines as a cultural evolution for protection against infectious diseases.

There is a book published by the CDC entitled "Epidemiology and Prevention of Vaccine-Preventable Disease" that is called the "Pink Book". Chemicals added to vaccines are called excipients and excipients that make the vaccine more efficacious, such as aluminum or alum, are called adjuvants. The CDC maintains an online appendix of the "Pink Book" titled "Vaccine Excipient & Media Summary" with a table of "Excipients Included in U.S. Vaccines by Vaccine". In order to keep current on vaccines that contain aluminum look for aluminum or alum containing vaccines in this table:

https://www.cdc.gov/vaccines/pubs/pinkbook/downloads/appendices/b/excipient-table-2.pdf

Aluminum in Vaccines

The aluminum adjuvant makes the vaccine more effective in creating an immunological response. The three most common aluminum containing adjuvants currently used are: aluminum hydroxide, aluminum phosphate, and alum. The following table gives a list of adjuvants used in vaccines and the amount of aluminum in each dose of vaccine. The average amount of aluminum per dose is 350µg. The maximum amount of aluminum per dose of vaccine is regulated at 0.850mg to 1.25mg in the U.S.[625,626].

Aluminum Containing Vaccines Given as 18 Vaccinations During First 72 Months				
Adjuvant	**Vaccine**	**Trade Name**	**Company**	**Aluminum/Dose (mg)**
Aluminum Hydroxide	DTaP[B]	Infanrix	GlaxoSmithKline	<0.625
	Hepatitis A	Harvrix	GlaxoSmithKline	0.25
	Hepatitis B	Engerix-B	GlaxoSmithKline	0.25
	Hib[A]	Ped Vax Hib	Merck and Co.	0.225
	DTaP[B]-Ipv[C] Hep.B	Pediarx	GlaxoSmithKline	<0.85
Aluminum Phosphate	PCV – Vacc. for Pneumococcus	Prevnar 13	Wyeth	0.125
	Hepatitis A	Vaqta	Merck and Co.	0.225
	Hepatitis A & B	Twinrix	GlaxoSmithKline	0.45
	Td[D] (adult)	Mass Biologic.	Mass. Dept.P.H.	0.45
	DTaP[B]	Daptacel	Aventis Pasteur	0.33
Alum	Hib[A]- Hepatitis B	Comvax	Merck and Co.	0.225
	Hepatitis B	Recombivax	Merck and Co.	0.5

A. Hib is for childhood meningitis, pneumonia, and epiglottitis. B. DTaP is for diphtheria, pertussis (a.k.a. whooping cough), and tetanus. C. IPV is inactivated polio vaccine. D. Td is a tetanus and diphtheria booster given every 10 years to adolescents and adults.

In 2002, Kieth et al. compared the amount of aluminum children received from a series of vaccinations under a then current schedule of vaccinations with aluminum absorbed from a diet of breastmilk and infant formula[627]. Aluminum absorbed from the gut, or muscle, into blood serum is bioavailable aluminum. The amount of bioavailable aluminum due to injections was modeled on an aluminum retention study done in 1992 with radioactive aluminum[628]. Kieth et al. concluded that the body burden of aluminum from vaccinations exceeded that from dietary sources. This work was revised by Mitkus in 2011 using the then current vaccination schedule and the same conclusion was reached[629].

Using radioactive aluminum as the adjuvant in vaccinations, it was shown with New Zealand white rabbits that aluminum is dissolved in the interstitial fluid, absorbed by the blood and distributed and retained by tissues and organs in the body including the brain[630]. This study simulates the 862μg of aluminum injected as vaccines in children at both 6 and 15 months. After vaccination of the rabbits with 850μg of aluminum hydroxide adjuvant, 17% was absorbed and 5.6% was excreted in the urine in 28 days. This means the bioavailability of the aluminum hydroxide adjuvant is 22.6% (e.g. 17%+5.6%). After vaccination with 850μg of aluminum phosphate as adjuvant, 51% was absorbed and 22% was excreted in the urine[630]. This means the bioavailability of aluminum phosphate adjuvant is 73% (e.g. 51%+22%). Also these data showed that 0.1μg (0.01%) of the aluminum from aluminum hydroxide adjuvant and 0.3μg (0.03%) of the aluminum from aluminum phosphate adjuvant ended up absorbed by the brain of the New Zealand white rabbits[630].

Unfortunately no study has measured aluminum absorption into blood serum and excretion in urine of human infants, after injection of 850μg of aluminum adjuvant into their skin and muscle. But the data on New Zealand white rabbits is relevant to humans. The dissolution of aluminum adjuvants into the muscular interstitial fluid (ISF) has been studied[630]. The weight of the white rabbits is similar to infants and rabbits and humans are both mammals. Therefore it is likely that similar percentages (i.e. 20-80%) of aluminum used as adjuvants in vaccines are bioavailable in infants and a small percentage is retained in the infant's brain as seen with the rabbit model.

Both Kieth and Mitkus concluded that the level of aluminum due to vaccination was below the minimum risk level (MRL) set by the government after a brief period following the injection and therefore vaccinations were safe for infants[627,629]. The current aluminum MRL of 1mg/day/kg of body weight as the maximum internal dose and chronic dose is established by the U.S. Agency for Toxic Substances and Diseases[631]. This MRL was established based upon minimal neurological testing with adult mice. The only neurological test performed on these mice was a delay in locating a platform in a water maze test[629]. Because of minimal neurological testing and testing with adult mice and not mice with developing brains, the aluminum MRLs should not be applied to infants.

The correlation between number of vaccinations and prevalence of autism

In 2011 Delong determined the relationship between the proportion of children receiving the recommended schedule of vaccines by age 2 to the prevalence of autism and speech or language impairment[632]. Data was used from each state in the U.S. from 2001 and 2007. A positive relationship was found between number of children receiving vaccinations and both autism and speech and language impairment. That is for every 1% increase in the number of children being vaccinated there were 680 more children having autism or speech and language impairment. Factors controlled for in this analysis were family income and ethnicity. Neither parental behavior nor access to care affected the results.

In 2011 Tomljenovic and Shaw looked at the prevalence of autism as a function of vaccination schedules in 7 western countries including the U.S.[633]. They found the following:

- Children from countries with the highest autism prevalence have the highest exposure to aluminum containing vaccines.
- The increase in exposure to aluminum adjuvants in the U.S. significantly correlates with the increase in autism prevalence in the U.S. over the last two decades.
- A significant correlation exists between the amount of aluminum administered to children, particularly at 3 to 4 months of age, and the current prevalence of autism in 7 western countries.

The correlation between vaccination schedules and prevalence of autism

There are 5 vaccines given in the first 72 months that contain an aluminum adjuvant. They are for hepatitis A and B; DTaP for diphtheria, whooping cough and tetanus; and PCV for pneumococcus. The current U.S. vaccination schedule of 18 vaccinations with the 5 vaccines containing an aluminum adjuvant is provided in the following table:

Current U.S. Vaccination Schedule by Vaccine and Aluminum (µg) per Dose							
Vaccine	**Birth**	**2 mo**	**4 mo**	**6 mo**	**15 mo**	**24 mo**	**72 mo**
Hepatitis B	250	250		250			
DTaP		375	375	375	375		375
Hib		112.5	112.5	112.5	112.5		
PCV		125	125	125	125		
Hepatitis A					250	250	
Total Al (µg)	250	862.5	612.5	862.5	862.5	250	375
Total Al (µg /kg bw)	73.5	172.5	107.5	113.5	78.4	19.8	19.3

Note: eight of the eighteen vaccinations are given from birth through 4 months of age. Two of these eight vaccinations (e.g. for PCV) have aluminum phosphate as adjuvant and two (e.g. for DTaP) can have either aluminum hydroxide or aluminum phosphate as adjuvant. The other two vaccinations (e.g. for Hepatitis B and Hib) have either aluminum hydroxide or alum (e.g. mixture of aluminum hydroxyphosphate sulfate and potassium aluminum sulfate) as adjuvants[626].

The vaccination schedule of seven western countries is provided in the following table along with the estimated aluminum exposure in micrograms per kilogram of body weight at different ages[633]. A range of exposures is given where DTaP and Hib are scheduled. The ASD prevalence was measured for the children's birth years as indicated. The vaccination schedule for each country corresponds to the schedule used during children's birth years used for the ASD prevalence study:

ASD Prevalence versus Schedule of First 6 Months of Aluminum (µg/kg bw) in Vaccines[633]								
Country	ASD prevalence/10,000	Birth	1 mo	2 mo	3 mo	4 mo	5 mo	6 mo
U.K.	157 (1994-99)	73.5	62.5	109-245	55.7-184	73.7-193	0	0
U.S.	110 (1990-2004)	73.5	0	109-245	0	51.8-171.1	0	71.7-161.2
Canada	65 (1987-98)	73.5	0	84-220	0	73.7-193	0	22.4-111.8
Australia	62.5 (1993-99)	73.5	0	84-220	0	73.7-193	0	55.3-144.7
Sweden	53.4 (1977-94)	0	0	0	32.1-160.4	0	25.4-126.9	0
Iceland	12.4 (1984-93)	0	0	0	32.1-160.4	0	25.4-126.9	0
Finland	12.2 (1979-94)	0	0	0	32.1-160.4	0	25.4-126.9	0

From this table it appears that scheduling vaccinations from birth to 4 months is highly correlated with higher ASD prevalence. Several milestones of human brain development occur during this time period including an increase of synapse development at birth, maximal growth of the hippocampus at 2 to 3 months[634], and amygdala maturation at 8 weeks[635]. The hippocampus is involved in memory storage and the amygdala regulates social interaction.

Specifically around 8 weeks of age, as the amygdala begins to mature, a normal infant becomes socially oriented. They will coo, goo, and phonate in response to smiling faces and will seek out the face of their care giver. These behaviors are attributed to the amygdala and the partially contiguous temporal lobe. The left amygdala can determine the direction someone else is looking and the right amygdale becomes active when making eye contact. Around 2 months of age the face detection neurons begin to develop in the amygdala and the infant will stare into the eyes of others and will recognize and orient toward familiar faces. These face recognition neurons are connected to temporal lobe neurons involved in auditory perception and social-emotional functioning triggering smiling and crying behavior. Frequently this development is not seen in autistic children.

Cures for Autism

By lowering your child's aluminum levels using high-dose vitamin D3 supplementation can be a cure for symptoms of autism. Doctor J.J. Cannell has recently published a series of anecdotal case reports of autism symptoms being minimized by the use of high dose vitamin D3 supplementation[326]. In order to see these improvements Doctor Cannell recommends sufficient D3 supplementation to maintain your child's serum level of vitamin D2 in the high-normal range. Your child's pediatrician should be involved in monitoring your child's serum level of vitamin D2 during high-level supplementation. Dr. Cannell recommends that autistic children receive regular vitamin D2 blood tests and start with the following dosage of vitamin D3 per day:

- Children weighing less than 33 pounds – 1,600 IU/day
- Children weighing 33-66 pounds – 3,300 IU/day
- Children weighing 66-100 pounds – 5,000 IU/day

After 3 months of supplementation at these levels of D3, Doctor Cannell recommends adjusting dosage of vitamin D3 accordingly to achieve vitamin D2 levels in the high-normal range[326].

There has been no published study of dissolved silica supplementation as a cure for symptoms of autism. However, there is reason to believe that dissolved silica may work to lower aluminum levels in autistic children and cure some symptoms of autism. The following is anecdotal information from a parent who has given his child silica rich water for 3 months:

"I have become fascinated with this subject and the unbelievable simplicity of drinking a silicon rich mineral water to remove aluminum from the body since discovering Prof Chris Exley's excellent work at the end of 2017. We have been using this on our 9 yr old son who has an ASD (Autism Spectrum Disorder) diagnosis and we have seen clear cognitive improvements with him after 3 months now. There have been improvements to his mood, his laughing. He is more happy and has more speech, asking significantly more questions (this is MASSIVE!), and more imaginative play".

Conclusion of Autism as a Mismatch Disease

In 2012 and 2015 two independent studies found that aluminum in the hair of autistic children was much higher than aluminum in the hair of non-autistic children[569,570]. In 2017 an analysis was performed on the brains of 5 individuals with confirmed ASD finding some of the highest aluminum levels in the brain yet recorded[571].

Four independent studies have found a correlation between baby formula usage and autism. Therefore we can conclude that autism is a mismatch disease. *Homo sapiens* evolved in an environment that required weaning at 3 years. The trend toward increased breast feeding beginning in 1971 has been associated with an increase in formula feeding in infants from 3 to 12 months of age. Also from 1980 to 2000 there was a 0 to 25% increase in market share taken by manufacturers of soy based baby formula that has been found in the U.K. and Canada to have very high levels of aluminum. Because both soy and non-soy based baby formula have significantly higher levels of aluminum than does breast milk, aluminum in the baby formula is very likely a causal factor of autism.

In 2015 it was found that children with ASD had significantly lower vitamin D2 (24nM) as compared with their non-ASD siblings (32nM)[290]. Since vitamin D lowers aluminum in children with high levels of aluminum, vitamin D deficiency results in higher aluminum levels in children. There has been an 18.6% decline in the level of vitamin D2 in the U.S. population from 1988 to 2004[302]. This is because UVB radiation from the sun is required to convert 7-dehydrocholesterol to vitamin D3 in our skin cells. But we use sunscreen and sunblock to protect ourselves from the increased risk of skin cancer. This increased risk is due to increased UV radiation resulting from the dysevolutionary practice of manufacturing chemicals that reduce ozone in the earth's atmosphere. Global dimming is due to the dysevolutionary practice of increasing air pollution. Therefore both increased global dimming and usage of sunscreen and sunblock act to lower our ability to produce vitamin D3 from 7-dehydrocholesterol resulting in higher levels of aluminum in our children.

Two studies found a significant correlation exists between the prevalence of ASD and the number of aluminum containing vaccinations administered as vaccines to infants from birth through 4 months of age[633] and 2 years of age[632]. The following table shows the monthly ingestion and vaccination sources of bioavailable aluminum during the first 4 months of an infant's life:

Bioavailable Aluminum (µg) During First 4 Months of Life in the U.S.					
Source	**1st Month**	**2nd Month**	**3rd Month**	**4th Month**	**Total Al**
Breastmilk[A]	3	3	3	3	12
Non-soy Formula[A]	13	13	13	13	52
Soy Formula[A]	39	39	39	39	156
Vacc–AlumHyd[B]	58[D]	83[E]	0	26[F]	167
Vacc–AlumPhos[C]	0	365[G]	0	365[G]	730

A. Aluminum in U.K., Spain, and Canadian formulas[384,385,393,403] and breastmilk[393,597] and bioavailable aluminum is 0.2% of ingested aluminum[391]
B. Aluminum hydroxide adjuvant 850µg injected results in 23% /month absorbed & urinated[630]
C. Aluminum phosphate adjuvant 850µg injected results in 73% /month absorbed & urinated[630]
D. Bioavailable aluminum in Hepatitus B with aluminum hydroxide (250µg x 0.23)
E. Bioavailable aluminum in Hepatitus B and Hib with aluminum hydroxide (362.5µg x 0.23)
F. Bioavailable aluminum in Hib with aluminum hydroxide (112.5µg x 0.23)
G. Bioavailable aluminum in PCV and DTaP with aluminum phosphate (500µg x 0.73)

The data in this table clearly agree with both Kieth in 2002[628] and Mitkus in 2011[629] who concluded that the body burden of aluminum from vaccinations exceeded that from dietary sources. The data in this table show that during the first four months of a child's life the amount of aluminum absorbed and urinated from vaccinations with aluminum containing vaccines is estimated to be more than five times higher than the amount of aluminum absorbed from ingested soy based baby formula. Therefore, since the increasing autism rate observed between 1980 and 2000 correlates with increasing baby formula usage during this same period, there is very little doubt that absorbed aluminum due to vaccinations is also a causal factor for autism and contributes to the increasing rate of autism.

Therefore the usage of baby formula is a cultural evolution in response to our dysevolutionary practice of shortening of weaning times and lengthening the period of formula feeding. The increased use of formula contributes to the rising rate of autism and makes autism a mismatch disease. Baby formula is not equivalent to mother's milk in the following four ways

- Higher aluminum concentration
- Low dissolvable silica
- Low PQQ
- Low vitamin D

The amount of aluminum in baby formula should be minimized and the level should be indicated on the container. Also fortification of formula with the nutrients PQQ and dissolvable silica should be required and the levels listed on the container. Until this is done the current manufacture, labeling, and use of baby formula is dysevolutionary.

Vaccinations are a cultural evolution in response to infectious diseases that are mismatch diseases. The addition of aluminum to vaccines is dysevolutionary and contributes to the rising rate of autism.

Autism is therefore a mismatch disease due to four factors:

- Increasing formula feeding and thereby increasing the infant's aluminum burden
- Decreasing vitamin D's aluminum protection due to global dimming
- Decreasing vitamin D's aluminum protection due to sunscreen and sunblock usage
- Increasing infant vaccinations and thereby increasing the infant's aluminum burden

Mesoamericans 5000 years ago responded to their dysevolutionary abandonment of hunting and gathering in favor of farming by chemically changing what they ingested to maintain their mental health. They created a chemical treatment of corn to make niacin bioavailable in order to avoid pellagra. Our culture must follow in their footsteps and change the way we manufacture and use baby formula, vitamin D supplementation, and vaccines in order to maintain our children's mental health and avoid the mismatch disease -- autism.

There exists in the world today a chemical environment that will lower the rate of autism. If you are not a believer look at the data in this table:

Current Autism Rate and AD Death Rate by Country		
Country	**Autism Rate (per 100,000)***	**AD Death Rate (per 100,000)****
United States	1470 (2014)	45.6
Iceland	1200 (2013)	34.1
Malaysia	160 (2008)	0.7
Singapore	100 (2001)	0.2

*Autism rate data from references 598-601, **AD death rate data 2016 worldlifeexpectancy.com

Given what is currently known about the neurotoxicity of aluminum there is enough data to conclude:

"Alzheimer's is a manifestation of accumulated aluminum in a mature brain and autism is a manifestation of aluminum in an immature developing brain."

Since aluminum can cause autism we should take steps to keep aluminum levels as low as possible in both formula and vaccines for the sake of the fetus and infant. In order to facilitate aluminum excretion by the mother and baby, mothers should keep serum silica and vitamin D levels as high as possible during pregnancy and beast-feeding. This will provide the fetus and newborn baby with sufficient levels of both silica and vitamin D.

The following recommendations are based upon currently available data:

1. Governments should fund research to find alternative adjuvants for vaccines that do not contain aluminum.
2. When possible do not have your infant vaccinated with more than one vaccine containing aluminum at the same time.
3. When a choice is available, as in the case with Hib and Hepatitis A and B, use vaccines with aluminum hydroxide and not aluminum phosphate or alum as an adjuvant.
4. Take a dissolved mineral orthosilicic acid (OSA) supplement during both pregnancy and breast feeding in order to increase serum silica levels and lower aluminum levels in the mother, fetus, and newborn infant (see Chapters 5 and 6).
5. Infants and children should also be given a dissolved mineral orthosilicic acid (OSA) supplement.
6. Take a vitamin D supplement (4,000 IU/day) during pregnancy and (6,000 IU/day) while breast feeding. Infants should be given 400 IU/day and children should be given 600 IU/day of vitamin D3. If baby formula is used it should have a sufficient level of vitamin D3 to correspond to 400 IU/day based upon the volume of formula the infant consumes in a day. Otherwise D3 supplementation is recommended, such as Baby D3 by California Gold Nutrition at 400 IU/drop.
7. All baby formula should be fortified with PQQ, and dissolvable silica
8. The amount of PQQ, and dissolvable silica should be listed as an ingredient on containers of baby formula
9. Governments should change the current standard for intravenous feeding solutions limiting the aluminum to less than 0.1μg/liter.
10. The current aluminum U.S. MRL standard should not be applied to human infants.

Conclusion of Prevent Alzheimer's, Autism, and Stroke

"We can alleviate physical pain but mental pain ... dementia is less accessible to treatment. It's connected to who we are – our personality, our character, our soul ..." Richard Eyre

This book is about what causes Alzheimer's, autism, and stroke and how you and your loved ones can avoid and prevent these terrible diseases. Based upon the latest scientific literature and annotated with references to that literature, this book introduces you to aluminum being the primary culprit that causes Alzheimer's, autism, and stroke. Specific methods are given for lowering your aluminum ingestion and enhancing your aluminum excretion. Secondary culprits such as genetics, vitamin and folic acid deficiency, LDL, triglycerides, atrial fibrillation, and lifestyle choices are also covered. A preventative system is proposed for individuals involving 7 supplements, 7 lifestyle choices, and a dissolved mineral that will prevent Alzheimer's, autism, and stroke. This is also a combination therapy that can reverse the cognitive decline in early stage Alzheimer's disease. Recently a combination therapy involving 6 of the 7 supplements and 2 of the 7 lifestyle choices was tested on a limited population of 10 Alzheimer's patients. The 9 early stage AD patients all showed improved cognition in the first 3 to 6 months of treatment. All six of the patients whose cognitive decline had a major impact on job performance returned to work during the study[536].

Alzheimer's, autism, and stroke may be thought of as both modern diseases and mismatch diseases. This is because these diseases resulted from behaviors and cultural practices that have changed both our environment and lifestyles making them more harmful than what our ancestors experienced during their evolution. Information is frequently the catalyst for cultural modification and hopefully the information in this book will facilitate a cultural change in behaviors that will ultimately prevent mismatch diseases, such as Alzheimer's, autism, and stroke. Individually and collectively we can change our culture and make the choice to prevent these mismatch diseases with the following recommendations:

Recommendations for Preventing Alzheimer's, Autism, and Stroke

Seven Supplements:

1. **PQQ:** Protect your brain during and after a stroke, increase the energy available in your brain, and enhance your memory and keep your brain young with more neurites by taking a PQQ supplement (20mg/day).

2. **CoQ10:** Protect your brain during and after a stroke from oxidative stress and increase its energy efficiency by taking a CoQ10 supplement (ubiquinone 200mg/day).

3. **Vitamin D3:** Lower aluminum levels in your blood and tissues and maintain healthy levels of glutathione and low levels of inducible nitric oxide synthase prior to age 71 with 600 IU or over age 71 with 2,000 IU's of supplemental D3. In order to protect the fetus and infant from aluminum, mothers are recommended to take 4,000 IU/day while pregnant and 6,000 IU/day of vitamin D3 while breastfeeding. Infants should be given 400 IU/day and children should be given 800 IU/day of vitamin D3. If baby formula is used it should have a sufficient level of vitamin D3 to correspond to 400 IU/day based upon the volume of formula the infant consumes, otherwise vitamin D3 supplementation is recommended.

4. **Taurine:** Protects your brain during and after a stroke and lowers the risk of stroke with a taurine supplement (500mg/day). Taurine crosses the blood-brain barrier and ameliorates the toxic effects of aluminum and other metals in the body.

5. **Vitamin K2-MK-4:** Prevents and possibly reverses aortic mitral valve calcification. Take a daily supplement of vitamin K2-MK-4 (500mcg/day) and vitamin K2-MK-7 (100mcg/day) for cardiovascular health. For osteoporosis take K2-MK-4 (5mg/day). Do not take these supplements if you are taking oral anticoagulants, like warfarin (a.k.a. Coumadin), that are vitamin K antagonists.

6. **B100 Supplement:** Keeps your homocysteine levels low (100mg/day of vitamin B6, 100mcg/day of vitamin B12, and 400mcg of folic acid). These are all found in a time-release B100 complex. In the case of vitamin B12 malabsorption, use sublingual absorption tablets containing B12, B6 (as pyridoxine hydrochloride), folic acid and biotin from Wonder Laboratory or get B12 shots from a doctor.

7. **5-MTHF (Methyl Folate):** Take 400mcg/day of 5-MTHF in order to keep your homocysteine levels low, even if you have the MTHFR gene that prevents your body from converting folic acid to methyl folate.

Seven Lifestyle Choices:

1. **Stop smoking** - in order to lower aluminum and homocysteine levels and risk of stroke.

2. **Decrease alcohol consumption** – in order to lower homocysteine levels and risk of stroke.

3. **Avoid aluminum ingestion**

    - **Avoid aluminum containing pharmaceuticals** – Read labels and lists of ingredients. Do not use antacids containing aluminum

    - **Filter your drinking water** - Use a Brita pour-through pitcher system with filter number OB03 to remove aluminum from your tap water.

    - **Avoid using aluminum cookware** – Use stainless steel and cast iron for cooking. Use non-stick aluminum foil with the non-stick surface against food or use a layer of plastic wrap between aluminum foil and food.

    - **Use aluminum free antiperspirants and astringents** - Use either Arm & Hammer's "Essentials" or Tom's of Maine "Original" deodorants that are both aluminum free. Use Epsom salts and avoid aluminum containing astringents for mild skin irritation.

- **Don't purchase and store beverages or food in aluminum containers** - as they will slowly add aluminum to the water and beverages. Purchase and store beverages and food in glass or plastic.

- **Avoid using soy-based infant formula** – Purchase non-soy based formula.

4. **Increase dissolved silica in your diet** – Eat food and drink beverages high in silica.

5. **Aerobically exercise** – Exercise for 40 minutes at least three times a week at 60 to 75% of your heart rate reserve for the following benefits:

- Results in the destruction and clean-up of amyloid plaque in the brain
- Increases neurogenesis in the dentate gyrus of the hippocampus resulting in larger hippocampal volume and increased memory
- Stimulates production of PYY that lowers aluminum absorption and accumulation.
- Reverses the effect of aluminum in the prefrontal cortex thereby improving working memory
- Increases aluminum excretion by perspiration facilitated by a diet including a mineral water with dissolved silicic acid.

6. **Avoid lack of sleep** – Get exposure to sunlight or blue light every day to maintain your circadian rhythm.

7. **Avoid head trauma** - Avoid head trauma by using walking and balance aids, wear a seat belt, wear a helmet on a bike, and remove obstacles on the floor of walkways.

Take the Dissolved Mineral OSA Daily:

Take three to four cups of high silica mineral water, such as Fiji Water or homemade Silicade. The recipe for Silicade is in Chapter 5. Or take a dissolved silica (OSA) supplement containing 10 to 34mg of silicon daily. For example take 5 drops of choline stabilized orthosilicic acid (a.k.a. Biosil) twice a day in a quarter cup of flavored liquid to increase aluminum excretion by your kidneys. Silica supplementation is also recommended for children.

Cultural and Governmental Changes:

1) Encourage your local community's water department to maintain at least 50mg/liter OSA (i.e. soluble silica) in drinking water. This will decrease aluminum accumulation in your and your children's brains. Silica also protects water pipes from corrosion (PQ Corp., Bulletin 37-3).

2) Encourage your local community's water department to cease adding fluoride to drinking water. This will both decrease aluminum corrosion while cooking in aluminum cookware and will decrease accumulation of aluminum in the brains of those who drink the water.

3) Encourage more government funded research to develop non-aluminum adjuvants for vaccines.

4) Have your child vaccinated with one vaccine at a time. This may require the use of the federal government's Vaccine Injury Compensation Program (VICP). In a landmark case in 2008 the Poling family was awarded damages under VICP when their daughter Hannah developed autism-like symptoms after the administration of vaccine.

5) When a choice is available, as in the case with Hib and Hepatitis A and B, use vaccines with aluminum hydroxide and not aluminum phosphate or alum as an adjuvant. Although all aluminum containing adjuvants are bioavailable, aluminum hydroxide has been shown to be less bioavailable than other aluminum adjuvants.

6) Encourage the labeling of all food and pharmaceutical products that contain aluminum as a food additive, inactive ingredient, or active ingredient. The warning label should both state that the product contains aluminum and that aluminum is a known neurotoxin causing Alzheimer's, autism, and stroke.

7) Encourage the labeling of all food, including baby formula, with the amount of aluminum per serving. This will allow producers of baby formula with low aluminum levels to differentiate their formula from other brands with higher aluminum levels.

8) Encourage the sale of baby formula fortified with dissolved or dissolvable silica, and PQQ as found in mother's milk. Producers of baby formula should find the addition of silica, and PQQ as a way to differentiate their baby formula from others on a crowded shelf of competing baby formulas in the market.

9) Encourage our government to change the current standard for intravenous feeding solutions (e.g. parenteral nutrition) used with premature babies, limiting the aluminum in these solutions to less than 0.1mcg/liter. This is the calculated average concentration of aluminum absorbed into the infant's blood when being fed breastmilk.

10) Encourage our government to adjust the current aluminum U.S. MRL standard to lower levels due to aluminum being a causal factor of Alzheimer's, autism, and stroke. Different MRL standards are required for infants and children, with developing brains, pregnant women, and other adults.

Miscellaneous Recommendations:

1) Get your homocysteine and B12 blood levels tested yearly.

2) Take zinc chelated with an amino acid (15mg/day) and N-acetylcysteine (NAC, 600mg/day) in order to keep your blood-brain barrier healthy by combating aluminum and increasing glutathione (see Appendix V).

3) Take a statin to lower your LDL and decrease the risk of stroke, if LDL or total serum cholesterol level is too high and you have not had a prior hemorrhagic stroke. Otherwise take chromium picolinate (200mcg/day) to lower your LDL.

4) Eat a diet high in omega-3 fatty acids, as described in the section on DHA in Chapter 3, and take a quarter gram per day of the omega-7 palmitoleic acid, if your serum triglyceride level is too high.

5) Take 1 to 2 grams of EPA supplement every day and a quarter gram per day of the omega-7 palmitoleic acid, if both your serum triglyceride and LDL levels are too high.

6) Take DHA (1 gram/day) or a mixture of DHA and EPA (1 gram/day), if your memory becomes impaired due to poor diet,

7) Use toothpaste not packed in aluminum lined tubes (i.e. Toms of Maine), or packed in tubes with a layer of plastic between the toothpaste and aluminum (i.e. Crest, Colgate).

8) Do not swallow toothpaste with fluoride during use.

9) Avoid using food products containing alum (i.e. some baking powders, baking mixes, shredded cheeses, and pickles).

10) Use homemade baking powder that contains less than 4mcg per teaspoon of aluminum. Made from cream of tartar, baking soda, and corn starch.

11) Use table salt, such as Morton, that is aluminum free.

12) Lower your stress and caffeine intake – 12oz. of coffee contains 200mg. of caffeine.

13) Lower aluminum intake by minimizing green and black tea and chocolate.

If you are like me and read the conclusion of books before reading the book, I suggest next reading the "Introduction" followed by the "Chapter Preview", as this will give you an overview and brief description of each chapter. Then read the detective story "Case of the Cloaked Assassin" in Chapter 1.

Appendix I

Dementia with Lewy Bodies and Parkinson's Disease

Clinically, dementia with Lewy bodies (DLB) is distinguished from AD by fluctuating cognition, prominent visual hallucinations, and Parkinson symptoms. It is distinguished from Parkinson's disease (PD), by cognitive or behavioral decline within one year of the appearance of Parkinson symptoms[636]. With periods of time much longer than a year, PD patients can develop PD dementia (PDD).

A pathological hallmark of both DLB and PD are large inclusions of aggregated α-synuclein peptides inside neurons. It has recently been found in patients with DLB that the amount of presynaptic accumulation of very small α-synuclein aggregates correlates with the extent of neurodegeneration or neurite loss[637]. PD is pathologically characterized by loss of neurons that produce dopamine in a specific region of the brain (e.g. ventral tier of the zona compacta of the substantia nigra)[638]. Aluminum accumulation in this brain region (e.g. substantia nigra) has been found to be associated with degeneration of neurons or neurite loss[639]. Also reduced glutathione (GSH) in this brain region has been found to be a biochemical characteristic in the brains of PD patients[640]. Low levels of GSH can be an indication of aluminum inhibition of the enzyme MS as discussed in Chapter 2.

In 2008 it was shown that exposure to a combination of the fungicide Maneb and herbicide Paraquat significantly increase the incidence of PD in people living in the Central Valley of California[641]. Three years later a case-control study nested in the Agricultural Health Study was used to show that exposure to just Paraquat or the pesticide Rotenone significantly increases the incidence of PD[642]. The mechanism is believed to involve irreversible and progressive neuorotoxicity of the substantia nigra region of the brain caused by all three of these commonly used agricultural chemicals[637,638,641,642]. This is particularly surprising as all three of these chemicals are considered safe to use even in residential areas.

Traumatic brain injury (TBI) with loss of consciousness is associated with risk of Lewy body accumulation, parkinsonism, and PD[643]. Simvastatin and atorvastatin have been shown to reduce functional neurological deficits after TBI. Simvastatin has also been found to reduce the risk of both dementia and Parkinson's disease by 50%[242]. This may be due to Simvastatin's ability to lower LDL levels in the blood and prevent vascular endothelial dysfunction as discussed in Chapter 2.

Chemically α-synuclein is similar to the Aβ peptide. Both are peptide products of a larger amyloid protein. Cells expressing α-synuclein production also have nonselective cation channels in the neuron's cell membrane. These results support the theory that in DLB and PD α-synuclein peptides on the neuronal cell membrane can form pore-like channels. Since these channels are nonselective they would allow calcium ions into the neurons that can lead to neuronal death[644]. Memantine is used to treat DLB by inhibiting the prolonged influx of calcium ions through these nonselective channels thereby preventing neuronal death[175].

Dissolved in the cytoplasm of neurons is 1% of α-synuclein that normally does not nucleate into aggregates. Evidence suggests that α-synuclein aggregation constitutes one of the first steps preceding Lewy body formation. Therefore antiaggregation strategies might be useful to prevent α-synuclein aggregate formation. Two such aggregation inhibitors have been recently identified *in vitro*: pyrroloquinoline quinone (PQQ) and cumin aldehyde[274,645].

Because both PQQ and cumin aldehyde are reactive toward amines, their ability to block aggregation indicates that amino acids with the free amines, such as the 15 lysine residues in α-synuclein, may be involved in α-synuclein aggregation. Aluminum reacts with free amine containing amino acids to form oligomeric protein complexes[17]. This could be the mechanism for neuron degeneration and loss observed with aluminum accumulation in PD[639]. This begs the question: Is aluminum involved in aggregation of α-synuclein resulting in DLB, PD, and PDD?

A 58 year old woman living in the Camelford area of Cornwall England was exposed to high levels of aluminum in her drinking water in July of 1988 and died 15 years later due to a rapidly progressive, fatal dementing illness. An autopsy showed Lewy bodies, dramatic Aβ peptide deposition in the cerebral cortical, a modest number of neurofibrillary tangles, and evidence of very high levels of aluminum content in affected brain regions[415]. This was the first autopsy-documented case of Lewy body and Alzheimer's disease-like neurodegeneration in a victim of aluminum exposure. It demonstrates not only a link between aluminum in drinking water and both Lewy bodies as well as AD, but also demonstrates that once aluminum is ingested it becomes permanently bound in the brain and is still present 15 years after ingestion.

Taurine has been found to ameliorate the effect of aluminum toxicity in animals (see "Mystery of How Taurine Protects Against Metal Toxicity" in Chapter 3. Since lower than normal levels of taurine are observed in Parkinson's disease patients, taurine supplementation is recommended for those patients[646,647].

Appendix II

Metabolic Dementia

Metabolic dementia is not caused by aluminum and unlike other dementias it can in most cases be cured or the symptoms relived. Metabolic dementia is discussed in this book because it demonstrates that when we know the cause of a dementia, getting a correct diagnosis and taking the prescribed cure does work to prevent or cure the dementia. By analogy with metabolic dementia, knowing that aluminum is the cause of Alzheimer's, autism, and stroke there is hope that we can also prevent these three diseases in by decreasing aluminum ingestion and increasing aluminum excertion. In this appendix the following five metabolic dementias are described:

- Pellagra - Chronic niacin deficiency leading to low metabolic energy production
- Hypoxia – Chronic low blood oxygen leading to low metabolic energy production
- Hyperammonemia - Ammonia metabolism imbalance
- Hypoglycemia - Control of blood sugar
- Hypercalcemia - Control of calcium levels in the blood
- Hypothyroidism - Control of thyroid hormone levels in the blood

Most of these factors can be controlled by avoiding alcohol and eating a balanced diet. In addition these factors can be controlled by taking drugs or supplements such as antibiotics to cure urinary tract infection, insulin injections for controlling blood sugar, calcimimetic drugs for controlling hyperparathyroidism, levothyroxine for hypothyroidism, and niacin for avoiding pellagra. Therefore metabolic dementia is preventable when it is correctly diagnosed and the prescribed cure taken as recommended.

Pellagra - A chronic niacin deficiency leads to a disease called pellagra. Pellagra is a disfiguring and mentally devastating disease that can be fatal. Niacin (a.k.a. vitamin B3, nicotinic acid) is required for your body's metabolism to produce energy from food. Niacin can be taken as a supplement and can also be found in many foods such as fish, chicken, turkey, pork, beef, peanuts, mushrooms, and potatoes.

Pellagra occurs in areas where people eat primarily corn (a.k.a. maize) as a staple food. This is because corn is very low in digestible niacin as 90% of the niacin is bound in a complex with hemicellulose. This complex is found in the germ and seed coat of the corn kernel. The germ is responsible for stored corn becoming rancid. In 1901 the Beall Degerminator was patented that could mill the corn removing the germ and seed coat from the kernels for improved storage. Corn was a staple food of the poor in the beginning of the 20th century in the southern part of the U.S. In this region of the U.S. between 1906 and 1940 mechanical corn milling resulted in 3 million people sickened by pellagra and more than 100,000 deaths due to pellagra.

In 1913 Casmir Funk wrote an article that suggested the new procedure for corn milling was causing pellagra but he was ignored[5]. The medical profession in the U.S. believed a toxin in corn was the cause of pellagra. It took 80 years after the connection between niacin deficiency and pellagra was discovered for the medical profession to finally abandon their toxin theory. There is a resistance to abandon theories in the face of scientific data when large egos or financial interests are at stake and this slows the adoption of new practices that can save lives.

In Mesoamerica, where corn was originally cultivated, a special cooking technique called nixtamalization was developed between 1500 to 1200 BC that became a vital part of the Aztec and Mayan cultures[550]. Nixtamalization uses an alkaline (i.e. basic pH) water solution to hydrolyze or release the niacin from corn meal. This made niacin bioavailable and allowed these cultures to avoid pellagra.

Hypoxemia – A reduction in oxygen supplied to any part of the body, including the brain, is called hypoxia. Chronic hypoxia is called hypoxemia and is a result of long term respiratory problems, such as chronic obstructive pulmonary disease (COPD). COPD is characterized by a persistent airflow limitation that is progressive and associated with an enhanced chronic inflammatory response in the airways and lungs to noxious particles and gases. COPD is a major risk factor for cognitive impairment. The risk of cognitive impairment has been found to increase by 10 fold as resting blood oxygen levels fall from 95% to 88%[648]. Regular use of supplementary oxygen therapy reduces this risk of cognitive impairment[648]. Two recent case control studies suggest that COPD is associated with reduced hippocampal and gray matter volumes in the brain[649,650]. Since oxygen is required for energy production in the brain, it is not surprising that low oxygen has a negative impact on brain function and neuronal survival.

Hyperammonemia - Disorders of ammonia metabolism can be due to cirrhosis of the liver or urinary tract infection and can result in confusion, brain edema, and neurological damage. In these hyperammonemia disorders excess ammonia in the blood crosses the blood-brain barrier and results in excess extracellular glutamate that stimulates excessive neurotransmission called excitotoxicity[651]. The most common cause of disorders of ammonia metabolism is alcoholism as 10-20% of chronic drinkers develop cirrhosis of the liver.

Hypoglycemia - In 2013 a 12 year study of 783 Americans aged 70-79 and who had no cognitive impairment in 1997 revealed that the risk of having dementia is doubled in older people with diabetes who experience frequent episodes of hypoglycemia or low blood sugar[652]. Blood sugar, like oxygen, is required by mitochondria in order to produce ATP that in the brain is fuel for neurotransmissions involved in cognition. An episode of hypoglycemia starves the mitochondria in neurons of both sugar and energy leading to metabolic dementia.

Hypercalcaemia - High levels of calcium in the blood due to hyperparathyroidism result in dementia. The four parathyroid glands are on the thyroid glands produce parathyroid hormone (PTH) that controls the amount of phosphorus and calcium in the blood. Asymptomatic hyperparathyroidism is common and the following conditions can cause hypercalcaemia or hyperparathyroidism[653]:

- Benign tumor on the parathyroid gland resulting in high levels of PTH
- Chronic kidney disease resulting in high aluminum levels and low vitamin D levels
- Low vitamin D particularly in the elderly
- High level vitamin D3 supplementation in infants (i.e. greater than 1,600 IU/day)[313]

In one person out of a 1,000 a benign tumor on a parathyroid gland called adenoma results in over-production of PTH that incorrectly signals a low blood calcium level[654]. In order to compensate the body mobilizes calcium from bones resulting in abnormally high levels of calcium in the blood, bone loss (osteoporosis), and kidney stones. Also, excess calcium crosses the blood-brain barrier and becomes toxic to neurons resulting in metabolic dementia with cognitive decline superimposed with acute delirium[655]. For people unable to have their parathyroid surgically removed a potential drug therapy is a calcimimetic such as cinacalcet (a.k.a. Sensipar or Mimpara) that mimics the action of calcium on tissues.

High levels of PTH also result in both enhanced gastrointestinal absorption of aluminum and aluminum accumulation in the brain and bones of rats[304,305]. These enhanced brain and bone levels of aluminum were found to be reversed by lowering PTH levels to normal[304,609]. Enhanced aluminum levels in the parathyroid gland[656] have been shown to ultimately inhibit PTH secretion and synthesis by the parathyroid gland of both rats and dogs in a dose dependent manner[300,657]. Since high levels of PTH are the marker for hyperparathyroidism, this negative feedback that controls PTH levels by aluminum may be the reason hyperparathyroidism is commonly asymptomatic. High aluminum levels can also inhibit the biosynthesis of vitamin D3 to active vitamin D. This leads to vitamin D3 resistant softening of the bones (osteomalacia)[301].

Hypothyroidism - The thyroid is stimulated by the thyroid stimulating hormone (TSH) to produce thyroxine (tetraiodothyronine T4). T4 is converted to small amounts of triiodothyronine (T3) that regulates the way energy is used in the body. In hypothyroidism T4 and T3 levels are low. These low levels of T3 and T4 can decrease the levels of glutathione and increase the levels of chemicals that are oxidizing (ROS). Also these low levels of T3 and T4 impair hippocampal neurogenesis, differentiation, and maturation of neuronal precursors, change synaptic transmission and neuroplasticity in the hippocampus, and account for the resulting memory impairment common in hypothyroidism[658-660]. Levothyroxine is a recommended drug for hypothyroidism. Also PQQ can ameliorate some of the effects of hypothyroidism induced metabolic dementia[659].

Appendix III

Hippocampal Sclerosis

Hippocampal sclerosis (HS) involves loss of pyramidal neurons and glial cell activation (a.k.a. gliosis) in the CA1 and subiculum of the hippocampus. Generally HS comes with temporal lobe epilepsy and severe memory loss. HS was first described in 1880 by Wilhelm Sommer[661]. HS is associated with hippocampal atrophy that can be detected by autopsy or MRI and has similar initial symptoms to Alzheimer's disease (AD). Also the rate of progression to dementia in both HS and AD are similar. Therefore HS is frequently misdiagnosed as AD. HS is found in 10% of individuals over 85 and in several studies the frequency of death due to HS has been shown to increase with age[662].

Loss of pyramidal neurons in the CA1 layer of the hippocampus can be the result of aluminum accumulation. Aluminum accumulation in the rat brain has been shown to have the greatest impact on pyramidal neuron death in the CA1 layer of the hippocampus[44]. The rate of aluminum accumulation in the brain increases with age in humans[28,29]. The hippocampus is a hot spot for aluminum accumulation as demonstrated in the following table:

Brain Aluminum Measurements from Humans with AD and Non-demented Controls[86]		
Regions of Brain Analyzed	**AD (mcg/g of brain tissue) Dry Weight**	**Controls (mcg/g brain tissue) Dry Weight**
Entorhinal Cortex	10.2 ± 9.0	1.5 ± 0.6
Hippocampus	4.9 ± 3.0	1.4 ± 0.6
Frontal Cortex (caudal)	6.8 ± 4.3	1.8 ± 0.6
Frontal Cortex (basal/ventral)	6.4 ± 2.9	2.5 ± 0.7

Xu et al. were the first to observe hot spots of aluminum accumulation in the brains of elderly suffering from dementia. Hot spots in human brains typically are in excess of 4mcg/g of aluminum[88]. Hot spots also contain a large number of pyramidal neurons with high levels of aluminum. Aluminum hot spots are not found in non-demented age-matched controls[88]. Both HS and AD have the same etiology with aluminum as causal factor in both cases. In 2011 Rusina et al. measured both aluminum and mercury in the hippocampus and associated visual cortex of 27 controls and 29 histologically-confirmed AD cases. They showed that there was a four-fold increase in aluminum levels in the hippocampus of the AD cases versus the controls. There was no difference in mercury levels between the AD cases and controls[87].

Glial cell activation is caused by some metal ions acting as physiological stressors in the brain by stimulating brain cells to produce oxidizing chemicals (a.k.a. ROS)[121,122]. The metal ions stimulate inducible nitric oxide synthase (iNOS) in microglial and astroglial cells of the brain to produce nitric oxide (NO) that reacts to produce ROS. This ROS can damage and kill neurons creating inflammation in the brain. The following table shows how much ROS is produced from a cell culture of human glial cells exposed to 50nM aqueous solutions of various common metal ions[58]. Aluminum tops the list as a generator of ROS by the brain's glial cells.

Metal Ion Induction of ROS by Human Glial Cells[58]	
Metal Sulfate	**Relative Induction of ROS**
Aluminum	10
Iron	6
Manganese	4.5
Zinc	4
Nickel	3.5
Lead	3.5
Gallium	3
Copper	3
Cadmium	3
Tin	2
Mercury	1.5
Magnesium	0
Sodium	0

Hippocampal atrophy can be caused by aluminum inducing ROS. This atrophy is seen in aluminum hot spots in the brain and it parallels aluminum accumulation in those regions of the brain as we age[86,94]. Some brain atrophy in the hippocampal complex and the frontal cortex (i.e. 0.3-0.6%) is common with age in healthy adults[93]. In 2009 Fjell et al. studied brain atrophy in people 60-91 years old. The study included 142 healthy participants and 122 with AD. The four areas of the brain found to significantly atrophy during one year in AD patients were the same areas found to be hot spots for aluminum accumulation. Also the rate of atrophy is much higher in AD brains than in healthy adult brains as shown in the following table[94].

Brain Atrophy in Humans with AD and Non-demented Controls During 1 Year[94]		
Regions of Brain Analyzed	**AD Longitudinal % Change**	**Controls Longitudinal % Change**
Entorhinal Cortex	-3.75	-0.55
Hippocampus	-2.42	-0.84
Frontal Cortex (caudal)	-1.60	-0.40
Frontal Cortex (ventral)	-1.06	-0.38

Note: these are the same brain regions found to be "hot spots" for aluminum accumulation[86]

The three hallmarks of hippocampal sclerosis (HS), loss of pyramidal neurons, glial cell activation, and hippocampal atrophy, can all be due to aluminum accumulation in the brain. This accumulation becomes faster as we age and accounts for why HS is seen in 10% of those over 85. The accelerated aluminum accumulation observed in elderly brains as compared with middle-age brains may be due to an increasing rate of gastrointestinal aluminum absorption with age in the elderly[28,29].

Appendix IV

Cerebral Amyloid Angiopathy

Cerebral amyloid angiopathy (CAA, a.k.a. congophilic angiopathy) is a disease in which Aβ peptide deposits form on the walls of blood vessels of the central nervous system (CNS) resulting in a hemorrhagic stroke usually confined to a particular lobe of the brain. This is the same Aβ peptide associated with Alzheimer's disease. Therefore these hemorrhages are usually more common in cases of AD. In fact CAA of variable extent is almost always found in cases of AD.

A woman living in the Camelford area of Cornwall England was exposed to high levels of alum in her drinking water in July of 1988 and died 15 years later at age 58 due to a rapidly progressing, fatal dementing illness. The aluminum concentration in her drinking water was 500 to 3,000 times higher than the maximum acceptable limit (e.g. 200mcg/L) under EU legislation. An autopsy showed dramatic Aβ peptide deposition in the cerebral cortical arterioles and capillaries in all the main lobes[415]. Only a few NFTs were observed in the transentorhinal and periamygdaloid cortex and hippocampus. The Aβ plaque was immunoreactive for Aβ protein but was diffuse rather than neuritic in nature. There were Lewy bodies observed in the locus coeruleus, parahippocampal gyrus, and amygdala. Also, aluminum was found at higher than normal levels in the affected brain regions[415]. For instance, four samples taken at various locations in the frontal lobe yielded aluminum levels of 3.24, 4.33, 5.71, and 11.01mcg/gr dry-weight. These values compare with 0 – 2mcg/gr dry-weight seen in normal brains. NFTs are hallmarks of AD and Lewy bodies are also observed in AD, particularly in early onset AD[663]. In this case the location of the Aβ peptide deposition in the vasculature was indicative of CAA, although no macroscopically visible hemorrhages were seen[415].

This is the first human case in which aluminum has been linked to CAA. There is animal data showing that aluminum accumulation in the brain does lead to Aβ peptide deposition in the CNS vascular system.

Appendix V

Blood-Brain Barrier's Role in Alzheimer's Prevention

The blood-brain barrier (BBB) protects the brain from blood-borne toxic molecules inside the vasculature (e.g. arteries, veins, and capillaries) from entering the space occupied by neurons. In the brain there is an extensive neurovasculature that comprises the BBB. This primarily consists of a capillary bed connected to the choroid plexus that regulates chemical transfer from the blood to the fluids of the brain. These brain fluids include interstitial and cerebrospinal fluids (CSF), the latter being produced by the choroid plexus. The BBB is made of cerebrovascular endothelial cells that are tightly wedged together in the walls of the vasculature and two additional cell types called astrocytes and microglial cells. Primary factors causing increased BBB permeability to blood-borne toxic molecules are:

- Aluminum[668-670]
- Traumatic Brain Injury (TBI)[671,672]

Aluminum chloride has been shown to increase the permeability of the BBB to lipophilic molecules[668]. Lipophilic molecules are more soluble in fat or hydrocarbon solvents than water. Also both acute and chronic traumatic brain injury has been shown to increase the permeability of the BBB[671,672].

Four factors that are not a cause but are associated with increased BBB permeability:

- Alzheimer's Disease[673]
- Vascular Disease – High Blood Pressure and Stroke[669]
- Ageing[674]
- Parkinson's Disease[675,676]

Aluminum is a causal factor of both Alzheimer's and vascular disease (see Chapters 1 and 2). Aluminum accumulates in the brain with age accounting for why aging is a non-causal factor associated with increased BBB permeability[674]. Traumatic brain injury and increased BBB permeability are associated with parkinsonism (see Appendix I)[643,675,676].

There are two ways aluminum disguises its self in order to cross the BBB:

- Bonding with lipophilic ligands
- Bonding with carrier proteins that have receptors on the BBB

In the blood lipophilic and non-lipophilic ligands have an affinity for aluminum. Examples of lipophilic ligands include medium and long chain fatty acids. Aluminum in the serum increases the permeability of the BBB allowing complexes of aluminum with lipophilic ligands, such as fatty acids, to enter the brain. An example of a carrier protein is transferrin that normally carries iron to the brain. Aluminum in the serum competes with iron for transferrin's two bonding sites. This allows aluminum, disguised as iron, to enter the brain. These factors allow slow accumulation of aluminum in the brain leading to Alzheimer's disease.

Aluminum increases the permeability of the BBB by decreasing the expression and production of F-actin, a protein for endothelial cell-to-cell adhesion, and occludin, a plasma-membrane protein located at tight-junctions between endothelium cells, both of which are required for BBB integrity. Zinc protects the integrity of the BBB in spite of aluminum by increasing the expression in the BBB of both F-actin and occludin. This was demonstrated by dosing simultaneously with both aluminum and zinc[670].

The primary factor slowing the accumulation of aluminum in the brain is orthosilicic acid. Orthosilicic acid can cross the BBB and chelate (i.e. complex with) aluminum forming aluminosilicates in both the serum and CSF. Aluminosilicates are non-lipophilic complexes that do not cross the BBB, even when the BBB's integrity has been impaired by aluminum. By forming these complexes, orthosilicic acid enhances the elimination of aluminum from the body by both urination and perspiration[36,515].

Reduced glutathione protects the brain and BBB from reactive oxygen species created in part by metal ions, such as aluminum. Aluminum is known to decrease the production of glutathione[578]. Reduced glutathione has been shown to be required for functional BBB integrity[677].

The permeability of the BBB can be decreased by supplementation of the following biochemicals and minerals that improve BBB integrity by either increasing glutathione in the brain or combating aluminum:

- o Biochemicals that Improve BBB Integrity by Increasing Glutathione[677]
    - Vitamin D[296]
    - N-Acetylcysteine (a.k.a. NAC)[677]
- o Mineral Supplements that Maintain BBB Integrity by Combating Aluminum[670,678]
    - Orthosilicic Acid[678]
    - Zinc[670]

Why Hemodialysis Patients Have High Levels of Serum Aluminum and a Low Risk of AD

There is a mystery as to why hemodialysis patients, who have high blood serum aluminum levels, do not get Alzheimer's disease. The solution is that orthosilicic acid can impede aluminum from crossing the BBB. There are two reasons:

- Aluminum must cross the BBB in order to cause Alzheimer's disease (see Chapter 1).
- Hemodialysis patients have both higher than normal serum aluminum and orthosilicic acid. The orthosilicic acid impedes aluminum from crossing the BBB[679-683]

Levels of Aluminum and Orthosilicic Acid in Serum and Cerebrospinal Fluid (CSF)		
Serum and CSF	Aluminum (mcg/Liter)	Orthosilicic Acid (mcg/Liter)
Normal Kidney Function		
Serum	<1	140 ± 40 (140 ± 14)
CSF	<1	235 ± 49
Hemodialysis Patients		
Serum	130 ± 8	4220 ± 630 (2190 ± 132)
CSF	5 ± 2	2580 ± 300

Data is from Van Landeghem[682] except for data in parenthesis from Roberts[680]

The data in this table shows that even though aluminum is much higher than normal, it is 25 fold lower in the CSF as compared with serum of those on hemodialysis. This shows that the BBB is working with orthosilicic acid to keep aluminum out of the brain. As the data in this table also shows, the level of orthosilicic acid is 15 fold higher than normal in the serum of those on hemodialysis. This results in chelation of the orthosilicic acid with aluminum forming non-lipophilic aluminosilicate that blocks aluminum from crossing the BBB. Since the kidneys of hemodialysis patients are not functioning correctly, aluminum, silicic acid, and aluminosilicate are not excreted by urination but are instead locally concentrated and deposited as aluminosilicates at the BBB.

In hemodialysis patients aluminum is found using laser microprobe mass analysis as deposits in the brain's vascular system, cytoplasm of choroidal epithelium cells, astrocytes, and microglial cells[684]. These aluminum containing deposits behave chemically like aluminosilicate[684] and are in a different location in the brain as compared with the aluminosilicate deposits found by x-ray microanalysis and nuclear magnetic resonance in the core of approximately 50% of Aβ plaques and neurofibrillary tangles that are seen as hallmarks of Alzheimer's disease[685,686]. This is because plaques and tangles are formed in and around neurons due to aluminum accumulation on the brain side of the BBB. High levels of serum orthosilicic acid impede aluminum from crossing the BBB by forming aluminosilicate that deposits on the blood side of the BBB.

The data in the table also shows that orthosilicic acid does cross the BBB as it is found at higher than normal levels in both the blood's serum and brain's CSF. Even though a small but higher than normal amount of aluminum is found in the CFS of hemodialysis patients, the higher than normal level of orthosilicic acid in the CFS protects the brain from this small amount of aluminum that does cross the BBB.

Possibly because of a history of traumatic brain injury or vascular disease, the BBB in a small number of patients (i.e. 4%) on hemodialysis does fail to protect the brain from aluminum crossing from the blood to the brain and quickly accumulating in the brain[687]. These patients suffer from dementia due to aluminum encephalopathy that can be fatal. This disease is much quicker to develop symptoms (i.e. 1 year or less) than Alzheimer's that takes 5 to 20 years before the first symptoms of cognitive impairment are observed. It is postulated that aluminum encephalopathy may involve aluminum altering brain calcium homeostasis by complexing with calmodulin[688]. The toxicity of aluminum on the brain side of the BBB is underscored by two patients who underwent routine brain surgery requiring bone cement. These cements contain labile aluminum and fluoride[689]. After the operations their CSF had 63-112 mcg/Liter of aluminum. They never regained consciousness and died 80-143 days after their operations[690].

Conclusion

The BBB working with orthosilicic acid protects the brain from aluminum preventing Alzheimer's disease and aluminum encephalopathy.

Without being aware of the roles played by the BBB and orthosilicic acid in protecting the brain from aluminum, many scientists incorrectly drew the conclusion that aluminum does not cause Alzheimer's because those on hemodialysis with high serum aluminum levels do not have the hallmarks of Alzheimer's[691]. This incorrect conclusion has resulted in a tragic lack of funding for research on how to prevent aluminum from causing Alzheimer's. Hopefully research efforts can be refocused while implementing a plan to prevent Alzheimer's by keeping the BBB functioning with glutathione, eliminating aluminum intake, and increasing orthosilicic acid intake.

Daily supplements that can be taken to help the BBB by increasing glutathione and combating aluminum are:

- Orthosilicic Acid – See Chapter 5
- Vitamin D – See Chapter 3
- Zinc – 15mg per day as an amino acid chelate
- N-Acetylcysteine (a.k.a. NAC) – 600mg per day

Appendix VI

Epidemiology Supporting Aluminum's Causal Role in Alzheimer's Disease

Epidemiological studies comparing the level of aluminum in drinking water to the relative risk of Alzheimer's disease support the contention that aluminum is a casual factor of Alzheimer's disease. Using epidemiology studies to find correlations between aluminum ingestion and Alzheimer's disease has been made difficult because there are many sources of aluminum in the human diet. Therefore it is surprising that correlations have been found between aluminum in drinking water and AD or dementia in the 7 largest epidemiology studies each involving more than 300 people with AD or dementia. The reason for this may be because aluminum in drinking water is more easily absorbed by the gastrointestinal tract than aluminum in food. It has been found that 0.3% of the aluminum in drinking water is absorbed, while only 0.1-0.2% of the aluminum in food is absorbed[391].

Epidemiology studies are only valid if the number of people with AD and/or dementia in the study is high enough to make the data statistically significant. Therefore the 13 epidemiology studies in the following table are listed in order of number of AD and/or dementia cases evaluated in each study. Note that there are 7 studies involving 300 or more cases of AD or dementia and all 7 of these studies found a greater risk of AD or dementia due to drinking water with higher aluminum levels. There are 6 studies involving approximately 100 or less cases of AD or dementia. With such a low number of cases it is not surprising that four of these studies (e.g. studies 8, 9, 12, and 13) found no statistically significant (NSS) relationship between aluminum in drinking water and the incidence of AD, dementia, or low cognition. For more details on these four studies see the notes at the end of the table.

Epidemiology Studies of Aluminum in Drinking Water (DW) and Alzheimer's Disease (AD)								
Study	No. of Cases AD/Dementia	Total No. People	Aluminum in DW mcg/liter	Relative Risk of AD/Dem.	Data Source	Country	Year of Publication	Ref.
1	3,736 D	1,224,558	<50	1.00	Death Certs.	Norway	1986-90	81, 692, 693
	9,545 D	2,494,345	50-200	1.17	"	"	"	"
	1,446 D	347,231	>200	1.37	"	"	"	"
2	598 AD	41,800	<67	1.00	Death Certs.	Ontario	1995	694, 695
	2,153 AD	145,000	68-200	0.82-1.01	"	"	"	"
	14 AD	1,000	>336	1.42-4.25	"	"	"	"
3	2,232 D	4,464	<10	1.0	Hospital Records	Ontario	1991	82
			10-100	1.13	"	"	"	"
			100-200	1.26	"	"	"	"
			>200	1.46	"	"	"	"
4	385 AD	680	<100	1.00	Autopsy Verified	Ontario	1995	75
			>100	1.70	"	"	"	"
			>125	3.60	"	"	"	"
			>150	4.40	"	"	"	"
			>175	7.60	"	"	"	"
5	371 D	870	<84.7	1.00	Cognition Tests	Ontario	1994	696
			>84.7	2.27	"	"	"	"
6	364 AD/455 D	1667	<100	1.00	Cognition Tests	France	2000-09	79
		216	>100	2.80/2.26	"	"	"	"
7	307 AD (<65)	1185	<20	1.00	CT Scans	U.K.	1989	80
			20-70	1.40	"	"	"	"
			80-110	1.60	"	"	"	"
			>110	1.70	"	"	"	"

Continued – Epidemiology Studies of Aluminum in Drinking Water (DW) and Alzheimer's Disease (AD)								
Study	No. of Cases AD/Dementia	Total No. People	Aluminum in DW mcg/liter	Relative Risk of AD/Dem.	Data Source	Country	Year of Publication	Ref.
8	106 AD (<75)			NSS	Clinically Diagnosed	U.K.	1997	697
9	105 AD (<65)		<100	NSS	Clinically Diagnosed	England	1995	426, 698
	4 AD (<65)		>100	"				
10	68 AD	4,700	12	1.00	NINCDS-ADRDA	Quebec	2000	77, 695
			>77	2.67	"	"	"	"
11	40 D			Weak Correlation	Death Certs.	Newfound-land	1991	79, 699, 700
12	None	800 (81-85)	4 - 98	NSS	Cognition Tests	Switzer-land	1991	701
13	None	386	3 Years of Exposure	NSS	Cognition Tests	U.K.	1997	702

NNS = Not statistically significant; AD = Alzheimer's disease; D = Dementia

Relative Risk of AD/Dementia: 1.00 = no added risk, 1.20 = 20% increased risk; 2.00 = twice the risk

Notes on Studies 7, 8, 9, 12, and 13

- Studies 7 (1989) and 8 (1997) were both carried out by the same group at South Hampton Hospital and published with the same lead author (e.g. C. N. Martyn)[80,697]. The positive correlation between high aluminum levels in drinking water and AD this group reported eight years earlier in study 7 was described and not retracted in study 8. With 200 fewer AD cases in study 8, they were unsuccessful in finding any correlation between high aluminum levels in drinking water and AD[697]. Seventy percent of the controls in study 8 were people with dementias and neurologic disorders, other than AD. The authors of study 8 point out that aluminum could also influence the course of these diseases in the controls resulting in a systematic error in study 8. In fact, in study 7 they reported a

higher relative risk (e.g. 1.1 - 1.2) of dementias, other than AD, in men 40-64 years of age exposed to aluminum levels in drinking water over 20mcg/liter[80].
- In study 9 only 4 cases of AD had been exposed to greater than 100mcg/liter of aluminum[426].
- In study 12 the participants only drank water with less that 100mcg/liter of aluminum[701].
- In study 13 elevated aluminum in drinking water was only ingested for 3 years[79,702].

Conclusion

In Chapter 1 of this book Hill's criteria was used to show that aluminum is a causal factor for AD. Epidemiological data supports both the strength and consistency of association between aluminum and AD. These two criteria are part of Hill's nine criteria for causality. From the results of the 7 largest epidemiology studies we can conclude, as did the World Health Organization, that "The positive relationship between aluminum in drinking-water and AD ... cannot be totally dismissed"[83]. Based upon this epidemiological data the World Health Organization recommended a maximum of 100mcg/liter of aluminum in drinking water in 1998 and 2003[83].

References

I would like to thank all the researchers referenced herein for their patience and persistence in making discoveries relevant to the subjects covered in this book. Without their research and the research of those who preceded them there would be no information on how to prevent Alzheimer's, autism, and stroke.

1. Alzheimer, A.; Uber eine eigenartige erkrankung der hirnrinde; Zentralbl Nervenheit Psychiatr; 30, 177179 (1907)
2. Exley, C., and Vickers, T.; Elevated brain aluminum and early onset Alzheimer's disease in an individual occupationally exposed to aluminum: a case report; J. Med. Case Reports; 8:41 (2014)
3. House, E., et al.; Aluminum, iron, and copper in human brain tissues donated to the Medical Research Council's cognitive functioning and ageing study; Metallomics; Jan. 4(1):56-65 (2012)
4. Alzheimer's Organization website 2015
5. Funk, C.; Studies on pellagra' The influence of the milling of maize on the chemical composition and nutritive value of the meal; J. Physiol.; 47:389-92 (1913)
6. Thompson, W.G.; Practical dietetics with special reference to diet in disease; D. Appleton and Co., New York (1895)
7. Humphry, G.M., Old Age: The results of information received respecting nearly nine hundred persons who had attained the age of eighty years, including seventy-four centenarians; MacMillan and Bowes, Cambridge, UK, 1889
8. Blansjaar, B.A., Thomassen, R., VanSchaick, H.W.; Prevalence of dementia in centenarians; Int. J. of Geriatric Psychiatry, 15(3):219-25 (2000)
9. Poirier, J., et al.; Apolipoprotein E and lipid homeostasis in the etiology and treatment of sporadic Alzheimer's disease; Neurobiol. of Aging; 35:S3-S10 (2014)
10. UN World Assembly on Ageing; World Population Ageing 1950-2050; Chapter IV – Demographic profile of the older population (2002)
11. Plassman, B.L., et al.; Prevalence of Dementia in the United States: The ageing, demographics, and memory study; Neuroepidemiology; 29:125-32 (2007)
12. Deane, R., et al.; apoE isoform-specific disruption of amyloid beta peptide clearance from mouse brain; J. Clin. Invest.; doi:10.1172/JCI36663

13. Nee, L.E., et al.; Dementia of the Alzheimer type: clinical and family study of 22 twin pairs; Neurology, Mar., 37(3):359-63 (1987)

14. Langergraber, K.E., et al.; Generation times in wild chimpanzees and gorillas suggest earlier divergence times in great ape and human evolution; PNAS; Sept.; 109(39):15716-15721 (2012)

15. Dahlgren, K.N., et al.; Oligomeric and fibrillary species of amyloid-β peptides differentially affect neuronal viability; J. Biol. Chem.; Aug., 277(35):3206-53 (2002)

16. Drago, D.; Aluminum modulates effects of beta-amyloid1-42 on neuronal calcium homeostasis and mitochondrial functioning and is altered in a triple transgenic mouse model of Alzheimer's disease; Rejuvenation Reas.; 11(5):861-871 (2008)

17. Mantyn, P.W., et al.; Aluminum, iron, and zinc ions promote aggregation of physiological concentrations of beta-amyloid peptide; J. Neurochem; Sep.; 61(3):1171-4 (1993)

18. Kuo, Y-M., et al.; Water-soluble Aβ (N-40, N-42) oligomers in normal and Alzheimer's disease brains; Feb., J. Biol. Chem.; 271(8):4077-81 (1996)

19. Arriagada P.V., et al.; Neurofibrillary tangles but not senile plaques parallel duration and severity of Alzheimer's disease; Neurology, 42:3 631 (1992)

20. Sun X-Y, et al.; Synaptic released zinc promotes tau hyperphosphorylation by inhibition of protein phosphatase 2A (PP2A); J Biolog Chem; 287,14:11174-82 (2012)

21. Mutter J, Curth, A, Naumann J, Deth R, Walach H; Does inorganic mercury play a role in Alzheimer's Disease? A systematic review and an integrated molecular mechanism; J Alzh Dis; 22:357-74 (2010)

22. Yamamoto, H., et al.; Dephosphorylation of tau factor by protein phosphatase 2A in synaptosomal cytosol fractions, and inhibition by aluminum; J. Neuroscience; 55:683-90 (1990)

23. Langui, D., et al.; Effects of aluminum chloride on cultured cells from rat brain hemispheres; 438(1-2):67-76 (1988)

24. Savory, J., et al.; Reversal by desferrioxamine of tau protein aggregates following two days of treatment in aluminum-induced neurofibrillary degeneration in rabbit – implications for clinical trials in Alzheimer's disease; Neurotoxicology; 19(2):209-14 (1998)

25. Leterrier, J.F., et al.; A molecular mechanism for the induction of neurofilament bundling by aluminum ions; J. Neurochemistry; 58(6):2060-70 (1992)

26. Crapper, D.R., Krishnan, S.S., Dalton, A.J.; Brain aluminum distribution in Alzheimer's disease and experimental neurofibrillary degeneration; Science, May, 180(4085):511-3 (1973)

27. Perl, D.P. and Brody, A.R.; Alzheimer's disease: X-ray spectrometric evidence of aluminum accumulation in neurofibrillary tangle-bearing neurons; Science; 208(4441), 297-99 (1980)

28. Shimizu, H., et al.; A correlative study of the aluminum content and aging changes of the brain in non-demented elderly subjects; Nihon Ronen Igakkai Zasshi; Dec.; 31(12)950-60 (1994)

29. Jansson, E.T.; Aluminum exposure and Alzheimer's disease; J. Alzheimer's Dis.; Dec.; 2(6)541-49 (2001)

30. Luo, Y., et al.; Altered expression of Abeta metabolism-associated molecules from D-galactose/AlCl(3) induced mouse brain; Mech. Ageing Dev. Apr.; 130(4):248-52 (2008)

31. Liang, R.F., et al.; Impact of sub-chronic aluminum-maltolate exposure on catabolism of amyloid precursor protein in rats; Biomed. Environ. Sci.; 26(6):445-52 (2013)

32. Liu, Q., et al.; Amyloid precursor protein regulates brain apolipoprotein E and cholesterol metabolism through lipoprotein receptor LRP1; Neuron; 56:66-78 (2007)

33. Pluta, R., et al.; Sporadic Alzheimer's disease begins as episodes of brain ischemia and ischemically dysregulated Alzheimer's disease genes; Mo. Neurobiol.; 48:500-515 (2013)

34. Forbes, W.F., and McLachlan, D.R.C.; Further thoughts on the aluminum-Alzheimer's disease link; J. Epidemiol. Community Health; 50:401-3 (1996)

35. Varner, J.A., et al.; Chronic administration of aluminum-fluoride or sodium-fluoride to rats in drinking water: alterations in neuronal and cerebrovascular integrity; Brian Res.; 784:284-8 (1998)

36. Bellia, J.P., Birchall, J.D., Roberts, N.B.; The role of silicic acid in the renal excretion of aluminum; Ann. Clin. Lab. Sci.; June, 26(3):227-33 (1996)

37. Exley, C., at. al.; Non-invasive therapy to reduce the body burden of aluminum in Alzheimer's disease; J. Alzheimer's Dis.; Sept., 10(1):17-24 (2006)

38. Davenward, S., et al.; Silicon-rich mineral water as a non-invasive test of the 'aluminum hypothesis' in Alzheimer's disease; J. Alzheimer's Dis.; 33(2):423-30 (2013)

39. Exley, C, Human Exposure to Aluminum; Environ. Sci.: Processes Impacts, 15:1807-16 (2013)

40. Divine, K.K., et al.; Quantitative particle-induced x-ray emission imaging of rat olfactory epithelium applied to the permeability of rat epithelium to inhaled aluminum; Chem. Res. Toxicol.; 12(7):575-81 (1999)

41. Sunderman, F.W. Jr.; Nasal toxicity, carcinogenicity, and olfactory uptake of metals; Annals Clin. Lab. Sci.; 31(1):3-24 (2001)

42. Zatta, P., et al.; Deposition of aluminum in brain tissues of rats exposed to inhalation of aluminum acetylacetonate; Neuroreport; Sept.; 4(9):1119-22 (1993)

43. Priest, N.D.; The biological behavior and bioavailability of aluminum in man, with special reference to studies employing aluminum-26 as a tracer: a review and study update; J. Environ. Monit,; 6:375-403 (2004)

44. Walton, J.R.; Cognitive deterioration and associated pathology induced by chronic low-level aluminum ingestion in a translational rat model provides and explanation of Alzheimer's disease, tests for susceptibility and avenues for treatment; Int. J. Alz. Dis.; 2012, Article ID 914947, 17 pages (2012)

45. Exley, C. and House, E.R.; Aluminum in the Human Brain; Monatsh Chem.; 42:357-63 (2011)

46. Morris, C.M., et al.; Comparison of the regional distribution of transferrin receptors and aluminum in the forebrain of chronic renal dialysis patients; J. Neurol. Sci.; Dec.; 94(1-3):295-306 (1989)

47. Trapp, G.A.; Plasma aluminum if bound to transferrin; Life Sci; 19:295-98 (1983)

48. Ohman, L.O., Martin, R.B.; Citrate as the main small molecule binding Al3+ in serum; Clin Chem; 40:598-601 (1994)

49. Bondy, S.C.; Prolonged exposure to low levels of aluminum leads to changes associated with brain ageing and neurodegeneration; Toxicology, Jan., 315:1-7 (2014)

50. Mirza, A., et al.; Aluminum in brain tissue in familial Alzheimer's disease (Preprint); J. Trace Elements in Medicine and Biology; Mar.; 40:30-36 (2017)

51. Edwardson, J.A., et al.; Effect of silicon on gastrointestinal absorption of aluminum; The Lancet; 342(8865):211-12 (1993)

52. Moore, P.B.; et al.; Absorption of aluminum-26 in Alzheimer's disease, measured using accelerator mass spectrometry; 11:66-69 (2000)

53. Taylor, G.A., et al.; Gastrointestinal absorption of aluminum in Alzheimer's disease: response to aluminum citrate; Age Ageing; Mar.; 21(2):81-90 (1992)

54. Virk, S. A., and Eslick, G.D.; Aluminum levels in brain, serum, and cerebrospinal fluid are higher in Alzheimer's disease cases than in controls: A series of meta-analyses; J. Alzheimer's Disease; 47(3):629-38 (2015)

55. Moreira, P.I., et al.; Mitochondrial dysfunction is a trigger of Alzheimer's disease pathophysiology; Biochim. Biophys. Acta; 1802:2-10 (2010)

56. Zatta, P., Lain E., Cagnolini C.; Effects of aluminum on activity of Krebs cycle enzymes and glutamate dehydrogenase in rat brain homogenate; Eur J Biochem; 267:3049-55 (2000)

57. Mailloux, R.J., et al.; Aluminum toxicity elicits a dysfunctional TCA cycle and succinate accumulation in hepatocytes; J. Biochem. Mol. Toxicol.; 20(4):198-208 (2006)

58. Pogue, A.I., et al.; Metal-sulfate induced generation of ROS in human brain cells: detection using an isomeric mixture of 5- and 6-carboxy-2',7'-dichlorofluoresein diacetate (carboxy-DCFDA) as a cell permeant tracer, Int. J. Mol.; 13:9615-26 (2012)

59. Scott, E.M., et al.; Purification and properties of glutathione reductase of human erythrocytes; J. Biol. Chem.; Dec.; 238:3928-33 (1963)

60. Yamamoto, Y., et al.; Aluminum toxicity is associated with mitochondrial dysfunction and production of reactive oxygen species in plant cells; Plant Physio.l; 128:63-72 (2002)

61. Braak, H., and Braak, E.; Neuropathological staging of Alzheimer-related changes; Acta Neuropathol.; 82:239-259 (1991)

62. Kahn, U.A.; et al.; Molecular drivers and cortical spread of lateral entorhinal cortex dysfunction in preclinical Alzheimer's disease; Nature Neuroscience; 17:304-11 (2014)

63. Scoville, W.B., and Milner, B.; Loss of recent memory after bilateral hippocampus lesions; J. Neurol. Neurosurg. Psychiat.; 20:11-21 (1957)

64. Willhite, C.C., et al.; Systematic review of potential health risks posed by pharmaceutical, occupational and consumer exposures to metallic and nanoscale aluminum, aluminum oxides, aluminum hydroxide and its soluble salts; Crit. Rev. Toxicol,; Oct.; Suppl. 44(S4):1-80 (2014)

65. Rogers, M.A.M. and Simon, D.G.; A preliminary study of dietary aluminum intake and risk of Alzheimer's disease; Age and Ageing; 28:205-9 (1999)

66. Yokel, R.A.; Aluminum in food – The nature and contribution of food additives; Univ. Kentucky, Pharmaceutical Sciences Faculty Publications; 31 (2012)

67. Tomljenovic, L.; Aluminum and Alzheimer's Disease: After a century of controversy, is there a plausible link?; J. Alzheimer's Disease, 23, 567-98 (2011)

68. WHO – Aluminum in Drinking Water WHO/HSE/WSH/10.01/13 (2010)

69. WHO – Joint FAO/WHO Expert Committee on Food Additives – Summary Report, July 4, 2011

70. Needleman, H.L.; The case of Deborah Rice: who is the Environmental Protection Agency protecting?; PLoS Biol. 6, e129, http://dx.doi.org/10.1371/journal.pbio.0060129

71. McLachlen, D. R. C., et al.; Intramuscular desferrioxamine in patients with Alzheimer's disease; The Lancet; 337(8753):1304-1308 (1991)

72. Hill, A.B.; The environment and disease: Association or causation?; Proc Royal Soc. Med B; 58:295-300 (1965)

73. Van Reekum, R.; et al.; Applying Bradford Hill's criteria for causation to neuropsychiatry: Challenges and opportunities; J. Neuropsychiatry Clin. Neurosci.; 13:318-25 (2001)

74. Walton, J.R.; Chronic aluminum intake causes Alzheimer's disease: Applying Sir Austin Bradford Hill's causality criteria; J. Alzheimer's Disease; 40:765-838 (2014)

75. McLachlan, D.R.C., et al.; Risk for neuropathologically confirmed Alzheimer's disease and residual aluminum in municipal drinking water employing weighted residential histories; Neurology, 46:401-5 (1996)

76. Rondeau, V., et al.; Aluminum and silica in drinking water and the risk of Alzheimer's disease or cognitive decline: findings from 15-year follow-up of the PAQUID cohort, Am. J. Epidemiol. 169:489-96 (2009)

77. Gauthier, E., et al.; Aluminum forms in drinking water and risk of Alzheimer's disease; Environ. Res.; 84, 236-46 (2000)

78. Bondy, S.C.; The neurotoxicity of environmental aluminum is still an issue; Neurotoxicology; 31:575-81 (2010)

79. Flaten, T.P.; Aluminum as a risk factor in Alzheimer's disease, with emphasis on drinking water; Brain Res. Bull.; May; 55(2):187-96 (2001)

80. Martyn, C.N., et al.; Geographic relation between Alzheimer's disease and aluminum in drinking water; Lancet, 1:59-62 (1989)

81. Flaten, T.P.; Geographical associations between aluminum in drinking water and death rates with dementia (including Alzheimer's disease),Parkinson's disease and amyotrophic lateral sclerosis in Norway; Environ. Geochem. Health; 12:152-167 (1990)

82. Neri, L.C., and Hewitt, D.; Aluminum, Alzheimer's disease, and drinking water; Lancet 338:390, (1991)

83. WHO – Joint FAO/WHO Expert Committee on Food Additives – Summary Report, July 4, 2011

84. Steinhausen, C., et al.; Investigation of the aluminum biokinetics in humans: a 26Al tracer study; Food Chem. Toxicol.; Mar.; 42(3):363-71 (2004)

85. De Sole, I.P., et al.; Possible relationship between Al/ferritin complex and Alzheimer's disease; Clin. Biochem.; 46:89-93 (2013)

86. Andrasi, E., et al.; Brain Al, Mg, and P contents of control and Alzheimer-diseased patients; J. Alzheimer's Dis.; 7:273-84 (2005)

87. Rusina, R., et al.; Higher aluminum concentrations in Alzheimer's disease after Box-Cox data transformation; Neurotox. Res.; 20, 329-33 (2011)

88. Xu, N., et al.; Brain aluminum in Alzheimer's disease using an improved GFAAS method; Neurotoxicology; 13:735-43 (1992)

89. Arnold, S.E., et al.; The topographical and neuroanatomical distribution of neurofibrillary tangles and neuritic plaques in the cerebral cortex of patients with Alzheimer's disease; Cereb. Cortex; 1, 103-116 (1991)

90. Hyman, B.T., et al.; Alzheimer's disease: Cell-specific pathology isolates the hippocampal formation; Science; 225:1168-70 (1984)

91. Van Hoesen, G.W., et al.; Entorhinal cortex pathology in Alzheimer's disease; Hippocampus; 1:1-8 (1996)

92. Gomez-Isla, T.; et al.; Profound loss of layer II entorhinal cortex neurons in very mild Alzheimer's disease; J. Neurosci.; 16:4491-4500 (1996)

93. Coffey, C.E., et al.; Quantitative cerebral anatomy of the aging human brain; Neurology; Mar.; 42(3):527 (1992)

94. Fjell, A.M., et al.; One-year brain atrophy evident in healthy aging; J. Neurosci.; Dec.; 29(48):15223-31 (2009)

95. Bauman, M.L., and Kemper, T.L.; The neurobiology of autism; John Hopkins University Press; Structural Brain Anatomy in Autism: What is the Evidence? Chapt. 9:121-35 (2005)

96. Papez, J.W.; A proposed mechanism for emotion; Arch Neuro. Psychiatry; 38:725-43 (1937)

97. Kawas, C., et al.; Multiple pathologies are common and related to dementia in the oldest-old: The 90+ study; Neurology; July 85(6) (2015)

98. Lukiw, W.J.; Nanomolar aluminum induces pro-inflammatory and pro-apoptotic gene expression in human brain cells in primary culture; J. Inorg. Biochem.; Sept.; 99(9):1895-8 (2005)

99. Sontage J-M, et al.; Folate deficiency induces in vitro and mouse brain region-specific downregulation of leucine carboxyl methyltransferase-1 and protein phosphatase 2A B subunit expression that correlate with enhanced tau phosphorylation; J Neurosci; 28:11477-87 (2008)

100. Vogelsberg-Ragaglia, V., et al.; PP2A mRNA expression is quantitatively decreased in Alzheimer's disease hippocampus; Exp. Neurol.; 168:402-12 (2001)

101. Zhang, L., et al.; Aluminum chloride impairs long-term memory and downregulates cAMP-PKA-CREB signaling in rats; Toxicology; Sep.; 323:95-108 (2014)

102. Wang, B.; et al.; Disturbance of intracellular calcium homeostasis and CaMKII/CREB signaling is associated with learning and memory impairments induced by chronic aluminum exposure; Neurotox. Res.; 26:52-63 (2014)

103. Pugazhenthi, S.; et al.; Downregulation of CREB expression in Alzheimer's brain and in AB-treated rat hippocampal neurons; Mol. Neuroddegen.; 6:60 (2011)

104. Sun, Z.Z., et al.; Alteration of Aβ metabolism-related molecules in predementia induced by AlCl3 and D-galactose; Age; 31:277-284 (2009)

105. Farasani, A., and Darbre, P.D.; Effects of aluminum chloride and aluminum chlorohydrate on DNA repair in MCF-10A immortalized non-transformed human breast epithelial cells; J. Inorg. Biochem.; Aug.; (2015)

106. Suberbielle, E.; DNA repair factor BRCA1 depletion occurs in Alzheimer's brains and impairs cognitive function in mice; Nature Comm.; Nov.; 1-14 (2015)

107. Huen, M. S. Y., et al.; BRCA1 and its toolbox for the maintenance of genome integrity; Nat. Rev. Mol. Cell Biol.; Feb.; 11(2):138-48 (2010)

108. Muratore, C. R., et al.; Age dependent decrease and alternative splicing of methionine synthase mRNA in human cerebral cortex and an accelerated decrease in autism; PLoS One; 8(2) (2013)

109. Tsunoda, M. and Sharma, R.P,; Modulation of tumor necrosis factor alpha expression in mouse brain after exposure to aluminum in drinking water; Arch. Toxicol.; Nov.; 73(8-9):419-26 (1999)

110. Miki, Y., et al.; A strong candidate for the breast and ovarian cancer susceptibility gene BRCA1; Science; Oct.; 266(5182):66-71 (1994)

111. Rosen, E.M., Fan, S., Goldberg, I.D.; BRCA1 and prostate cancer; Cancer Invest.; 19(4):396-412 (2001)

112. Jensen-Jarolim, E.; Aluminum in allergies and allergen immunotherapy; World Allergy Organization J.; 8(7)1-6 (2015)

113. Makesbery, W.R., et al.; Brain trace elements concentrations in aging; Neurobiol. Aging; 5:19-28 (1984)

114. Makesbery, W.R., et al.; Instrumental neutron activation analysis of brain aluminum in Alzheimer's disease and aging; Ann. Neurol.; 10:511-16 (1981)

115. James, G.W.B.; The treatment of senile insanity. I. Pre-senile mental disorders; Alzheimer's dementia; Lancet ii, 820-21 (1926)

116. Rothschild, D.; Alzheimer's disease. A clinicopathologic study of five cases; Am. J. Psychiatry; 91:485-519 (1934)

117. National Center for Health Statistics; Death rates by 10-year age groups and age-adjusted death rates for 113 selected causes, race and sex: United States, 1979-98. CDC/NCHS, National Vital Statistics System, Table HIST001R (2003), at www.cdc.gov/nchs/data/statab/hist001r.pdf Accessed 11/3/2015.

118. Tejada-Vera, B.; Mortality from Alzheimer's disease in the United States. Data for 2000 and 2010. NCHS data brief, no. 116. National Center for Health Statistics, Hyattsville, MD (2013)

119. Cullen, J.M., and Allwood, J.M.; Mapping the global flow of aluminum: from liquid to end-use goods; Environ. Sci. Technol.; Apr.; 47(7):3057-64 (2013)

120. Flaten, T.P.; Geographical associations between aluminium in drinking water and death rates with dementia (including Alzheimer's disease), Parkinson's disease and amyotrophic lateral sclerosis in Norway; Environ. Geochem. Health; 12:152-167 (1990)

121. Zhang, Y. Rosenberg, P.A.; The essential nutrient pyrroloquinoline quinone may act as a neuroprotectant by suppressing peroxynitrite formation; Eur J Neurosci; Sep.; 16(6):1015-24 (2002)

122. El-Aleem, S.A., et al.; Upregulation of the inducible nitric oxide synthase in rat hippocampus in a model of Alzheimer's disease: A possible mechanism of aluminum induced Alzheimer's; Egypt. J. Histol. 32(1):173-180 (2008)

123. Siegel, N., and Haug, A.; Aluminum-induced inhibition of calmodulin-regulated phosphodiesterase activity: Enzymatic and optical studies; Inorg. Chim. Acta; 79:230-231 (1983)

124. Hebb, D.O.; The Organization of Behavior; "The first stage of perception: growth of the assembly"; Introduction and Chapter 4; Wiley, N.Y.; pp xi-xix and 60-78 (1949)

125. Dan, Y., and Poo, M.-M.; Spike timing-dependent plasticity: from synapse to perception; Physiol. Rev.; 86:1033-48 (2006)

126. Julka, D., and Gill, K.D.; Altered calcium homeostasis – a possible mechanism of aluminum-induced neurotoxicity; Biochimica Biophysica Acta; 1315:47-54 (1996)

127. Levi, R., et al.; Immuno-detection of aluminum and aluminum induced conformational changes in calmodulin-implications in Alzheimer's disease; Mol. Cell. Biochem.; 189:41-6 (1998)

128. Herzig, S., and Neumann, J.; Effects of serine/threonine protein phosphatases on ion channels in excitable membranes; Physiol. Rev.; 80:173-210 (2000)

129. Cordeiro, J.M., et al.; Aluminum-induced impairment of Ca2+ modulatory action on GABA transport brain cortex nerve terminals; J. Inorg. Biochem.; Sep.; 97(1):132-42 (2003)

130. Pennington, J.A., and Schoen, S.A.; Estimates of dietary exposure to aluminum; Food Addit. Contam.; Jan.-Feb.; 12(1):119-28 (1995)

131. Yokel, R.A., et al.; Aluminum bioavailability from basic sodium aluminum phosphate, an approved food additive emulsifying agent, incorporated in cheese; Food Chem. Toxicol.; June; 46(6):2261-66 (2008)

132. Walton, J.R.; Evidence for participation of aluminum in neurofibrillary tangle formation and growth in Alzheimer's disease; J. Alzheimer's Disease; 22:65-72 (2010)

133. Gong, C-X; et al.; Phosphorylation of micro-tubule associated protein tau is regulated by protein phosphatase 2A in mammalian brain. Implications for neurofibrillary degeneration in Alzheimer's disease; J. Biol. Chem.; 275:5535-44 (2000)

134. Murphy, M.P., and LeVine III, Harry; Alzheimer's disease and the B-Amyloid Peptide; J. Alzheimer's Dis.; 19(1):311- 28 (2010)

135. Buxbaum, J.D., et al.; Protein phosphorylation inhibits production of Alzheimer amyloid B/A4 peptide, Proc. Natl. Acad. Sci. U.S.A.; Oct.; 90:9195-98 (1993)

136. Cochran, M., Elliott, D.C., Brennan, P., Chawtur, V.; Inhibition of protein kinase C activation by low concentrations of aluminum; Clin. Chim. Acta; 194:167-172 (1990)

137. Robinson, S.R., and Bishop, G.M.; Abeta as a bioflocculant: Implications for the amyloid hypothesis of Alzheimer's disease; Neurobiol. Aging; 23, 1051-71 (2002)

138. Muma, N.A., and Singer, S.M.; Aluminum-induced neuropathology: Transient changes in microtubule-associated proteins; Neurotoxicology and Teratology; Nov.-Dec., 18(6):679-90 (1996)

139. Medana, I.M., and Esiri, M.M.; Axonal damage: A key predictor of outcome in human CNS diseases, Brain, 126:515-30 (2003)

140. Stokin, G.B., et al.; Axonopathy and transport deficits early in the pathogenesis of Alzheimer's disease; Science; 307:1282-88 (2005)

141. Montgomery, J., et al.; Gleaming, white, and deadly: using lead to track human exposure and geographic origins in the Roman period in Britain; Roman Diasporas, J. Roman Archeol.; Suppl. 78:199-226 (2010)

142. Crisponi, G., et al.; Human diseases related to aluminum overload; Monatsh. Chem.; 142:331-340 (2012)

143. Walton, J.R.; Cognitive deterioration and related neuropathology in older people with Alzheimer's disease could result from life-long exposure to aluminum compounds; Chapter 2; Aging and vulnerability to environmental chemicals: Age-related disorders; Issues in Technology 16; Weiss, B., editor, RCS Publishing (2013)

144. Doty, R.L., et al.; Olfactory dysfunction in three neurodegenerative diseases; Geriatrics; Aug.; 46 Suppl. 1:47-51 (1991)

145. Hawkes, C.; Olfaction in neurodegenerative disorder; Mov. Disord.; Apr.; 18(4):364-72 (2003)

146. Bonanni, E., et al.; Daytime sleepiness in mild and moderate AD disease and its relationship with cognitive impairment; J. Sleep Res.; 14:311-17 (2005)

147. Ciulla, M.E., et. al; Episodes of fall asleep during day time in an elder woman with vascular dementia: Impact on cerebral ischemic tolerance and utility of ECG Holter monitoring; The Open Cardiovascular Med. J.; 4:189-91 (2010)

148. Brambilla-Perrot, B.; The management of arrhythmic sincope; Minerva Medica; 100:195-211 (2009)

149. Walton, J.R.; Brain lesions comprised of aluminum-rich cells that lack microtubules may be associated with the cognitive deficit of Alzheimer's disease; Neurotoxicology; 30:1059-69 (2009)

150. Maruyama, M., et al.; Imaging of tau pathology in a tauopathy mouse model and in Alzheimer patients compared to normal controls; Neuron; Sept.; 79:1094-1108 (2013)

151. Higuchi, M., et al.; 19F and 1H MRI detection of amyloid beta plaques in vivo; Nat. Neurosci.; Apt.; 8(4):527-33 (2005)

152. Iqbal, K., et al.; Cytosolic abnormally hyperphosphorylated tau but not paired helical filaments sequester normal MAPs and inhibit microtubule assembly; J. Alzheimers Dis. Aug. 14(4):365-70 (2008)

153. Hoover, B.R., et al.; Tau mislocalization to dendritic spines mediates synaptic dysfunction independently of neurodegeneration; Neuron; 68(6); 1067-81 (2010)

154. Nixon, R.A., et al.; Aluminum inhibits calpain-mediated proteolysis and induces human neurofilament proteins to form protease-resistant high molecular weight complexes; J. Neurochem., Dec. 55(6):1950-9 (1990)

155. Shea, T.B. and Husan, T.; Inhibition of proteolysis enhances aluminum-induced perikaryal neurofilament accumulation but does not enhance tau accumulation; Mol. Chem. Neuropathology, 26:195 (1995)

156. Sontag E, Hladik C, Montgomery L, Luangpirom A, Mudrak, I, Ogis E, White C.L.; Downregulation of protein phosphatase 2A carboxy methylation and methyltransferase may contribute to Alzheimer's disease pathogenesis; J Neuropathol Exp Neurol; 63:1080-91 (2004)

157. Sontag E, et al.; Protein phosphatase 2A methyltransferase links homocysteine metabolism with tau and amyloid precursor protein regulation; J Neurology; 27:2751-59 (2007)

158. Seshadri S., et al.; Plasma homocysteine as a risk factor for dementia and Alzheirmer's Disease; New Engl J Med; 346:7, 476-83 (2002)

159. Spalding K.L. et al.; Dynamics of hippocampal neurogenesis in adult humans; Cell, 153:1219-27 (2013)

160. Frisone, G.B., et al.; Mapping local hippocampal changes in Alzheimer's disease and normal ageing with MRI at 3 Tesla; Brain, 131,3266-76 (2008)

161. Kril, J.J., et al.; Neuron loss from the hippocampus of Alzheimer's disease exceeds extracellular neurofibrillary tangle formation; Acta. Neuropathologica; April, 103, 4:370-76 (2002)

162. Rao, M.V., et al.; J. Neurosci.; Specific calpain inhibition by calpastatin prevents tauopathy and neurodegeneration and restores normal lifespan in tau P301L mice; J. Neurosci.; Jul. 9:34(28):9222-34 (2014)

163. Johnson, J.W., and Ascher, P.; Glycine potentiates the NMDA response in cultured mouse brain neurons; Nature; 325:529-31 (1987).

164. Han, N.-L. R., et al.; Comparison of taurine- and glycine-induced conformational changes in the M2-M3 domain of the glycine receptor; J. Biol. Chem.; 279:19559-65 (2004)

165. Horning, M.S., and Tombley, P.Q.; Zinc and copper influence excitability of rat olfactory bulb neurons by multiple mechanisms; J. Neurophysiol., 86:1652-60 (2001)

166. Hosie, A.M., et al.; Zinc-mediated inhibition of GABA(A) receptors: discrete binding sites underlie subtype specificity; Nat. Neurosci.; Apr.; 6(4):362-9 (2003).

167. Woodin, M.A., et al.; Coincidence pre- and postsynaptic activity modifies GABAergic synapses by postsynaptic changes in Cl- transporter activity; Neuron; Aug.; 39(5):807-20 (2003)

168. Bannai, H., et al.; Activity-dependent tuning of inhibitory neurotransmission based on GABAAR diffusion dynamics; Neuron; 62:670-82 (2009)

169. Deshpande, A., et al.;A role for synaptic zinc in activity-dependent Aβ oligomer formation and accumulation at excitatory synapses; J Neurosci; April 29(13):4004-15 (2009)

170. Lipton, S.A., et al.; Neurotoxicity associated with dual actions of homocysteine at the N-methyl-D-asparate receptor; Proc Natl Acad Sci; May 94:5923-28 (1997)

171. Lipton, S.A., Rosenberg P.A.; Excitatory amino acids as a final common pathway for neurologic disorders; N Engl Med; March 330:613-22 (1994)

172. Globus, M. Y.-T., Busto, R., Martinez, E., Valdés, I., Dietrich, W. D. and Ginsberg, M. D.; Comparative Effect of Transient Global Ischemia on Extracellular Levels of Glutamate, Glycine, and γ-Aminobutyric Acid in Vulnerable and Nonvulnerable Brain Regions in the Rat; J Neurochem, 57: 470–478 (1991)

173. Takeda, A.; Insight into glutamate excitotoxicity from synaptic zinc homeostasis; Int. J. Alzheimer's Disease; ID 491597 (2011)

174. Simon, R.P., Swan J.H., Griffiths T., Meldrum B.S.; Blockade of N-methyl-D-aspartate receptors may protect against ischemic damage in the brain; Science Nov. 16; 226(4676):850-2 (1984)

175. Lipton, S.A.; Paradigm shift in neuroprotection by NMDA receptor blockade: memantine and beyond; Nat Rev Drug Disc; Feb. 5:160-170 (2006)

176. Paula-Lima, A.C., et al.; Activation of GABAA receptors by taurine and muscimol blocks the neurotoxicity of beta-amyloid in rat hippocampal and cortical neurons; Neuropharmacology, 49(8):1140-8 (2005)

177. Louzada, P.R., et al.; Taurine prevents the neuorotoxicity of beta-amyloid and glutamate receptor agonists – activation of GABA receptors and possible implications for Alzheimer's disease and other neurological disorders; FASEB J.; 18,511-8 (2004)

178. Malinow, R.; AMPA receptor trafficking and long-term potentiation; Phil. Trans. R. Soc. Lond. B; 358:707-14 (2003)

179. Sun, P., et al.; Differential activation of CREB by Ca2+/calmodulin-dependent protein kinases type II and type IV involves phosphorylation of a site that negatively regulates activity; Genes Dev.; 8:2527-39 (1994).

180. Tokumitsu, H., et al.; Activation mechanisms for Ca2+/Calmodulin-dependent protein kinase IV; J. Biol. Chem.; 269(46):28640-47 (1994)

181. Silva, A.J., et al.; CREB and memory; Annu. Rev. Neurosci.; 21:127-49 (1998)

182. Bourtchuladze, R., et al.; Deficient long-term memory in mice with a targeted mutation of the cAMP-responsive element-binding protein; Cell; Oct.; 79(1):59-68 (1994)

183. Carlyle, B.C.; cAMP-PKA phosphorylation of tau confers risk for degeneration in ageing association cortex; PNAS; April; 111(13):5036-41 (2014)

184. Sengupta, A., et al.; Phosphorylation of tau at both Thr 231 and Ser 262 is required for maximal inhibition of its binding to microtubules; Arch. Biochem. Biophys.; Sep.; 357(2):299-309 (1998)

185. Braitwaite, S.P.; et al.; Protein phosphatases and Alzheimer's disease; Prog. Mol. Biol. Transl. Sci.; 106:343-379 (2012)

186. Available at: http://www.who.int/mediacentre/factsheets/fs310/en/

187. Available at: http://www.uhnj.org/stroke/stats.htm

188. Available at: http://ninds.nih.gov/disorders/stroke/stroke_rehabilitation.htm

189. Available at: http://en.wikipedia.org/wiki/Tissue_plasminogen_activator

190. Uh J., Yezhuvath U., Cheng Y., Lu H.; in vivo vascular hallmarks of diffuse leukoaraiosis; J Magn Reson Imaging; Jul; 32(1):184-90 (2010)

191. Schenk C., Wuerz T., Lerner A.J.; Small vessel disease and memory loss: what the clinician needs to know to preserve patient's brain health; Curr Cardiol Rep; Dec; 15(12):427 (2013)

192. Grueter B.E., Schulz U.G.; Age-related cerebral white matter disease (leukoaraiosis) a review; Postgrad Med J; Feb; 88(1036):79-87 (2012)

193. Baezner H., Blahak C., Poggesi A., et al.; Association of gait and balance disorders with age-related white matter changes: the LADIS study; Neurology; Mar 18; 70(12):935-42 (2008)

194. Hassan A., Hunt B.J., O'Sullivan M., et al.; Homocysteine is a risk factor for cerebral small vessel disease, acting via endothelial dysfunction; Brain.: Jan;127(Pt 1): 212-9 (2004)

195. Austin, R.C., Lentz, S.R., and Werstuck; Role of hyperhomocysteinemia in endothelial dysfunction and atherothrombic disease; Cell Death and Differentiation; 11:S56-S64 (2004)

196. Steinberg, D.; Low density lipoprotein oxidation and its pathobiological significance; J. Biol. Sci.; Aug.; 272(34):20963-6 (1997)

197. Gaballa, I.F., et al.; Dyslipidemia and disruption of L-carnitine in aluminum exposed workers; Egyptian J. Occup. Med.; 37(1):33-46 (2013)

198. Wald D.S., Law M., Morris J.K., Homocysteine and cardiovascular disease: evidence on causality from a meta-analysis. BMJ; 325(7374):1202 (2002)

199. Ji Y., et al.; Vitamin B supplementation, homocysteine levels and the risk of cerebrovascular disease: a meta-analysis; Neurology (2013)

200. Perry I.J., Refsum H., Morris R.W., Ebrahim S.B., Ueland P.M., Shaper A.G., Prospective study of serum total homocysteine concentration and risk of stroke in middle-aged British men. Lancet; 346:1395-8 (1995)

Note: This decade long study of 5661 men 40-69 year of age shows that 107 men who had a stroke also had an average 2.8µM/L higher level of homocysteine as compared with men who did not have a stroke. These results compliment a study that showed a 10% decreased risk of recurrent stroke over a 2 year period with an average 3µM/L decrease in homocysteine levels resulting from vitamin supplementation[201].

201. Toole J.F., Malinow M.R., Chambless L.E., Spence J.D., Pettigrew L.C., Howard V.J., Sides E.G., Wang C.H., Stampfer M.; Lowering homocysteine in patients with ischemic stroke to prevent recurrent stroke, myocardial infarction, and death; JAMA; 291: 565–575 (2004)

Note: An alternate conclusion based upon the data in this paper is that a 3µM/L drop in homocysteine due to B12 (6µg), B6 (200µg), and folic acid (20µg) daily supplementation resulted in 10% lower risk of recurrent stroke and a 16% lower risk of death on average among 1853 patients with non-disabling cerebral infarction and higher level (e.g. 100 fold) supplementation is excessive, as these levels resulted in an insignificantly lower risk of 2% and 7% respectively with only a 2µM/L additional drop in homocysteine

202. Censori B., Partziguian T., Manara O., Poloni M.; Plasma homocysteine and severe white matter disease; Neurol Sci; Oct.; 28(5):259-63 (2007)

203. Sachdev P., Parslow R., Salonikas C., et al.; Homocysteine and the brain in midadult life: evidence for an increased risk of leukoaraiosis in men; Arch Neurol; Sep. 61(9): 1369-76 (2004)

204. Mailloux, R.J., Lemire, J., and Appanna, V.D.; Hepatic response to aluminum toxicity: dyslipidemia and liver diseases; Exp. Cell Res.; Oct.; 317(16):2231-8 (2011)

205. Lemire, J., et al.; The disruption of L-carnitine metabolism by aluminum toxicity and oxidative stress promotes dyslipidemia in human astrocytic and hepatic cells; Toxicol. Lett. Jun.; 203(3):219-26 (2011)

206. Waly, M., et al.; Activation of methionine synthase by insulin-like growth factor-1 and dopamine: a target for neurodevelopmental toxins and thimerosal; Mol. Psychiatry 9, 358-70 (2004)

207. Waly, M. I-A., and Deth, R.; Neurodevelopmental toxins deplete glutathione and inhibit folate and vitamin B12-dependent methionine synthase activity – a link between oxidative stress and autism; FASEB J; 22:894 1 (2008)

208. Kurth, T., et al.; Body mass index and the Risk of Stroke in Men; Ach Intern. Med.; Dec., 162:2557-62 (2002)

209. Chuang, Y-F, et al.; Midlife adiposity predicts earlier onset of Alzheimer's dementia, neuropathology and presymptomatic cerebral amyloid accumulation; Mol. Psychiatry; Sept. (2015)

210. Bramble, D.M., and Lieberman, D.L.; Endurance running and the evolution of Homo; Nature, 432, 345-52 (2004)

211. With low CBS activity the brain can still make some glutathione and taurine because cystathionine levels in the human cortex are 40 times higher than other tissues [665,666]. High cystathionine levels in the brain may counteract the low activity of the enzyme CBL that converts cystathionine to cysteine. CBL's enzyme activity is 100 times lower in the brain than in the liver[667].

212. Lever, M., et al.; Betaine and trimethylamine-N-oxide as predictors of cardiovascular outcomes show different patterns in diabetes mellitus: An observational study; PLOS; DOI:10.1371 (2014)

213. Kirke, P.N., et al.: Impact of the MTHFR C677T polymorphism on risk of neural tube defects: case-control study; BMJ, 328:1535-6 (2004)

214. Herbert V., ed. Vitamin B12 deficiency. London: Royal Society of Medicine Press; Vitamin B12- An overview 1-81 (1999)

215. Pennypacker L.C., Allen R.H., Kelly J.P., Matthews L.M., Grigsby J., Kaye K., et al. High prevalence of cobalamin deficiency in elderly outpatients; J Am Geriatr Soc.; 40:1197–204 (1992)

216. Karnaze D.S., Carmel R.; Low serum cobalamin levels in primary degenerative dementia: do some patients harbor atypical cobalamin deficiency states? Arch Intern Med; 147:429—431 (1987)

217. Huang Y., et al.; Prehypertension and the Risk of Stroke: A Meta-analysis; Neurology; March 12, (2014)

218. Clarke R., Refsum H., Birks J., et al.; Screening for vitamin B12 and folate deficiency in older people; Am J Clin Nutr;77:1241–7 (2003)

219. Willems, F.F., et al.; Pharmacokinetic study on the utilization of 5-methyltetrahydrofolate and folic acid in patients with coronary artery disease; British J Pharmacol., 141, 825-30 (2004)

220. Lamers, Y., et al.; Red blood cell folate concentrations increase more after supplementation with [6S]-5-methyltetrahydrofolate than with folic acid in women of childbearing age; Am J Clin Nutr; 84:156-61 (2006)

221. Detopoulou P., et al.; Dietary choline and betaine intakes in relation to concentrations of inflammatory markers in healthy adults: the Attica Study; Am J Clin Nutr; 87:424-30 (2008)

222. Yang, H.T., et al.; Efficacy of folic acid supplementation in cardiovascular disease prevention: and updated meta-analysis of randomized control trials; Eur. J. Intern. Med.; 23(8)745-54 (2012)

223. Craig S.A.; Betaine in human nutrition; Am J Clin Nutr; 80:539-49 (2004)

224. De Bree, A., et al.; Lifestyle factors and plasma homocysteine concentrations in a general population sample; Am. J. Epidemiology; 154(2):150-4 (2001)

225. Xiao, Y., et al.; Dietary protein and plasma total homocysteine, cysteine concentrations in coronary angiographic subjects; Nutr. J.; 12:144-54 (2013)

226. Haddad, E.H., et al.; Dietary intake and biochemical, hematological, and immune status of vegans compared with nonvegetarians; Am. J. Clin. Nutr.; 70(suppl):586S-93S (1999)

227. Kenyon, S.H., et al.; The effect of ethanol and its metabolites upon methionine synthase activity in vitro; Alcohol; May; 15(4):305-9 (1998)

228. Bleich, S., et al.; Moderate alcohol consumption in social drinkers raises plasma homocysteine levels – a contradiction of the French Paradox?; Alcohol Alcoholism; 36(3):189-92 (2001)

229. Thein S.S., Hamidon B.B., Teh H.S., Raymond A.A.; Leukoaraiosis as a predictor for mortality and morbidity after an acute ischemic stroke: Singapore Med J; May; 48(5): 396-9 (2007)

230. Li H., Xu G., Xiong Y., et al.; Relationship between cerebral atherosclerosis and leukoaraiosis in aged patients: Results from DSA; J. Neuroimaging; Sep. 3 (2013)

231. Stuhlinger, M.C., et al.; Homocysteine impairs the nitric oxide synthase pathway – Role of asymmetric dimethylarginine; Circulation; 104:2569-75 (2001)

232. Welch N.G., Loscalzo J.; Homocysteine and atherosclerosis; N Engl J Med; 338:1042-50 (1998)

233. Mizrahi, E.H., et al.; Further evidence of interrelation between homocysteine and hypertension in stroke patients: a cross-sectional study; IMAJ, Vol. 5, 791-94 (2003)

234. Amarenco, P.; Lipid management in the prevention of stroke – review and updated meta-analysis of statins for stroke prevention; Lancet, 8(5):453-63 (2009)

235. Elkind, M., et al.; Lipid-lowering agent use at ischemic stroke onset is associated with decreased mortality; Neurology; July; 65(2):253-58 (2005)

236. Blanco, M., et al.; Statin treatment withdrawal in ischemic stroke; Neurology; Aug.; 69(9):904-10 (2007)

237. Leitersdorf, E.; Cholesterol absorption inhibition – filling an unmet need in lipid-lowering management; European Heart J Supplements; 3 (supplement E) E17-E23 (2001)

238. Davidson, M.H.; Ezetimibe coadministered with simvastatin in patients with primary hypercholesterolemia; J. Am. Coll. Cardiol.; Dec. 18; 40(12):2125-34 (2002)

239. Glossmann, H.H.; Origin of 7-dehydrocholesterol (provitamin D) in the skin; J. Investigative Dermat.; 130:1239-41 (2010)

240. Anagnostis, P., et al.; Comparative effect of Atorvastatin and Rosuvastatin on 25-hydroxy-vitamin D levels in non-diabetic patients with dyslipidaemia: A prospective random open-label pilot study; Open Cardio. Med. J.; 8:55-50 (2014)

241. Rejnmark, L., et al.; Simvastatin does not affect vitamin D status, but low vitamin D levels are associated with dyslipidemia: Results from a randomized, controlled trial; Internat. J. Endocrin.; 2010, Article ID 957174 (2010)

242. Wolozin, B., et al.; Simvastatin is associated with a reduced incidence of dementia and Parkinson's disease; BMC Medicine; 5:21-31 (2007)

243. Betterman, K., et al.; Statins, risk of dementia and cognitive function: Secondary analysis of the Ginkgo Evaluation of Memory Study (GEMS); J Stroke Cerebrovasc. Dis.; Aug.; 21(6):436-444 (2012)

244. Newman, H.A.I., et al: Serum chromium and angiographically determined coronary artery disease; Clin Chem; 24:541-544 (1978)

245. Simonoff, M., et al: Low plasma chromium in patients with coronary artery and heart diseases; Biol Trace Element Res; 6:431-439 (1984)

246. Press, R.I., et al.; The effect of chromium picolinate on serum cholesterol and apolipoprotein fractions in human subjects; West J. Med., Jan.; 152:41-5 (1990)

247. Armitage, J. et al.; The HPS2-THRIVE Collaborative Group. Effects of extended release niacin and laropiprant in high-risk patients; N Engl J Med; 371:203-12 (2014)

248. Bruckert, E., et al.; Meta-analysis of the effect of nicotinic acid alone or in combination on cardiovascular events and atherosclerosis; Atherosclerosis; June; 210(2):353-61 (2010)

249. Lisak, M., et al.; Hypertriglyceridemia as a possible independent risk factor for stroke; Acta. Clin. Croat.; Dec; 52(4):458-63 (2013)

250. Rubins, H.B., et al.; Reduction in stroke with Gemfibrozil in men with coronary heart disease and low HDL cholesterol; Circulation; 103:2828-2833 (2001)

251. Munoz-Aguirre, P., et al.; The effect of vitamin D supplementation on serum lipids in postmenopausal women with diabetes: A randomized controlled trial; Clin. Nutr.; Oct.; 34(5):799-804 (2015)

252. Harris, W.S.; n-3 Fatty acids and serum lipoproteins: human studies; A. J. Clin. Nutr.; 65(suppl.):1645S-54S (1997)

253. Bernstein, A.M., et al.; "Purified palmitoleic acid for the reduction of high-sensitivity C-reactive protein and serum lipids: a double-blinded, placebo controlled study; J. Clin. Lipidol.; 8(6):612-7 (2014)

254. Wei, M.J.; Effects of eicosapentaenoic acid versus docosahexanoic acid on serum lipids: a systematic review and meta-analysis; Curr. Atheroscler. Rep.; Dec.; 13(6):474-83 (2011)

255. Kawahara, M., Kato-negishi, M.; Link between aluminum and the pathogenesis of Alzheimer's Disease: The integration of the aluminum and amyloid cascade hypotheses; Internat J Alz Disease; 2011:1-17; Article ID 276393 (2011)

256. Wolf, P.A., Abbott, R.D., Kannel, W.B.; Atrial fibrillation as an independent risk factor for stroke – the Framingham Study; Stroke, 22:983-88 (1991)

257. Figueiredo, J.C., et al.; Folic acid and risk of prostate cancer: Results from a randomized clinical trial; J. Natl. Cancer Inst; 101:432-5 (2009)

258. Lee, J.E., et al.; Are dietary choline and betaine intakes determinants of total homocysteine concentrations?; Am. J. Clin. Nutr.; 91:1303-10 (2010)

259. Niculescu, M.D., et al.; Diet, methyl donors and DNA methylation – interactions between dietary folate, methionine and choline; J. Nutr.; 132:2333S-5S (2002)

260. E.J. Corey and A. Tramontano; Total synthesis of the quinonoid alcohol dehydrogenase coenzyme (1) of methylotrophic bacteria; J. Am. Chem. Soc.; 103(18):5599-5600 (1981)

261. Hara, H., Hiramatsu, H., Adachi, T.; Pyrroloquinoline quinone is a potent neuroprotective nutrient against 6-hydroxydopamine-induced neurotoxicity; Neurochem Res; Mar. 32(3):489-95 (2007)

262. Nunome, K., et al.; Pyrroloquinoline quinone prevents oxidative stress-induced neuronal death probably through changes in oxidative status of DJ-1; Biol Pharm Bull; Jul.; 31(7):1321-6 (2008)

263. Hirakawa, A., Shimizu, K., Fukumitsu, H., Furukawa, S.,; Pyrolloquinoline quinone attenuates iNOS gene expression in the injured spinal cord; Biochem Biophys Res Commun; 378:308-312 (2009)

264. Rucker, R,, Chowanadisai, Nakano, M.; Potential physiological importance of pyroloquinoline quinone; Alt Med Rev; 14(3):268-77 (2009)

265. Ouchi, A., Nakano, M., Nagaoka, S., Mukai, K.; Kinetic study of the antioxidant activity of pyrroloquinolinequinol (PQQH(2), a reduced dorm of pyrrolocholinequinone) in micellar solution; J. Agric Food Chem; Jan 57(2):450-6 (2009)

266. Chowanadisai, W., et al.; Pyrroloquinoline quinone stimulates mitochondrial biogenesis through cAMP response element-binding protein phosphorylation and increased PGC-1a expression; J Biol Chem; Jan. 285(1):142-52 (2010)

267. Onyango, I.G., et al.; Regulation of neuron mitochondrial biogenesis and relevance to brain health; Biochim Biophys Acta; Jan.; 1802(1):228-34 (2010)

268. Murase, K., Hattori, A., Kohno, M., Hayashi, K.; Stimulation of nerve growth factor synthesis/secretion in mouse astroglial cells by coenzymes; Biochem Mol Biol Int; Jul.; 30(4):615-21 (1993)

269. Harris, C., et al.; Dietary pyrroloquinoline quinone (PQQ) alters indicators of inflammation and mitochondrial-related metabolism in human subjects; J. Nutr. Biochem.; 24:2076-84 (2013)

270. Nakani, M., Ubukata, K., Yamamoto, T., Yamaguchi, H.; Effect of pyrroloquinoline quinone (PQQ) on mental status of middle-aged and elderly persons; Food Style; 21 13(7):50-3 (2009)

271. Jensen, et al.; The putative essential nutrient pyrroloquinoline quinone is neuroprotective in a rodent model of hypoxic/ischemic brain injury; Neuroscience; Sept. 62(2):399-406 (1994)

272. Zhang, Y., Feustel, P.J., Kimelberg, H.K.; Neuroprotection by pyrroloquinoline quinone (PQQ) in reversible middle cerebral artery occlusion in the adult rat; Brain Res; June; 1094(1):200-6 (2006)

273. Kim, J., et al.; Pyrroloquinoline quinone inhibits the fibrillation of amyloid proteins; Prion; 4(1):26-31 (2010)

274. Kobayashi, M., et al.; Pyrroloquinoline quinone (PQQ) prevents fibril formation of alpha-synuclein; Biochem. Biophys. Research Comm; Oct., 349(3):1139-44 (2006)

275. Nakano, M., et al.; Acute and subchronic toxicity studies of pyrroloquinoline quinone (PQQ) disodium slat (BioPQQTM) in rats; Reg. Toxicol. Pharmacol.; Oct.; 70(1):107-121 (2014)

276. Nakano, M., et al.; Genotoxicity of pyrroloquinoline quinone (PQQ) disodium salt; Reg Tox Pharm; 67:189-97 (2013)

277. Kumazawa, T., et al.; Levels of pyrroloquinoline quinone in various foods; Biochem J; 307:331-3 (1995)

278. Noji, N., et al,; Simple and sensitive method for pyrroloquinoline quinone (PQQ) analysis in various foods using liquid chromatography/electrospray-ionization tandem mass spectrometry; J Agric Food Chem; Sep.; 55(18):7258-63 (2007)

279. Mitchell, A.E., Jones, A.D., Mercer, R.S., Rucker R.B.; Characterization of pyrroloquinoline quinone amino acid derivatives by electrospray ionization mass spectrometry and detection in human milk; Anal Biochem; May; 269(2):317-25 (1999)

280. Rodriguez, J.I., and Kern, J.K.; Evidence of microglial activation in autism and its possible role in brain underconnectivity, Neuron Glia Biology, 7(2-4):205-13 (2011)

281. Drubin, D.G., et al.; Nerve growth factor-induced neurite outgrowth in PC12 cells involves the coordinate induction of microtubule assembly and assembly-promoting factors; J Cell Biol; Nov.; 101:1799-1807 (1985)

282. Murase, K., Hattori, A., Kohono, M., Hayashi, K.; Stimulation of nerve growth factor synthesis/secretion on mouse astroglial cells by coenzymes, Biochem Mol Biol Int; Jul., 30(4):615-21 (1993)

283. Urakami, T., Tanaka, A., Yamaguchi, K., Tsuji, T., Niki, E.; Synthesis of esters of coenzyme PQQ and IPQ, and stimulation of nerve growth factor production; Biofactors, 5(3):139-46 (1995-1996)

284. Ren, Z., et al.; Mechanisms of brain injury with deep hypothermic circulatory arrest and protective effects of coenzyme Q10; J Thorac Cardiovasc Surg; Jul.; 108(1) 126-33 (1994)

285. Dumont, M., Kipiani, K., Yu, F.; Coenzyme Q decreases amyloid pathology and improves behavior in transgenic mouse model of Alzheimer's disease; J Alzheimers Dis.; 27(1):211-23 (2011)

286. Lopez-Lluch, G., et al.; Is coenzyme Q a key factor in ageing? Mech Ageing Dev; Apr. 131(4):225-35 (2010)

287. Deichmann, R., Lavie, C., Andrews, S.; Coenzyme Q10 and statin-induced mitochondrial dysfunction; Oschner J; 10:16-21 (2010)

288. Hosoe, K., Kitano, M., Kishida, H., et al.; Study on safety and bioavailability of ubiquinol (Kaneka QH(trade mark)) after single and 4-week multiple oral administration to healthy volunteers; Regul Toxicol Pharmaco; Aug 17, 2006

289. Azik, F.M., et al.; A different interaction between parathyroid hormone, calcitriol, and serum aluminum in chronic kidney disease; a pilot study; Int. Urol. Nephrol.; 43:467-470 (2011)

290. Fernell, E., et al.; Autism spectrum disorder and low vitamin D at birth: a sibling control study; Molecular Autism; 6:3 (2015)

291. Morales, E., et al.; Vitamin D in pregnancy and attention deficit hyperactivity disorder-like symptoms in childhood; Epidemiology; Jul.; 26(4):458-65 (2015)

292. Littlerjohns, T.J., et. al; Vitamin D and the risk of dementia and Alzheimer's disease; Am. Acad. Neurology; 1-9 Published Online (2014)

293. Miller, J.W., et al.; Vitamin D status and rates of cognitive decline in a multiethnic cohort of older adults; JAMA Neurology, Sep. (2015)

294. Buell, J.S., et al, 25-Hydroxyvitamin D, dementia, and cerebrovascular pathology in elders receiving home services; Neurology, 74:18-26 (2010)

295. Daubail, B., et al: Serum 25-hydroxyvitamin D predicts severity and prognosis in stroke patients; Eur J Neurol; Jan 20(1):57-61 (2013)

296. Garcion, E., et al,; New clues about vitamin D functions in the nervous system; Trends in Endocrine Metab; 13(3):100-105 (2002)

297. Muir, S. W., et al.; Effect of vitamin D supplementation on muscle strength, gait, and balance in older adults; J. Am. Geriatrics Soc.; 59(12):2291-2300 (2011)

298. Cannell, J.J., Autism and vitamin D; Med. Hypotheses; 70(4):750-9 (2008)

299. Voet, D. and Voet, J.G.; Biochemistry. Vol. 1; Biomolecules, mechanism of action, and metabolism, 3rd. ed., 663-64, John Wiley & Sons (2004)

300. Robertson, J.A., et al.; Animal model of aluminum induced osteomalcia: role of chronic renal failure; Kidney Int.; 23:327-35 (1983)

301. Goodman, W.G., et al.; Parenteral aluminum administration in the dog II. Induction of osteomalcia and effect on vitamin D metabolism; Kidney Int.; 25:370-75 (1984)

302. Adit, A., et al.; Demographic differences and trends of vitamin D insufficiency in the US population, 1988-2004; Arch. Intern. Med. 169(6):626-632 (2009)

303. Alfrey, A.C., et al.; Metabolism and toxicity of aluminum in renal failure; Am. J. Clin. Nutr.; 33:509-1516 (1980)

304. Mayor, G.H., et al.; Parathyroid hormone-mediated aluminum deposition and egress in the rat; Kidney Int.; Jan.; 17(1):40-4 (1980)

305. Constantini, S.; Distribution of aluminum following intraperitoneal injection of aluminum lactate in the rat; Pharmacol. Oxicol.; Jan.; 64(1):47-50 (1989)

306. Hirschberg, R., et al.; Organ distribution of aluminum in uremic rats: influence of parathyroid hormone and 1,25-dihydroxyvitamin D3; Miner Electrolyte Metab.; 11(2):106-10 (1985)

307. Quarles, L.D., et al.; Aluminum deposition at the osteoid-bone interface; J. Clin. Invest.; May; 75:1441-47 (1985)

308. Drueke, T.; et al.; Oral aluminum administration to uremic, hyperparathyroid, or vitamin D-supplemented rats; Nephron; 39:10-17 (1985)

309. Ittel, T.H.; et al.; Enhanced gastrointestinal absorption of aluminum in uraemia: Time course and effect of vitamin D; Nephrol. Dial. Transplant; 3(5):617-623 (1988)

310. Adler, A.A. and Berlyne, G.M.; Duodenal aluminum absorption in the rat: effect of vitamin D; Gastrintest. Liver Physiol.; 12:G209-G213 (1985)

311. Cox, K.A. and Dunn, M.A.; Aluminum toxicity alters the regulation of calbindin-D28k protein and mRNA expression in chick intestine; Am. Soc. Nutritional Sci.; Nov.; 2007-13 (2001)

312. Gross, M.L., et al.; Severe vitamin D deficiency in 6 Canadian First Nation formula-fed infants; Int. J. Circumpolar Health; Apr.; 72:20244 (2013)

313. Gallo, S., et al.; Effect of different dosages of oral vitamin D supplementation on vitamin D status in healthy, breastfed infants: a randomized trial; JAMA; 309(17):1785-92 (2013)

314. Casey, C. F., et al.; Vitamin D supplementation in infants, children, and adolescents; Am. Family Physician; Mar.; 81(6):745-48 (2010)

315. Wagner, G.L., et al.; High-dose D3 supplementation in a cohort of breastfeeding mothers and their infants: a 6-month follow-up pilot study; Breastfeed. Med.; Summer 1(2):59-70 (2006)

316. Hollis B.W., et al.; Vitamin D supplementation during pregnancy: double-blind, randomized clinical trial of safety and effectiveness; J. Bone Miner. Res.; Oct.; 26(10):2341-57 (2011)

317. Institute of Medicine, Food and Nutrition Board. Dietary Reference Intakes for Calcium and Vitamin D. Washington, DC: National Academy Press, 2010. http://ods.od.nih.gov/factsheets/VitaminD-HealthProfessional/

318. Turetaky, A., et al.; Low serum vitamin D is independently associated with larger lesion volumes after ischemic stroke; J. Stroke Cerebrovasc. Dis.; 24(7):1555-63 (2015)

319. Park, K.Y., et al.; Serum vitamin D status as a predictor of prognosis in patients with acute ischemic stroke; Cerebrovasc. Dis.; 4(1-2):73-8 (2015)

320. Tompkins, A.J., et al; Mitochondrial dysfunction in cardiac ischemia-reperfusion injury: ROS from complex I, without inhibition; Biochim Biophys Acta; 1762:223-231 (2006)

321. Chen, X.M., Chen, H.S., Xu, M.J., Shen, J.G.; Targeting reactive nitrogen species: a promising therapeutic strategy for cerebral ischemia-reperfusion injury; Acta Pharmacol Sin; Jan 34(1):67-77 (2013)

322. Balden, R., Selvamani, A., Sohrabji, F.; Vitamin D deficiency exacerbates experimental stroke injury and dysregulates ischemia-induced inflammation in adult rats; Endocrinology; May 153(5):2420-36 (2012)

323. Mosekilde, L.; Vitamin D and the elderly; Clin. Endocrinol. (Oxf.); Mar.; 62(3):265-81 (2005)

324. Atlas, E., et al.; Comparison between daily supplementation doses of 200 versus 400 IU of vitamin D in infants; Eur. J.Pediatr.; Aug.; 172(8):1039-42 (2013)

325. Houghton, L.A., and Vieth, R.; The case against ergocalciferol (vitamin D3) as a vitamin supplement; Am. J. Clin. Nutr.; 84:694-7 (2006)

326. Cannell, J.J.; Autism causes prevention and treatment; Sunrise River Press (2015)

327. London, G.M., et al.; Arterial calcifications and bone histomorphometry in end-stage renal disease; J. Am. Soc. Nephrology; 15:1943-51 (2004)

328. Kudo, H., et al; Quantitative analysis of glutathione in human brain tumors; J Neurosurg, Apr 72(4):610-5 (1990)

329. Kumazawa, T., et al; Trace levels of pyrroloquinoline quinone in human and rat samples detected by gas chromatography/mass spectrometry; Biochem Biophys Acta; Dec 1156(1):62-6 (1992)

330. Zhang, Y., Rosenberg, P.A.; The essential nutrient pyrroloquinoline quinone may act as a neuroprotectant by suppressing peroxynitrite formation; Eur J Neurosci, Sep 16(6):1015-24 (2002)

331. Zhang, Q., et al; Pyrroloquinoline quinone protects rat brain cortex against acute glutamate induced neurotoxicity; Neurochem Res; Aug 38(8):1661-71 (2013)

332. Benrabh, H., et al.; Taurine transport at the blood-brain barrier: an in vivo brain perfusion study; Brain Res.; 692:57-65 (1995)

333. Miller, T.J., et. al.; Developmental changes in organic osmolytes in prenatal rat tissues; Comp. Biochem. Physiol. Part A. Mol. Integr. Physiol.; Jan.; 125(1):45-56 (2000)

334. Banay-Schwartz, et al.; Changes with aging in the levels of amino acids in rat CNS structural elements. II. Taurine and small neutral amino acids; Neurochem. Res.; 14:563-570 (1989)

335. Gebara, E., et al.; Taurine increases hippocampal neurogenesis in aging mice; Stem Cell Res.; May; 14(3):369-79 (2015)

336. Yamori, Y., et al.; Taurine as the nutritional factor for the longevity of the Japanese revealed by a world-wide epidemiological survey; Taurine 7, Vol 18, Azuma, J., Schaffer, S.W., Ito, T. (Eds.), Springer, Chapter 2, p13-25 (2009)

337. Menzie, J., Prentice, H., Wu, J.-Y.; Neuroprotective mechanisms of taurine against ischemic stroke; Brain Sci., 3, 877-907 (2013)

338. Kumari, N., Prentice, H., Wu, J.-J.-Y.; Taurine and its neuroprotective role; Taurine 8, Vol. 1: The nervous system, immune system, diabetes, and the cardiovascular system, El Idrissi, A, L'Amoreaux W.J. (Eds.), Springer, Chapter 2, p19-27 (2013)

339. El Idrissi, A.; Taurine increases mitochondrial buffering of calcium: role in neuroprotection; Amino Acids, 34, Feb. 2:321-28 (2008)

340. Ricci, L., et al.; Protection by taurine of rat brain cortical slices against oxygen glucose deprivation-and-reoxygenation-induced damage; Eur. J. Pharmacol.; Oct 25:621(1-3):26-32 (2009)

341. Flora, S.J.S., et al.; Combined administration of taurine and monoisoamyl DMSA protects arsenic induced oxidative injury in rats; Oxidative Med. Cell. Long.; 1;1 39-45 (2008).

342. Flora, S.J.S., et al.: Combined administration of taurine and meso 2,3-dimercaptosuccinic acid in the treatment of chronic lead intoxication in rats; Hum. Exp. Toxicol.; April 23:4 157-166 (2004).

343. Kahtani, M.A.; Renal damage mediated by oxidative stress in mice treated with aluminum chloride: protective effects of taurine; J. Biol. Sci.; 10(7):584-95 (2010).

344. Abdel-Moneim, A.M.; Effects of taurine against histomorphological and ultrastructural changes in the testes of mice exposed to aluminum chloride; Arh. Hig. Rada Toksikol; 64:405-414 (2013)

345. Opinion of the Scientific Committee on Food – Additional information on "energy" drinks; SCF/CS/PLEN/ENDRINKS/16 Final (2003)

346. Trautwein, E.A. and Hayes, K.C.; Taurine concentrations in plasma and whole blood in humans: estimation of error from intra- and inter-individual variation and sampling technique; Am. J. Clin. Nutr.; 52:758-64 (1990)

347. USDA Handbook No. 8

348. Pasantes-Morales, H., Lopez, I., Ysunza, A.; Taurine content in breast milk of Mexican women from urban and rural areas; Arch. Med. Res.; Spring: 26(1):47-52 (1995)

349. El-Sayed, W. M.; et al.; Prophylactic and therapeutic effects of taurine against aluminum-induced acute hepatotoxicity in mice; J. Hazard Mater.; Aug.; 192(2):880-6 (2011)

350. Barasch, E., et al.; Clinical significance of calcification of the fibrous skeleton of the heart and aortosclerosis in community dwelling elderly – The Cardiovascular Health Study – CHS; Am. Heart J.; Jan; 151(1):39-47 (2006)

351. Novaro, G.M., et al.; Plasma homocysteine and calcific aortic valve disease; Heart, 90:802-3 (2002)

352. Fusaro, M., et al.; Vitamin K, Veretebral fractures, vascular calcifications, and mortality – Vitamin K Italian - VIKI – dialysis study; J. Bone and Mineral Res.; Nov.; 27(22):2271-78 (2012)

353. Geleijnsa, J.M., et al.; Dietary intake of menaquinone is associated with a reduced risk of coronary heart disease – The Rotterdam Study; The J. of Nutrition; 3100-5 (2014)

354. Shurgers, L.J.; et al.; Regression of warfarin-induced medial elastocalcinosis by high intake of vitamin K in rats; Blood; 109(7):2823-31 (2006)

355. Knapen, M.H., et al.; Menaquinone-7 supplementation improves arterial stiffness in healthy postmenopausal women. A double-blind randomized clinical trial; Thromb. Haemost.; May; 113(5):1135-44 (2015)

356. Gallieni, M., and Fusaro, M.; Vitamin K and cardiovascular calcification in CKD – is patient supplementation on the horizon?; Kidney International; 86:232-34 (2014)

357. Shea, M.K. and Holden, R.M.; Vitamin K status and vascular calcification – Evidence from observational and clinical studies; Adv. Nutr.; 3:158-65 (2012)

358. Vermeer, C.; Vitamin K – the effect on health beyond coagulation – an overview; Food and Nutr. Res.; 56:5329-35 (2012)

359. Koitaya, N., et al.; Low-dose vitamin K2 (MK-4) supplementation for 12 months improves bone metabolism and prevents forearm bone loss in postmenopausal Japanese women; J. Bone Miner. Meta.; Mar.; 32(2):142-50 (2014).

360. Schurgers, L.J., et al.; Post-translational modifications regulate matrix Gla protein function – importance for inhibition of vascular smooth muscle cell calcification; J. Thrombosis Haemostasis; 5:2503-11 (2007)

361. Theuwissen, E., et al.; The role of vitamin K in soft-tissue calcification; Adv. Nutr.; 3:166-73 (2012)

362. Caluwe, R., et al.; Vitamin K2 supplementation in haemodialysis patients – a randomized dose-finding study; Nephrol. Dial. Transplant 0:1-7 (2013)

363. Heap, L.C., Peters, T.J., Wessely, S.; Vitamin B status in patients with chronic fatigue syndrome; J Royal Soc Med; 92:183-5 (1999)

364. http://en.wikipedia.org/wiki/Vitamin_B12_deficiency

365. Gomm, W., et al.; Association of proton pump inhibitors with risk of dementia – A pharmacoepidemiological claims data analysis; JAMA Neurol.; Feb. 15, published online (2016)

366. Dharmarajan, T.S., et al.; Do acid lowering agents affect vitamin B12 status in older adults?; J. Am. Med. Dir. Assoc.; Mar.; 9(3):162-7 (2008)

367. Bahasher, H.; Methylcobalamin versus cyanocobalamin; The Association of Physicians of India; Chapter 139 (2011)

368. Van Asselt, D.Z.B.; et al.; Nasal absorption of hydroxycobalamin in healthy elderly adults; Br. J. Clin. Pharacol.; 45:83-8 (1998)

369. Izumi, K., et al.; Mecobalamin improved pernicious anemia in an elderly individual with Hashimoto's disease and diabetes mellitus; Nihon Ronen Igakkai Zasshi; 50(4):542-5 (2013)

370. Singh, M.; Essential fatty acid, DHA, and human brain; Indian J. Pediatrics, 72:239-42 (2205)

371. Spector, A.A.; Essentiality of fatty acids; Lipids,; 34(1):S1-S3 (1999)

372. Yurko-Mauro, K.; Beneficial effects of docosahexaenoic acid on cognition in age-related cognitive decline; Alzheimer's & Dementia; Nov., 6(6):456-64 (2010)

373. Astarita, G., et al.; Deficient liver biosynthesis of docosahexaneoic acid correlates with cognitive impairment in Alzheimer's disease; PLoS ONE; 5(9):1-8 (2010)

374. Quinn, J.F. et al.; Docosahexaenoic acid supplementation and cognitive decline in Alzheimer's disease – a randomized trial; JAMA; Nov.; 304(17):1903-11 (2010)

375. http://www.dhaomega3.org/Overview/Dietary-Sources-of-Omega-3-Fatty-Acids

376. Li, D., et al.; Alpha-Linolenic acid content of commonly available nuts in Hangzhou; Int. J. Vitam. Nutr. Res.; 76(1):18-21 (2006)

377. http://en.wikipedia.org/wiki/Alpha-Linolenic_acid

378. Brand, A., et al.; Metabolism of cysteine in astroglial cells: hypotaurine and taurine; J. Neurochem.; 71(2): 827-32 (1998)

379. Stipanuk, M.H., Ueki, L.; Dealing with methionine/homocysteine sulfur: cysteine metabolism to taurine and inorganic sulfur; J. Inherit. Metab. Dis.; 34(1):17-32 (2011)

380. Lord, R.S., Fitzgerald, N.D.; Significance of low plasma homocysteine; Metametrix Clinical Lab., Dept. Sci. and Education, Norcross, GA (2006)

381. Ghandforoush-Sattari, M., et al.; Changes in plasma concentration of taurine in stroke; Neurosci. Lett., June 8; 496(3):172-5 (2011)

382. Shaw, C.A., and Tomljenovic; Aluminum in the central nervous system (CNS): toxicity in humans and animals, vaccine adjuvants, and autoimmunity; Immunol. Res.; 56:304-16 (2013)

383. Mullan, N., and Yasko, A.; Aluminum toxicity in mitochondrial dysfunction and ASD; Autism Sci. Digest; J. Autismone; 5:22-29 (2013)

384. Burrell, S.-A., and Exley, C.; There is (still) too much aluminum in infant formulas; BMC Pediatrics; 10(63):1-4 (2010)

385. Chuchu, N., et al.; The aluminum content of infant formulas remains too high; BMC Pediatrics; 13:162:1471-31 (2013)

386. Flarend, R., et al.; A preliminary study of the dermal absorption of aluminum from antiperspirants using aluminum-26; Food Chem. Toxicol.; Feb.; 39(2):163-8 (2001)

387. Bassioni, G., et al.; Risk assessment of using aluminum foil in food preparation; Int. J. Electrochem. Sci.; 7:4498-4509 (2012)

388. Muller, M., Ankr, M., Illing-Gunther, H.; Availability of aluminum from tea and coffee; Z. Lebensm Unters Forsch A; 205:170-73 (1997)

389. Barcena-Padilla, D.A., et al.; Aluminum contents in dry leaves and infusions of commercial black and green tea leaves: effects of sucrose and ascorbic acid added to infusions; Natural Resources, 2, 141-45 (2011)

390. Matsushima, F., Meshitsuka, S., Nose, T.; Nihon Eiseigaku Zasshi, Oct. 48(4):864-72 (1993)

391. Yokel, R.A. and McNamara, P.J.; Aluminum toxicokinetics: an updated minireview; Pharmacol. Toxicol.; 88:159-167 (2001)

392. Stahl, T., Taschan, H., Brunn, H.; Aluminum content of selected foods and food products, Environ. Sci. Europe; 23:37 (2011)

393. Fernandez-Lorenzo, J.R., et al.; Aluminum contents of human milk, cow's milk and infant formulas; J. Ped. Gastroenterol. Nutr.; 28:270-275 (1999)

394. Yokel, R.A. and Florence, R.L.; Aluminum bioavailability from approved food additive leavening agent acidic sodium phosphate, incorporated into a baked good is lower than from water; Toxicol.; 227:86-93 (2006)

395. Hem, J.D.; Graphical methods for studies of aqueous aluminum hydroxide, fluoride, and sulfate; Geological water-supply paper 1827-B, U.S. Dept. of Interior, U.S. Gov. Printing Office, Washington (1968)

396. U.S. Code of Federal Regulations 21CFR82.51 and 21CFR82.1051; Listing of certified provisionally listed colors and specifications; Lakes FD&C and D&C (2015)

397. Stevens, L., et al.; Amounts of artificial food dyes in foods and sweets commonly consumed by children; Clin. Pediatr.; Apr. 24; published online (2014)

398. Stevens, L., et al.; Amounts of artificial food colors in commonly consumed beverages and potential behavioral implications for consumption in children; Clin. Pediatr.; 53:133-140 (2014)

399. Gupta, R.K., et al.; Adjuvant properties of aluminum and calcium compounds; Pharm. Biotechnol.; 6:229-48 (1995)

400. He, Q, et al.; Calcium phosphate nanoparticle adjuvant; Clin. Diag. Lab. Immunology; Nov.; 7(6):899-903 (2000)

401. Petrovsky, N. and Aguilar, J.C.; Vaccine adjuvants: current state and future trends; Immunol. Cell Biol.; 82:488-496 (2004)

402. Flarend, R.E, et al.; In vivo absorption of aluminum-containing vaccine adjuvants using 26Al; Vaccine; Aug.-Sept.; 15(12-13):1314-8 (1997)

403. Dabeka, R., et al.; Lead, cadmium, and aluminum in Canadian infant formulae, oral electrolytes, and glucose solutions; Food Addit. Contam.; June; 28(6):744-53 (2011)

404. Kazi, T.G., et al.; Determination of toxic elements in infant formulae by using electrothermal atomic absorption spectrometer; Food Chem. Toxicol.; 47:1425-29 (2009)

405. Hawkins, N.M., et al.; Potential aluminum toxicity in infants fed special infant formula; J. Ped. Gastroenterol. Nutr.; 19:377-81 (1994)

406. Chuchu, N., et al.; The aluminum content of infant formulas remains too high; BMC Pediatrics; 13:162:1471-31 (2013)

407. Anane, R., et al.; Bioaccumulation of water soluble aluminum chloride in the hippocampus after transdermal uptake in mice; Arch. Toxicol.; 69(8):568-71 (1995)

408. Graves, A.B., et al.; The association between aluminum-containing products and Alzheimer's disease; J. Clin. Epidemiology; 43(1):35-44 (1990)

409. Wulff-Zottele, C., et al.; Sulphate fertilization ameliorates long-term aluminum toxicity symptoms in perennial ryegrass; Plant Physiol. Biochem.; Oct. 83:88-99 (2014)

410. Waldman, J.; Rust: The longest war; Simon & Schuster, Inc. (2014)

411. Verissimo, M.I.S., et al.; Aluminum migration into beverages: Are dented cans safe?; Sci. Tot. Environ.; Nov.; 405(1-3):385-88 (2008)

412. Seruga, M., et al.; Aluminum content of soft drinks from aluminum cans; Z. Lebensm. Unters. Forsch.; 198:313-16 (1994)

413. Seruga, M., et al.; Aluminum content of beers; Z. Lebensm. Unters. Forsch.; A 204:221-26 (1997)

414. Rondeau, V., et al.; Relation between aluminum concentrations in drinking water and Alzheimer's disease: an 8-year follow-up study; Am. J. Epidemiol. 152:59-66 (2000)

415. Exley, C., Esiri, M.M.; Severe cerebral congophilic angiopathy coincident with increased brain aluminum in a resident of Camelford, Cornwall, UK; J Neurosurg Psychiatry; 77:877-879 (2006)

416. Whittier, J.; The value of tap water: A comparison of bottled, filtered, and tap water using the MWRA as a case study; Environ. Management I Harvard Extension School; Dec. 19 (2007). Judith Whittier was employed as a chemist by the Massachusetts Water Resource Authority

417. Crouse, D.N., Unpublished research performed by the author (2016)

418. Al-Muhtaseb, S.A., El-Naas, M.H., Abdallah, S.; Removal of aluminum from aqueous solutions by adsorption on date-pit and BDH activated carbons; J. Hazardous Mat.; 158:300-7 (2008)

419. Ekstrom, T.; Leaching of Concrete; Lund Institute of Technology – Division of Building Materials (2001)

420. Berend, K., and Trouwborst; T.; Cement-mortar pipes as a source of aluminum; J. AWWA, (7)91:91-100 (1999)

421. Miller, R.G., et al.; The occurrence of aluminum in drinking water, J. Am. Water Works Assoc.; 78:84 (1984)

422. Lettermann, R.D. and Driscoll, C.T.; Survey of residual aluminum in filtered water; J. Am. Water Works Assoc.; 80:154 (1988)

423. Cech, I. and Montera, J.; Spatial variation in total aluminum concentrations in drinking water supplies; Water Res.; 34:2703 (2000)

424. Srinivasan, P.T., et al.; Aluminum in drinking water: an overview; Water SA; Jan.; 25(1):47-56 (1999)

425. Strekopytov, S., and Exley, C.; The formation, precipitation and structural characterization of hydroxyaluminosilicates formed in the presence of fluoride and phosphate; Polyhedron, 24:1585-92 (2005)

426. Taylor, G.A., et al.; Alzheimer's disease and the relationship between silicon and aluminum and water supplies in northern England; J. Epidemiology and Community Health; 49:323-28 (1995)

427. Schneider, C., et al.; The solubility of a hydroxyaluminosilicate; Polyhedron; 23:3185-91 (2004)

428. Dobrzynski, D.; Chemistry of neutral and alkaline waters with low Al3+ activity against hydroxyaluminosilicate HASB solubility. The evidence from ground and surface waters of the Sudetes Mtns.; Aquat. Geochem.; 13:197-210 (2007)

429. Srinivasan, P.T., et al.; Aluminum in drinking water: and overview; Water SA, 25:47 (1999)

430. Nogaro, G., et al.; Aluminum sulfate (alum) application interactions with coupled metal and nutrient cycling in a hypereutropic lake ecosystem; Environ. Pollution; May; 176:267-74 (2013)

431. Culp, R.L. and Stolenberg, H.A.; Fluoride reduction at La Crosse, Kan.; J. Am. Water Works Assoc.; 50:427 (1958)

432. Maier, F.J.; Defluoridation of municipal water supplies; J. Am. Water Works Assoc.; 45:874 (1953)

433. Ahemad, S.N. and Chaudhari, S.; Innovative method for domestic defluoridation of water; Proc. International Workshop on fluoride in drinking water – held in Bopal; p220 (2001)

434. http://www.cdc.gov/fluoridation/faqs/

435. Beltran-Aguilar, E.D., et al.; Prevalence and severity of dental fluorosis in the United States, 1999-2004; NCHS Data Brief, No. 93 (2010)

436. Griffin, S.O., et al.; Effectiveness of fluoride in preventing caries in adults, J. Dent. Res.; 86(5):410-415 (2007)

437. Marinho, V.C. et al.; Fluoride toothpastes for preventing dental caries in children and adolescents; Cochrane Database Syst. Rev.; 1:CD002278 (2003)

438. Marinho, V.C. et al.; Fluoride mouth rinses for preventing dental caries in children and adolescents; Cochrane Database Syst. Rev.; 3:CD002284 (2003)

439. Kandergan, K.; Groups stirring fluoride debate; Boston Globe; Jan 31, (2015)

440. Experiments performed at the Medical Research Endocrinology Dept., Newcastle upon Tyne, England, and the Physics Dept. of the Univ. of Ruhana, Sri Lanka, showed that fluoridated water at 1 ppm, when used in cooking in aluminum cookware, concentrated the aluminum up to 600 ppm, whereas water without fluoride did not. Science news 131:73 (1983)

441. Cottrell, von T. L.; The strengths of chemical bonds; Butterworths Publications Ltd.; London; 2 (1958). Table 4.11 Bond dissociation energies

442. McBride, W. J. et al.; Radiofluorination using aluminum-fluoride (Al18F); EJNMMI Res.; 3:36 1-12 (2013)

443. Varner, J. A., et al.; Chronic administration of aluminum-fluoride or sodium-fluoride to rats in drinking water – alterations in neuronal and cerebrovascular integrity; Brain Res.; 784:284-98 (1998)

444. Choi, A.L., et al.; Developmental fluoride neurotoxicity: A systematic review and meta-analysis; Environ. Health Perspectives; 120(10):1362-68 (2012)

445. Sun, M.M., et al.; Measurement of intelligence by drawing test among children in the endemic area of Al-F combined toxicosis (in Chinese); J. Guiyang Med. College; 16(3):204-6 (1991)

446. Proposed HHS recommendation for fluoride concentration in drinking water for prevention of dental caries; U.S. Dept. HHS; Fed. Reg. 76(9) Jan. 13 (2011)

447. Patten, J., et al.; Oral absorption of radioactive fluoride and iodide in rats; Arch. Oral Biol.; 23:215-17 (1978)

448. Neafsey, E.J., and Collins, M.A.; Moderate alcohol consumption and cognitive risk; Neuropsychiatric Disease and Treatment; 7:465-484 (2011)

449. Sripanyakorn, S., et al.; The silicon content of beer and its bioavailability in healthy volunteers; British J. Nutrition; 91:403-9 (2004)

450. James, B.R., et al.; An 8-hyrdroxyquinoline method for labile and total aluminum in soil extracts; Soil Sci. Soc. Am. J.; 47:893-97 (1983)

451. Jacqmin-Gadda, H., et al.; Components of drinking water and risk of cognitive impairment in the elderly; Epidemiol.; May; 7(3):281-5 (1996)

452. Jugdaohsingh, R., et al.; Oligomeric but not monomeric silica prevents aluminum absorption in humans; Am. J. Clin. Nutr.; 71:944 (2000)

453. Jugdaohsingh, R., et al.; High-aluminum-affinity silica is a nanoparticle that seeds secondary aluminosilicate formation; PLOS; Dec. 13, (2013)

454. Belles, M., et.al; Silicon reduces aluminum accumulation in rats – relevance to the aluminum hypothesis of Alzheimer disease; Alzheimer Dis. Assoc. Disord.; Jun; 12(2) 83-7 (1998)

455. Carlisle, E.M., and Curran, M.J.; Effect of dietary silicon and aluminum on silicon and aluminum levels in rat brain; Alzheimer Dis. Assoc. Disord.; 1(2):83-9 (1987)

456. Davenward, S., et al.; Silicon-rich mineral water as a non-invasive test of the 'aluminum hypothesis' in Alzheimer's disease; J. Alzheimer's Dis.; 33(2):423-30 (2013)

457. Brzezinski, M., et al.; Silica production and the contribution of diatoms to new and primary production in the central North Pacific, Mar. Ecol. Prog. Ser., 167;89-104 (1998)

458. Weigden, C.H. van der; Cahiers of Geochemistry – Silicon II: marine biogenic silica (2007)

459. http://www.worldlifeexpectancy.com/cause-of-death/alzheimers-dementia/by-country/

460. Kaasalainen, H., and Stefansson, A.; The chemistry of trace elements in surface geothermal waters and steam, Iceland; Chemical Geology; 330-331:60-85 (2012)

461. Jacqmin-Gadda, H., et al.; Components of drinking water and risk of cognitive impairment in the elderly; Am. J. Epidemiol.; 139:48-57 (1994)

462. Select committee on GRAS substances – SCOGS-61, NTIS Pb 301-402/AS (1979)

463. Iler, R.K.; Soluble silicates; ACS Symposium Series, 194(7):95-114 (1982)

464. Alexander, G.B.; The reaction of low molecular weight silicic acids with molybdic acid; J. Am. Chem. Soc.; 75:5655-57 (1975)

465. Taylor, P.D., et al.; Soluble silica with high affinity for aluminum under physiological and natural conditions; J. Am. Chem. Soc.; 119, 8852-56 (1997)

466. Kozisek, F.; Health risks from drinking demineralized water; National Institute of Public Health, Czech Republic; Chapter 12; Water, sanitation, and health protection and the human environment; W.H.O.; Geneva (2005)

467. Demadis, K., et al.; Catalytic effect of magnesium ions on silicic acid polycondensation and inhibition strategies based on chelation; Industrial Eng. Chem. Research; 51:9032-40 (2012)

468. Sheikholeslami, R., et al.; Desalination and the environment water shortage – Pretreatment and the effect of cations and anions on prevention of silica fouling; Desalination; Sept.; 139(1-3):83-95 (2001)

469. Sripanyakorn, S., et al.; The comparative absorption of silicon from different foods and food supplements; Br. J. Nutr.; Sept.; 102(6):825-34 (2009)

470. Jurkic, L.M., et al.; Biological and therapeutic effects of ortho-silicic acid and some ortho-silicic acid-releasing compounds: New perspectives for therapy; Nutrition & Metabolism; 10:2 (2013)

471. Richman, E.L., et al.; Choline intake and risk of lethal prostate cancer: incidence and survival; Am. J. Clin. Nutr.; 96:855-63 (2012)

472. Aguilar, F., et al.; Calcium silicate and silicon dioxide/silica acid gel added for nutritional purposes to food supplements; EFSA J.; 1132:1-24 (2009)

473. Aguilar, F., et al.; Choline-stabilized orthosilicic acid added for nutritional purposes to food supplements; EFSA J.; 948:1-23 (2009)

474. Fede, C., et al.; The toxicity outcomes of silica nanoparticles (Ludox) is influenced by testing techniques and treatment modalities; Anal. Bioanal. Chem.; 404:1789-1802 (2012)

475. Drueke, T.D.; Intestinal absorption of aluminum in renal failure; Nephrol. Dial. Transplant; 17[Suppl. 2]:13-16 (2002)

476. Rusanen, M.; Smoking, pulmonary and heart diseases and the risk of cognitive impairment and dementia: an epidemiological approach; Dissertations in Health Sci; 152 (2013)

477. Newhouse, P., et al.; Nicotine treatment of mild cognitive impairment; Neurology J; 78:91-101 (2012)

478. http://en.wikipeida.org/wiki/Nicotine

479. Report Brief – Ending the tobacco problem: a blueprint for the nation; Inst. Med.; May (2007)

480. Exley, C., et al.; Aluminum in tobacco and cannabis and smoking-related disease; Am. J. Med.; 118:276 (2006)

481. Dean, K., et al.; Sustainability of Brita Filters; Sustainability Science Group Project, Univ. Vermont; Dec. 6, (2010)

482. Verd Vallespir, S., et al.; Association between calcium content of drinking water and fractures in children; An. Esp. Pediatr.; Dec.; 37(6):461-5 (1992)

483. Jugdaohsingh, R.; Silicon and bone health; J. Nutr. Health Aging; 11(2):99-110 (2007)

484. Jugdaohsingh, R., et al.; Dietary silicon is positively associated with bone mineral density in men and premenopausal women; J. Bone Mineral Res.; 19(2): 297-307 (2004)

485. Reffitt, D.M., et al.; Orthosilicic acid stimulates collagen type 1 synthesis and osteoblastic differentiation in human osteoblast-like cells in vitro; Bone; Feb.; 32(2):127-135 (2003)

486. Van Dyck, K., et al.; Indications of silicon essentiality in humans – Serum concentrations in Belgian children and adults, including pregnant women; Biological Trace Element Res.; 77:25-32 (2000)

487. Tanaka, T., et al.; Silicon concentrations in maternal serum and breastmilk in the postpartum period; Nihon Eiseigaku Zasshi; Oct.; 45(4):919-25 (1990)

488. Kaufmann, K.; Silica: The Forgotten Nutrient; Alive Books (1993)

489. Jugdaohsingh, R., et al.; Dietary silicon intake and absorption; Am. J. Clin. Nutr.; 75(5):887-93 (2002)

490. Dietzel, M.; Dissolution of silicates and the stability of polysilicic acid; Geochimica et Cosmochimica Acta; 64(19):3275-81 (2000)

491. European Food Safety Authority; EFSA J.; 950:1-12 (2009)

492. DeFina, L. F., et al.; The association between midlife cardiorespiratory fitness levels and later-life dementia – A cohort study; Ann. Intern. Med.; 158(3):162-68 (2013)

493. Martins, C., et. al; Effects of exercise on gut peptides, energy intake, and appetite; J. Endocrin.; 193:251-58 (2007)

494. Berg, B.M., et. al; Peptide YY administration decreases brain aluminum in the Ts65Dn Down Syndrome mouse model; Growth, Development, Aging (GDA); 64(1-2):3-19 (2000)

495. Broom, D.R., et. al; Influence of resistance and aerobic exercise on hunger, circulating levels of acylated ghrelin, and peptide YY in healthy males; Am. J. Physiol. Regul. Integr. Comp. Physiol.; 296:R29-35 (2009)

496. Jones, T.E., et al.; Long-term exercise training in overweight adolescents improves plasma peptide YY and resistin; Obesity; 17(6):1189-95 (2009)

497. Martins, C., et. al; The effects of exercise-induced weight loss on appetite-related peptides and motivation to eat; J. Clin. Endocrinol. Metab.; 95:1609-16 (2010)

498. Batterham, R., et al.; Critical role of peptide YY in protein-mediated satiation and body-weight regulation; Cell Metabolism; Sept., 4:223-33 (2006)

499. Batterham, R., et al.; Inhibition of food intake in obese subjects by peptide YY3-36; New England J. Med.; Sept., 349(10):941- (2003)

500. Stokes, K.; Growth hormone responses to sub-maximal and sprint exercise; Growth Hormone IGF Res.; 13:225-38 (2003)

501. Ribeiro, L., et al.; Impact of acute exercise intensity on plasma concentrations of insulin, growth hormone, and somatostatin; Acta Med. Port.; May-Jul.; 17(3):199-204 (2004)

502. Wideman, L., et al.; Synergy of l-arginine and GHRP-2 stimulation of growth hormone in men and women – modulation by exercise; Am. J. Physiol.; 279(4):R1467-77 (2000)

503. Maesako, M., et al.; Continuation of exercise is necessary to inhibit high fat diet-induced B-amyloid deposition and memory deficit in amyloid precursor protein transgenic mice; PLOS one; 8(9)1-10 (2013)

504. Rosser, M. N., et al.; Reduced amounts of immunoreactive somatostatin in the temporal cortex in senile dementia of Alzheimer type; Neurosci. Let.; 20(3):373-77 (1980)

505. Arnsten, A.F.T.; Stress signaling pathways that impair prefrontal cortex structure and function; Nat. Rev. Neurosci.; 32:267-87 (2009)

506. Resveratrol, a popular supplement for improved mitochondrial and cardiac function, inhibits PDE4A allowing the concentration of cAMP to rise and for this reason it can't be recommended[664].

507. Wang, M., et al.; Neuronal basis of age-related working memory decline; Nature; Jul.; 476(7359):210-3 (2011)

508. Bracken, R. M., et al.; Plasma catecholamine and norepinephrine responses to brief intermittent maximal intensity exercise; Amino Acids; 36:209-217 (2009)

509. Trapp, E. G., et al.; Metabolic response of trained and untrained women during high-intensity intermittent cycle exercise; Am. J. Physiol. Regul. Integr. Comp. Physiol.; 293:R2370-75 (2007)

510. Silverman, H G. and Mazzeo, R. S.; Hormonal responses to maximal and submaximal exercise in trained and untrained men of various ages; J. Gerontology; Biol. Sci.; 51A(1):B30-B37 (1996)

511. Bondareff, W., et al.; Loss of neurons of origin of the adrenergic projection to cerebral cortex (nucleus locus ceruleus) in senile dementia; Neurology; Feb.; 32(2):164-8 (1982)

512. Michalski, B., et al.; Brain-derived neurotropic factor and TrkB expression in the "oldest-old", the 90+ study: correlation with cognitive status and levels of soluble amyloid-beta; Neurobiology of aging; (2015)

513. Erickson, P.S., et al.; Neurogenesis in the adult human hippocampus; Nature; 4(11):1313-17 (1998)

514. Erickson, K. I., Exercise training increases size of hippocampus and improves memory; PNAS; 108(7):3017-22 (2011)

515. Minshal, C., Nadel, J., Exley, C.; Aluminum in human sweat; J. Trace Elem. Med. Biol.; 28: 87-88 (2014)

516. Exley, C.; Aluminum toxicity: a major threat to brain health; Alzheimer's and Dementia Summit; Hosted by J. Landsman; July 31 (2016)

517. Xie, L., et al.; Sleep drives metabolite clearance from the adult brain; Science; Oct.; 342(6156) (2013)

518. Olmo, N.D., et al.; Taurine-induced synaptic potentiation and the late phase of long-term potentiation are related mechanistically; Neuropharmacology; 44(1):26-39 (2003)

519. Pizzorusso, T., et al.; Brain-derived neurotrophic factor causes cAMP response element-binding protein phosphorylation in absence of calcium increases in slices and cultured neurons from rat visual cortex; J. Neuroscience; 20(8):2809-18 (2000)

520. Luo, J., et al.; Increases in cAMP, MAPK activity, and CREB phosphorylation during REM sleep – Implications for REM sleep and memory consolidation; J. Neuroscience; 33(15):6460-68 (2013)

521. Liguori, C., et al.; Orexinergic system dysregulation, sleep impairment, and cognitive decline in Alzheimer disease; JAMA Neurol.; Oct. (2014)

522. Drago, D., et al.; Potential pathogenic role of β-amyloid$_{1-42}$-aluminum complex in Alzheimer's disease; Int. J. Biochem. & Cell Biol.; 40:731-46 (2008)

523. More, S.S., et al.; Early detection of amyloidopathy in Alzheimer's mice by hyperspectral endoscopy; Invest. Ophthalmol. Vis. Sci.; 57:3231-38 (2016)

524. LaMorgia, C., et al.; Melanopsin retinal ganglion cell loss in Alzheimer's disease; Ann. Neurol.; 79:90-109 (2016)

525. Figueiro, M. G., et al.; Tailored lighting intervention improves measures of sleep, depression, and agitation in persons with Alzheimer's disease and related dementia living in long-term care facilities; Clin. Interventions Aging; 9:1527-1537 (2014)

526. Leng, Y., et al.; Sleep duration and risk of fatal and nonfatal stroke; Neurology; 84:1-8 (2015)

527. Abe, T., et al.; Sleep duration is significantly associated with carotid artery atherosclerosis incidence in a Japanese population; Atherosclerosis; 217:509-13 (2011)

528. Khawaja, O., et al.; Sleep duration and risk of atrial-fibrillation (from the Physician's Health Study); Am. J. Cardiol.; 111:547-551 (2013)

529. Gardner, R. C., et al.; Dementia risk after traumatic brain injury vs nonbrain trauma – The role of age and severity; JAMA Neurol.; Oct.; (2014)

530. McKee, A. C.; et al.; The spectrum of disease in chronic traumatic encephalopathy; Brain; 1-22 (2012)

531. Gillette-Guyonnet, S., et al.; Cognitive impairment and composition of drinking water in women: findings of the EPIDOS study; Am. J. Clin. Nutr.; 81:897-902 (2005)

532. Domingo, J.L., et al.; Citric, malic and succinic acids as possible alternatives to desferoxamine in aluminum toxicity; J. Toxicol. Clin. Toxicol.; 26(1-2):67-79 (1988)

533. Domingo J.L., et al.; Comparative effects of several chelating agents on the toxicity, distribution and excretion of aluminum; Hum. Toxicol.; May; 7(3):259-62 (1988)

534. Llobet, J.M., et al.; Acute toxicity studies of aluminum compounds: antidotal efficacy of several chelating agents; Pharmacol. Toxicol.; Apr.; 60(4):280-3 (1987)

535. Penniston, M.D., et al.; Quantitative assessment of citric acid in lemon juice, lime juice, and commercially-available fruit juice products; J. Endourol.; Mar.; 22(3);567-70 (2008)

536. Bredesen, D.E.; Reversal of cognitive decline: A novel therapeutic program; Aging; 6(9):707-17 (2014)

537. Wang, J. M., et al.; Allopregnanolone reverses neurogenic and cognitive deficits in mouse model of Alzheimers disease; PNAS; 107(14):6498-6503 (2010)

538. Irwin, R. W., et al.; Neuroregenerative mechanisms of allopregnanolone in Alzheimer's disease; Frontiers Endocrin.; 2:117:1-14 (2012)

539. Marx, C., et al.; The neurosteroid allopregnanolone is reduced in prefrontal cortex in Alzheimer's disease" Biol Psychiatry; 60(12):1287-94 (2006)

540. http://en.wikipedia.org/wiki/Cholinergic

541. Poly, C., et al.; The relation of dietary choline to cognitive performance and white matter hyper-intensity in the Framingham offspring cohort; Am J Clin Nutr; 94:1585-91 (2011)

542. Knobel, M.; Approach to a combined pharmacologic therapy of childhood hyperkinesis; Behav. Neuropsychiatry; Mar. 6(1-12):87-90 (1974)

543. http://en.wikipedia.org/wiki/Meclofenoxate

544. http://en.wikipedia.org/wiki/Galantamine

545. Masters, C. L., and Beyreuther, K.; Alzheimer's centennial legacy: prospects for rational therapeutic intervention targeting the Aβ amyloid pathway; Brain, 129:2823-39 (2006)

546. Bramble, D.M., and Jenkins, F.A.; Mammalian locomotor-respiratory integration; Science, 262, 235-40 (1993)

547. Bramble, D.M., and Lieberman, D.L.; Endurance running and the evolution of Homo; Nature, 432, 345-52 (2004)

548. Carrier, D.R.; The energetic paradox of human running and hominid evolution; Current Anthropology, 25:483-95 (1984)

549. Cordain, L., et al.; The paradoxical nature of hunter-gatherer diets: meat-based, yet non-atherogenic; European J. Clin. Nutrition; 56(Suppl. 1):S42-S52 (2002)

550. Staller, J.E. and Carrasco, M.; Pre-Columbian foodways: Interdisciplinary approaches to food, culture, and markets in ancient Mesoamerica; Berlin, Springer-Verlag p317 (2009)

551. http://www.poweredbyosteons.org/2012/01/lead-poisoning-in-rome-skeletal.html

552. Kientz, M.A. and Dunn, W.; A comparison of the performance of children with and without autism on the sensory profile; Am. J. Occupational Therapy; 51:530-37 (1997)

553. Carper, R.A., et al.; Cerebral lobes in autism: early hyperplasia and abnormal effects; Neuroimage; Aug.; 16(4):1038-61 (2002)

554. Courchesne, E. and Pierce, K.; Why the frontal cortex in autism might be talking only to itself: local over-connectivity but long-distance disconnection; Curr. Opin. Neurobiol.; Apr.; 15(2):225-30 (2005)

555. Hernandez, R.N., et al.; Autism spectrum disorder in fragile X syndrome: a longitudinal evaluation; Am. J. Med. Genetics; Part A 149A:1125-37 (2009)

556. Baron-Cohen, S.; The facts: autism and Asperger syndrome; Oxford University Press, N.Y. (2008)

557. Lee, R.B.; What hunters do for a living, or how to make out on scarce resources; In Lee, R.B., DeVore, I., eds. Man the hunter. Chicago: Aldine Publishing Co., 30-48 (1968)

558. Mitani, N. and Ma, J.F.; Uptake of silicon in different plant species; J. Exp. Botany; 56(414):1255-1261 (2005)

559. Luxwolda, M.F.; Traditionally living populations in East Africa have a mean serum 25-hydoxyvitamin D concentration of 115 nmol/l; Br. J. Nutr.; 108(9):1157-61 (2012)

560. Luxwolda, M.F., et al.; Vitamin D status indicators in indigenous populations in East Africa; Eur. J. Nutr.; 52(3):1115-25 (2013)

561. Harvey, E.L. and Fuller, D.Q.; Investigating crop processing using phytolith analysis: the example of rice and millets; J. Archaeological Sci.; 32:739-752 (2005)

562. Milton, K.; Hunter-gatherer diets – a different perspective; Am. J. Clin. Nutr.; 71:665-7 (2000)

563. CDC – Breastfeeding among U.S. children born 2001-2011, CDC national immunization survey (2011)

564. Mothers Survey, Ross Products Division, Abbott Laboratories (2002)

565. Gilbert-Barness, E., et al.; Aluminum toxicity; Arch Pediatr. Adolesc. Med.; 152:511-512 (1998)

566. Sorenson, J.R.J., et al.; Aluminum in the environment and human health; Environ. Health Perspectives; 8:3-95 (1974) - See top of page 44 and page 49 in this paper

567. Kobayashi, K., et al.; 26Al tracer experiment by accelerator mass spectrometry and its application to the studies of amyotrophic lateral sclerosis and Alzheimer's disease; Proc. Japan Acad.; 66 Ser. B, 189-192 (1990)

568. D'Eufemia, P., et al.; Abnormal intestinal permeability in children with autism; Acta Paediatr.; Sep.; 85(9):1079-9 (1996)

569. Blaurock-Busch, E., et al.; Toxic metals and essential elements in hair and severity of symptoms among children with autism; Maedica, J. Clin. Med.; 7(1):30-48 (2012)

570. Mohamed, F.E.B., et al.; Assessment of hair aluminum, lead, and mercury in a sample of autistic Egyptian children: Environmental risk factors of heavy metals in autism; Behavioral Neurology; Article ID 545674:1-9 (2015)

571. Mold, M., et al.; Aluminum in Brain Tissue in Autism; J. Trace Elements in Med. Biol.; Accepted Manuscript p1-23 (2017)

572. McCaddon, A., et al.; Total serum homocysteine in senile dementia of the Alzheimer type; Int. J. Geriaty. Psychiatry; Apr.; 13(4):235-9 (1998)

573. Gottfries, C.G., et al.; Early diagnosis of cognitive impairment in the elderly with the focus on Alzheimer's disease; J. Neural Transm.; 105(8-9):773-86 (1998)

574. Clarke R., et al.; Folate, vitamin B12, and serum total homocysteine levels in confirmed Alzheimer disease, Arch. Neurol.; Nov.; 55(11):1449-55 (1998)

575. Ghanizadeh, A.; Increased glutamate and homocysteine and decreased glutamine levels in autism: A review and strategies for future studies of amino acids in autism; 35(5):281-86 (2013)

576. Morrison, L.D., et al.; Brain s-adenosylmethionine levels are severely decreased in Alzheimer's disease; J. Neurochem.; Sept.; 67(3):1328-31 (1996)

577. James, S.J., et al.; Metabolic biomarkers of increased oxidative stress and impaired methylation capacity in children with autism; Am. J. Clin. Nutr.; 80:1611-7 (2004)

578. Ansari, M.A. and Scheff, S.W.; Oxidative stress in the progression of Alzheimer disease in the frontal cortex; J. Neuropathol. Exp. Neurol.; Feb.; 69(2):155-167 (2010)

579. Tu, W.-J., et al.; Application of LC-MS/MS analysis of plasma amino acid profiles in children with autism; J. Clin. Biochem. Nutr.; Nov.; 51(3):248-249 (2012)

580. Ali, A., et al.; Hyperhomocysteinemia among Omani autistic children: a case-control study; Acta Biochemica Polonica; 58(4):547-551 (2011)

581. Pasca, S.P., et al.; High levels of homocysteine and low serum paraoxonase-1-arylesterase activity in children with autism; Life Sci.; Apr.; 78(19):2244-48 (2006)

582. Ghanizadeh, A.; Increased glutamate and homocysteine and decreased glutamine levels in autism: A review and strategies for future studies of amino acids in autism; Disease Markers; 35(5):281-86 (2013)

583. Rossignol, D.A., and Frye, R.E.; Mitochondrial dysfunction in autism spectrum disorders a systematic review and meta-analysis; Mol. Psychiatry; 17:290-314 (2012)

584. Swegert, C.V., et al.; Effect of aluminum-induced Alzheimer like condition on oxidative energy metabolism in rat liver, brain, and heart mitochondria; Mech. Ageing Dev.; Dec.; 112(1):27-42 (1999)

585. Robertson, C.E., et al.; Reduced GABAergic action in the autistic brain; Current Biology; 26:80-5 (2016)

586. Bogdashina, O.; Sensory perceptual issues in autism and Asperger Syndrome – Different sensory experiences – different perceptual worlds; Jessica Kingsley Publishers; London (2003)

587. Trombley, P.Q.; Selective modulation of GABAA receptors by aluminum; Am. Physiol. Soc.; 80:755-761 (1998)

588. Galanopoulou, A.S.; Dissociated gender-specific effects of recurrent seizures on GABAA signaling in CA1 pyramidal neurons: Role of GABAA receptors; J. Neurosci.; Feb.; 28(7):1557-67 (2008)

589. CDC, Morbidity and mortality weekly report, Prevalence of autism spectrum disorders – Autism and developmental disabilities monitoring network, 14 sites, United States (2008)

590. Hertz-Picciotto, I, and Delwiche, L.; The rise of autism rate and the role of age at diagnosis; Epidemiology; 20(1):84-90 (2009)

591. Fomon, S.J.; Infant feeding in the 20th century: formula and beikost; Am. Soc. Nutri. Sci.; J. Nutr. 131:409S-420S (2001)

592. Shurtleff, W., and Aoyagi, A.; History of Soymilk and other non-dairymilks; (2013)

593. Schultz, S., et al.; Breastfeeding, infant formula supplementation, and autistic disorder – the results of a parent survey; Internat. Breastfeeding J.; I:16:1-7 (2006)

594. Al-Farsi, Y.M.; et. al.; Effect of suboptimal breast-feeding on occurrence of autism: a case-control study; Nutrition; Jul.; 28(7-8):e27-32 (2012)

595. Shafai, T., et al.; The association of early weaning and formula feeding with autism spectrum disorders; Breastfeeding Medicine; 9(5):275-6 (2014)

596. Tanoue, Y., and Oda, S.; Weaning time of children with infantile autism; J. Autism dev. Disord.; Sep; 19(3):425-34 (1989)

597. Baxter, M.J., et al.; Aluminum levels in milk and infant formulae; Food Addit. Contam.; Sept-Oct.; 8(5):653-60 (1991)

598. CDC; Morbidity and Mortality Weekly Report – Surveillance Summaries; 63(2) March 28 (2014)

599. Saemundsen, E., et al.; Prevalence of autism spectrum disorders in an Icelandic birth cohort; DMJ Open; Jun. 20; 3(6) (2013)

600. Neik, T.T., et al.; Prevalence, diagnosis, treatment and research on autism spectrum disorders (ASD) in Singapore and Malyasia; International J. Spec. Ed.; 26(3):1-10 (2014)

601. Bernard-Opitz, V., et al.; Epidemiology of autism in Singapore: findings of the first autism survey; Internat. J. Rehab. Research; 24:1-6 (2001)

602. Cheslack-Postava, K., et al.; Increased risk of autism spectrum disorders at short and long interpregnancy intervals in Finland; J. Am. Acad. Adolescent Psyc.; 53(10):1074-81.e4 (2014)

603. Mostsafa, G.A., and Al-Ayadhi, L.Y.; Reduced serum concentrations of 25-hydroxy vitamin D in children with autism: Relation to autoimmunity; J. Neuroinflammation; 17(9):201 (2012)

604. Ginde, A.A., et al.; Demographic differences and trends of vitamin D insufficiency in the US population; 1988-2004; Arch. Intern. Med.; 169(6):626-32 (2009)

605. Skaaby, W.B., et al.; Prospective population-based study of the association between serum 25-hydroxyvitamin-D levels and the incidence of specific types of cancer; Cancer Epidemiol. Biomarkers Prev.; 23:1220-29 (2014)

606. Grant, W.B.; Why the prospective population-based study in Denmark did not find an association of 25-hydroxyvitamin D levels with cancer incidence rates; CEBP EPI-14-0530 (2014)

607. Code of Federal Regulations 21CFR107.100; Nutrient specifications; April (2015)

608. Hershberg, R.; et al.; Organ distribution of aluminum in uremic rats: influence of parathyroid hormone and 1,25-dihydroxyvitamin D3; Miner Electrolyte Metab.; 11:106-110 (1985)

609. Mayor, G.H., et al.; Impaired renal function and aluminum metabolism; Fed. Proc.; Oct.; 42(13):297-83 (1983)

610. Burnatowska-Hledin, M.A., et al.; Aluminum, parathyroid hormone, and osteomalacia; Spec. Top. Endocrinol. Metab.; 5:201-26 (1983)

611. Klein, G.L., et al.; Serum levels of 1,25-dihyroxyvitamin D in children receiving parenteral nutrition with reduced aluminum content; J. Pediatr. Gastroenterol. Nutr.; Feb.; 4(1):93-6 (1985)

612. Stanhill, G. and Cohen, S.; Global dimming; a review of the evidence for a widespread and significant reduction in global radiation with discussion of its probable causes and possible agricultural consequences; Agric. For. Meteorol.; (4)107:255-78 (2001)

613. Brody, R.; What's new in sun-care products; A tanless society by the year 2000; NY Times Business Day, July 24, (1988)

614. Notes on U.S. sun-care market for the year 2000; Soap and Cosmetics; April 76(4):44 (2000)

615. Notes on major brands of sunscreens and sunblocks for the year 2002; Chain Drug Review; June; 24(11):256 (2002)

616. Thomas, L. and Lim, H.W.; Focus on: sunscreens; J. Drugs Dermatology; 2:174 (2003)

617. Blencowe, H., et al.; National, regional, and worldwide estimates of preterm birth rates in the year 2010 with time trends since 1990 for selected countries: a systematic analysis and implications; Lancet; 379:2162-72 (2012)

618. Kunzniewicz, M.W., et al.; Prevalence and neonatal factors associated with autism spectrum disorders in preterm infants; J. Pediatrics; 164(1):20-25 (2014)

619. Sviridov, N.K.; Aluminum in human pathology; Lab. Delo. 12:699 (1966)

620. Unanyan, G.S.; Levels of copper, manganese, silicon, aluminum, and magnesium in the colostrum, intermediate and mature milk of mothers, and in mature and premature babies; Zh. Eksp. Klin. Med.; 7(6):96 (1967); Chem. Abstr. 69:34003 (1968)

621. Unanyan, G.S.; Characteristics of the level of the trace elements copper, manganese, silicon, aluminum, and magnesium in the blood of premature babies and in their mothers' milk; Zh. Eksp. Klin. Med.; 9(1):38 (1969)

622. Grebennikov, E.P.; Content of copper, silicon, aluminum, titanium, and magnesium in the blood of newborns; Pediatriya (Moscow) 38(10):29 (1960)

623. U.S. Code of Federal Regulations, 21CFR201.323 Aluminum in large and small volume parenterals used in total parenteral nutrition (2014)

624. Taylor, L., et al.; Vaccines are not associated with autism – An evidence-based meta-analysis of case-control and cohort studies; Vaccine; 32(29):3623-29 (2014)

625. U.S. Code of Federal Regulations; 21CFR610.15; Part 610 – General biological products standards; Subpart B – General provisions; Sec. 610.15 Constituent material.

626. CDC Pinkbook of excipients in vaccines: http://www.cdc.gov/vaccines/pubs/pinkbook/downloads/appendices/B/excipient-table-2.pdf

627. Kieth, L.S., et al.; Aluminum toxicokinetics regarding infant diet and vaccinations; Vaccine; May; 20 Suppl. 3:S13-7 (2002)

628. Redhead, K., et al.; Aluminum-adjuvated vaccines transiently increase aluminum levels in murine brain tissue; Pharmacol. Toxicol.; Apr.; 70(4):278-80 (1992)

629. Mitkus, R.J., et al.; Updated aluminum pharmacokinetics following infant exposures through diet and vaccination; Vaccine; Nov.; 29(51):9538-43 (2011)

630. Hem, S.L.; Elimination of aluminum adjuvants; Vaccine; May; 20 Suppl. 3:S40-3 (2002)

631. MRL's, U.S. Dept. Health Human Serv., Agency for toxic substances and disease registry (2013)

632. Delong, G.; A positive association found between autism prevalence and childhood vaccination uptake across the U.S. population; J. Toxicol. Environ. Health A; 74(14):903-16 (2011)

633. Tomljenovic, L., and Shaw, C.A.; Do aluminum vaccine adjuvants contribute to the rising prevalence of autism?; J. Inorg. Biochem.; 105:1489-99 (2011)

634. Avishi-Eliner – Stressed-out or in (utero)?; Trends Neurosci.; 25(10):518-24 (2002)

635. Rhawn, J.; Neuropsychiatry, Neuropsychology, and Clinical Neuroscience; third ed. Lippincott Williams & Wilkins; (1996) http://brainmind.com/EmotionalBrainDevelopment4.html

636. http://en.wikipedia.org/wiki/Dementia_with_Lewy_bodies

637. Kramer, M.L., Schulz-Schaeffer; Presynaptic synuclein aggregates, not Lewy bodies, cause neurodegeneration in dementia with Lewy bodies; J. Neuroscience, Feb. 27(6):1405(2007)

638. Fearnley, J.M. and Lees, A.J.; Ageing and Parkinson's disease: substantia nigra regional selectivity; Brain; 114:2283-301 (1991)

639. Good, P.F., et al.; Neuromelanin-containing neurons of the substantia nigra accumulate iron and aluminum in Parkinson's disease. A LAMMA study; Brain Res.; 593:343-6 (1992)

640. Jenner, P., et al.; Oxidative stress as a cause of nigral cell death in Parkinson's disease and incidental Lewy body disease; Ann. Neurol.; 32:882-7 (1992)

641. Costello, S., et al.; Parkinson's disease and residential exposure to Maneb and Paraquat from agricultural applications in the central valley of California; Am. J. Epidemiol.; 169(8):919-26 (2009)

642. Tanner, C. M., et al.; Rotenone, Paraquat, and Parkinson's disease; Environ. Health Perspect.; 119:866-72 (2011)

643. Crane, P.K.; et al.; Association of traumatic brain injury with late-life neurodegenerative conditions and neuropathological findings; JAMA Neurol.; Sept.; 73(9):1062-1069 (2016)

644. Tsigelny, I.F., et al.; Dynamics of alpha-synuclein aggregation and inhibition of pore-like oligomer development by beta-synuclein; FEBS J., Apr., 274(7):1862-77 (2007)

645. Dina, M., Farhang, A.; The inhibitory effects of cumin aldehyde on amyloid fibrillation and cytotoxicity of alpha-synuclein; Modares J of Med Sci (Pathobiology); Spring; 15(1):60-45 (2012)

646. Zhang, L., et. al; Reduced plasma taurine level in Parkinson's disease; association with motor severity and levodopa treatment; Int. J. Neurosci.; May 23:1-24 (2015).

647. Engelborghs, S., et. al; Amino acids and biogenic amines in cerebrospinal fluid of patients with .Parkinson's disease; Neurochem. Res.; Aug., 28(8):1145-50 (2003)

648. Thakur, N., et al.; COPD and cognitive impairment: the role of hypoxemia and oxygen therapy; Int. J. Chronic Obstructive Pulmonary Dis.; 5:263-9 (2010)

649. Li, J. and Fei, G.H.; The unique alterations of hippocampus and cognitive impairment in chronic obstructive pulmonary disease; Respir. Res.; 14:140 (2013)

650. Zhang, H., et al.; Reduced regional gray matter volume in patients with chronic obstructive pulmonary disease – a voxel-based morphometry study; Am. J. Neuroradiol.; 34:334-9 (2013)

651. Albrecht, J.; Role of ammonia in the pathogenesis of hepatic encephalopathy; Hepatic Encephalopathy, Mullen, K.D., Prakash, R.K. (Eds.), Springer, Chapter 2, p7-17 (2012)

652. Yaffe, K., et al.; Association between hypoglycemia and dementia in a biracial cohort of older adults with diabetes mellitus; JAMA Intern. Med., 173(14):1300-06 (2013)

653. Fraser, W.D.; Hyperparathyroidism; Jul.; 374(9684):145-58 (2009)

654. http://en.wikipedia.org/wiki/Hyperparathyroidism

655. Seccareccia, D.; Cancer-related hypercalcaemia; Canadian Family Physician, March, 56:244-46 (2010)

656. Cann, C.E., et al.; Aluminum uptake by the parathyroid glands; J. Clin. Endocrin Metab.; 49:543-45 (1979)

657. Diaz-Corte, C., et al.; Effect of aluminum load on parathyroid hormone synthesis; Nephrol. Dial. Transplant; 16:742-45 (2001)

658. Desouza, L.A., et al.; Thyroid hormone regulates hippocampal neurogenesis in the adult rat brain; Mol. Cell. Neurosci.; 29, 414-26 (2005)

659. Kumar, N., Kar, A.; Pyrroloquinoline quinone has the potential to ameliorate PTU induced lipid peroxidation and oxidative damage in mice; Int. J. Pharm. Pharmaceutical Sci.; 6(2):880-885 (2014)

660. Ambrogini, P., et al.; Thyroid hormones affect neurogenesis in the dentate gyrus of adult rat; Neuroendocinolgy; 81(4):244-53 (2005)

661. Sommer, W.; Erkrankung des Ammon's horn als aetiologis ches moment der epilepsien; Arch. Psychiatr. Nurs.; 10:631-75 (1880)

662. Nelson, P.T., et al.; Alzheimer's disease is not "brain aging": neuropathological, genetic, and epidemiological human studies; Acta Neuropathol.; May 121(5):571-87 (2011)

663. Giasson, B.I., et al.; Parkinson's disease, dementia with Lewy bodies, multiple system atrophy and the spectrum of diseases with alpha synuclein inclusions; The neuropathology of dementia; 2nd Editon; Cambridge University Press; 353-7 (2004)

664. Park, S.-J., et al.; Resveratrol ameliorates ageing-related metabolic phenotypes by inhibiting cAMP phosphodiesterases; Cell; 148(3):421-433 (2012)

665. Vitvitsky, V., et al.; A functional transsulfuration pathway in the brain links to glutathione homeostasis; J. Biolog. Chem. 281(47) 35785-93 (2006)

666. Tallen, H.H., et al.; L-Cystathionine in human brain; J. Biol. Chem.; 230:707-16 (1958)

667. Finkelstein, J.D.; Methionine metabolism in mammals; J. Nutr. Biochem.; May, 1:228 (1990)

668. Banks, W.A., and Kastin, A.J.; Aluminum alters the permeability of the blood-brain barrier to some non-peptides; Neuropharmacology; may; 24(5):407-12 (1985)

669. Kaya, M., et al.; Effect of aluminum on the blood-brain barrier permeability during nitric oxide-blockade-induced chronic hypertension in rats; Biol. Trace Elem. Res.; Jun.; 92(3):221-30 (2003)

670. Song, Y., et al.; Effects of acute exposure to aluminum on blood-brain barrier and the protection of zinc; Neurosci. Lett.; Nov.; 445(1):42-6 (2008)

671. Chadobski, A., et al.; Blood-brain barrier pathophysiology in traumatic brain injury; Transl. Stroke Res.; Dec.; 2(4):492-516 (2011)

672. Price, L., et al.; Chapter 4 Blood-brain barrier pathophysiology following traumatic brain injury; Translational research in traumatic brain injury; Laskowitz, D., and Grant, G. Editors; Boca Raton, FL, CRC Press/Taylor and Francis Group (2016)

673. Mooradian, A.D.; Effect of aging on the blood-brain barrier; Neurobiology of Aging; 9:31-9 (1988)

674. Farrall, A.J. and Wardlaw, J.M.; Blood-brain barrier: ageing and microvascular disease - - systematic review and meta-analysis; Neurobiol. Aging; Mar.; 30(3):337-52 (2009)

675. Kortekaas, R., et al.; Blood-brain barrier dysfunction in parkinsonian midbrain in vivo; Ann. Neurol.; 57:176-9 (2005)

676. Gray, M.T. and Woulf, J.M.; Striatal blood-brain barrier permeability in Parkinson's disease; J. Cerebral Blood Flow and Metab.; 35:747-50 (2015)

677. Agarwal, R., and Shukla, G.S.; Potential role of cerebral glutathione in the maintenance of blood-brain barrier integrity in rat; Neurochem. Res.; Dec.; 24(12):1507-14 (1999)

678. Exley, C.; Hydroxyaluminosilicate formation in solutions of low total aluminum concentration; Polyhedron; 11(15):1901-7 (1992)

679. Hosokawa, S., et al.; Trace elements and complications in patients undergoing chronic hemodialysis; Nephron.; 55(4):375-9 (1990)

680. Roberts, N.B., and Williams, P.; Silicon measurements in serum and urine by direct current plasma emission spectrometry; Clin. Chem.; 36(8):1480-85 (1990)

681. D'Haese, P.C., et al.; Increased silicon levels in dialysis patients due to high silicon content in drinking water, inadequate water treatment procedures, and concentrate contamination: A multicenter study; Nephrol. Dial. Transpant; 10(10):1838-44 (1995)

682. Van Landeghem, G.F., et al.; Aluminum speciation in cerebrospinal fluid of acutely aluminum-intoxicated dialysis patients before and after desferrioxamine treatment; a step in the understanding of the element's neurotoxicity; Nephrol. Dial. Transpant; 12:1692-98 (1997)

683. Parry, R.; et al.; Silicon and aluminum interactions in hemodialysis patients; Nephron. Dial. Transplant; 13(7):1759-62 (1998)

684. Reusche, E., and Seydel, U.; Dialysis associated encephalopathy light and electron microscopic morphology and topography with evidence of aluminum by laser microprobe analysis; Acta Neuropathol.; 86:249 (1993)

685. Candy, J.M., et al.; Aluminosilicates and senile plaque formation in Alzheimer'e disease; Lancet; Feb.; 1(8477):354-7 (1986)

686. Moretz, R.C., et al.; Microanalysis of Alzheimer's disease NFT and plaques; Envriron. Geochem. Health; March; 12(1):15-6 (1990)

687. Schreeder, M.T, et al.; Dialysis encephalopathy and aluminum exposure: an epidemiological analysis; J Chronic Dis.; 36(8)581-93 (1983)

688. Farnell, B.J., et al.; Calcium metabolism in aluminum encephalopathy; Exp. Neurol.; April.; 88(1):68-83 (1985)

689. Sidhu, S.K. and Nicholson, J.W.; A review of glass-ionomer cements for clinical dentistry; J. Funct. Biomater.; 7(3):16 (2016)

690. Hantson, P., et al.; Fatal encephalopathy after otoneurosurgery procedure with an aluminum containing biomaterial; J. Toxicol. Clin. Toxicol.; 33(6):645-8 (1995)

691. Shirabe, T., et al.; Autopsy case of aluminum encephalopathy; Neuropathology; Sep.; 22(3):2016-10 (2002)

692. Flaten, T.P.; An investigation of the chemical composition of Norwegian drinking water and its possible relationships with the epidemiology of some diseases. Dept. of Chem.; Norwegian Univ. Sci. and Tech., Trondheim, Norway (1986)

693. Vogt, T.; Water quality and health: Study of a possible relation between aluminum in drinking water and dementia. Sosiale og Okonomiske Studier no. 61. Oslo: Statistics Norway (1986)

694. Forbes, W.F., et al.; Geochemical risk factors for mental functioning, based upon the Ontario Longitudinal Study of Aging (LSA) V. Comparison of the results, relevant to aluminum water concentrations, obtained from LSA and death certificates mentioning dementia; Can. J. Aging; 14:642-56 (1995)

695. Canadian Study of Health and Aging Group; The incidence of dementia in Canada in 1991; Neurology; July; 55(1):66-73 (2000)

696. Forbes, W.F., and Agwani, N.; Geochemical risk factors for mental functioning, based upon the Ontario Longitudinal Study of Aging (LSA) III. The effects of aluminum-containing compounds; Aging 13:488-98 (1994)

697. Martyn, C.N., et al.; Aluminum concentrations in drinking water and risk of Alzheimer's disease; Epidemiology; 8:281-86 (1997)

698. Forster, D.P., et al.; Risk factors in clinically diagnosed presenile dementia of the Alzheimer's type: A case-control study in northern England; J. Epidemiol. Community Health; 49:253-58 (1995)

699. Frecker, M.F.; Dementia in Newfoundland: identification of a geographical isolate?; J. Epidemiol. Community Health; 45:307-11 (1991)

700. Doll, R.; Review: Alzheimer's disease and environmental aluminum; Age Aging; 22:138-53 (1993)

701. Wettstein, A.; et al.; Failure to find a relationship between mnestic skills of octogenarians and aluminum in drinking water; Int. Arch. Occup. Environ Health 63:97-103 (1991)

702. Wood, D.J., et al.; Bone mass and dementia in hip fracture patients from areas with different aluminum concentrations in water supplies; Age Aging; 17:415-19 (1988)

Printed in Great Britain
by Amazon